C0-BVA-272

A Guide to Medical Mathematics

A Guide to
Medical Mathematics

D. A. Franklin, B.A. M.Sc.
Director, Computing Unit for
Medical Sciences, St Bartholomew's Hospital
London, England

G. B. Newman, M.A. M.B.C.S.
Lecturer in Mathematics
The Middlesex Hospital Medical School
London, England

A HALSTED PRESS BOOK

JOHN WILEY AND SONS

NEW YORK

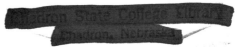

First published 1973

LIBRARY OF CONGRESS CATALOGING IN PUBLICATION DATA

Franklin, D A
A guide to medical mathematics.

A Halsted Press book
Bibliography: p
1. Medicine—Mathematics.
I. Newman, G. B., joint author.
II. Title. [DNLM: 1. Mathematics 2. Medicine. QA37.2 F831g 1973]
R707.F7   510'.2'461   73-15859

ISBN 0-470-27520-0

Printed in Great Britain

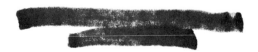

Contents

Preface

'... Mathematics ... set up by the universities as a golden calf when the cult of the classic gods became unprofitable, has now matured into a sacred cow which as often as not gets in the way of scientific traffic. I am all for the exaltation of mathematics as an art, an æsthetic experience only slightly more difficult than modern music ... but in sciences less abstract than physics, in particular in biology, mathematics proper is seldom useful and certainly not essential.'

Professor P.G.H.Gell, 1968. Quoted in *Lancet* **i**, p. 273, 1969.

'... Thus techniques are available which could turn biology, including of course, medicine, into a mathematical science ....'

Professor J.A.B.Gray, *British Medical Bulletin* **24**, p. 188, 1968.

This book is intended for the medical research worker and student whose study of mathematics stopped at an early stage in his career. There is no doubt that one can become a highly successful doctor with little knowledge of formal mathematics. However, the student will find the mathematical content of his courses increasing, and the research worker is often confronted with a paper which seems full of incomprehensible formulae.

Although parts of medical mathematics are straightforward, the range of knowledge required is often very large. The human body is probably the most complex mechanism being studied by scientific methods today, and so the medical research worker may often have to make use of techniques which involve reading specialized mathematical texts. Some of the difficulty for the medical worker may lie in interpreting the strange collections of symbols and words used by authors of mathematical work. We have therefore given at least as much priority to explaining the language as we have to explaining the techniques of mathematics.

The mathematical topics covered in this book are those which in the authors' experience most frequently occur in medical work. It is unlikely that any one individual worker will in fact meet all the topics mentioned. There is no detailed discussion of computing and statistics, for which there are many books already available; however, the mathematical methods and notation often assumed by the authors of these books are included. We are particularly aware that the use of computers in medicine is increasing and that much of the computation may be done using programmable calculators or computers and their associated libraries of programs. We have tried to indicate the kind of information required by these programs, the methods they use and the precautions that sometimes have to be taken when solving a problem by these methods. In many places we use statistical or computing examples to illustrate the mathematical methods. We consider co-ordinate geometry in considerable detail, but we have not included a chapter on Euclidean geometry or the classical study of volumes and areas of simple shapes. To some extent this is now covered by co-ordinate geometry or the calculus, and it has been our experience that medical workers are often much better at appreciating the properties of flat and solid shapes than some more mathematically oriented scientists.

Each chapter represents a reasonably self-contained topic and may be read on its own. A reference is given to the appropriate chapter and section, where it is felt that the reader may be missing some essential knowledge of preceding topics. The * sign is used to indicate multiplication for reasons given on page 6. The sections are numbered with the chapter number and section number; thus Section 11.3. The formulae in the book are numbered in a similar fashion but enclosed in brackets, i.e. (11.3) refers to a formula and not a section. Sections of the Appendix are labelled with the appropriate section of the main text.

We have tried to take as many as possible of the worked examples from the medical literature. This has not always been easy, for the published work is usually either very simple or extraordinarily complicated. We have not given any exercises for the reader to do himself; we were quite frankly informed by our medical colleagues that they would not consider doing them anyway, and in any case we feel that the best exercises are probably to be found in the reader's own work. In some textbooks the exercises are used to present additional facts which the author does not wish to demonstrate in detail; in this book we have included a large amount of such material additional to the main text in the Appendix, and the reader who feels in need of exercising his powers might try proving any of the mathematical relationships given there.

To cover the very wide range of mathematical knowledge required in medicine we have started simply with arithmetic and algebra although we have moved fairly fast through these to a variety of other subjects. The Appendix contains many formulae which are not discussed in the main chapters, and it is our hope that the book may form a suitable reference even if the reader has had to consult more specialized texts. Many of these formulae may be used directly for computation; in other cases the formulae may be intended to put some mathematical expression or phrase in its context. It may often help, for example, to know that the Bessel functions are solutions of a particular differential equation without necessarily knowing what the functions are or what their values might be.

The Medlars medical bibliography holds roughly the same number of papers in the category, **mathematical formulae essential to the research,** as are noted under the heading **depression.** Some of our medical colleagues might find more than mere coincidence in this suspicious statistic, but we hope that this book will go some way to protect them from people who occasionally seem determined to blind them with mathematical jargon.

Although this book has been devoted to an exposition of mathematical notation and methods, it is as well to keep in mind the role of mathematics in a practical subject such as medicine. The use of mathematics in these circumstances is an attempt to quantify our ideas and to deduce consequences from observations. Frequently this involves simplification of the physical situation, and the result and predictions must therefore be checked by experiment and measurement. The ultimate test in any situation is always the extent to which the mathematical handling of symbols and values enables us to correctly describe and predict the behaviour of real medical processes.

Acknowledgments

We would like to thank the many authors and publishers from whose papers we have taken examples. Many of our colleagues, friends, and family gave us advice and help; we are particularly grateful to Mr N.G.Brown, Mr A.Datta, Dr Patricia Fraser, Dr Mary Kellerman, Mr A.Todd Pokropek, and Miss Barbara Smolny, for their help. Our thanks also go to Miss Joan Berhman for Fig. 10.2, to Mr H.Oldman who drew many of the diagrams, to Mrs Sally Franklin who typed a large part of the manuscript, and to the many other typists who suffered for a short time the horrors of preparing a mathematical text. Our families also participated in most of the difficulties of preparation without the compensatory pleasures, and we would also like to record our thanks for the patience of our printers and publishers.

Note

For reasons given on page 6, the ∗ sign is used to indicate multiplication throughout this book.

Chapter 1
Mathematical Symbols and their Uses

1.1   Introduction

In this chapter we shall consider some of the symbols used in mathematics and the way in which they are used. It is often the collection of strange and unfamiliar symbols which deters the reader from mathematical work, but the reason for the introduction of mathematical symbols should be to simplify written representation of our work. Sometimes these symbols are used for no apparent reason; this tends to give a quite false air of exactness to the work and is to be deplored. There is no advantage in representing the total amount of fluid excreted by the kidney by the symbols:

$$\int C_k(t)\, dt$$

unless these symbols are to be used separately elsewhere in the text, or an analogy is being drawn to other processes represented by the same symbols. The same mathematical symbols may represent many different processes, enabling useful analogies to be drawn between them. The ordinary numbers themselves are symbols, and can represent measurements of different types, orders or rankings, or convenient codes such as the chapter numbers or page numbers in this book.

Mathematical notation and rules can be considered in the abstract, just as rules for manipulating symbols. However, mathematics has developed in the real world, and so the rules have usually been developed to explain some physical behaviour of the world around us; as a result the abstract handling of these symbols (*pure mathematics*) often has important applications in science, commerce or engineering (*applied mathematics*).

Mathematical notation is a shorthand for writing complicated processes in a very brief way; compare e.g. the simple symbol '−' for subtraction and the actual physical processes it represents. It comes as some surprise to discover that mathematical notation is often ambiguous and personal. The mathematician develops his own personal collection of squiggles and alphabets to handle a particular problem; even the simple process of multiplication does not have a satisfactory and accepted notation, and the reader of an article containing mathematics will have to use the context of the problem to follow the symbolic formulae. Fortunately the advent of mathematical languages for use on digital computers has done much to improve the situation. These machines require at the present time an unambiguous representation of formulae by means of a limited and predetermined set of symbols.

1.2   Representation of numbers

The reader is assumed to be familiar with the conventional decimal notation for numbers. However, in some modern applications of arithmetic it is necessary to consider various alternative notations and make some comment on the accuracy with which a number may be represented and handled in calculations. Numbers were first used to indicate the exact order which an object or event occupies in a series, and most of the problems arise in using them to represent measurements which are always limited by the accuracy of our instruments or calculating devices.

1.2.1   Number bases

The decimal notation provides a representation of a number using the ten symbols **0, 1, 2, 3, 4, 5, 6, 7, 8, 9**. We note that each position to the left of the decimal point represents units, tens, hundreds, etc., and each position to the right of the decimal point represents tenths, hundredths, thousandths, etc.

100's	10's	1's		$\frac{1}{10}$	$\frac{1}{100}$	$\frac{1}{1000}$	$\frac{1}{10000}$
	2	2	· 5	6	2		5

Such a system has ten symbols, and each position represents 10 times the size of the previous position in the number; it is said to be in *base 10*.

It is possible to propose other systems which may be more convenient under certain circumstances. The most popular of these is the *binary* system (base 2); this system is useful because it can represent numbers by the use of only two symbols: **0** and **1**. Its main advantages are in electronic or mechanical representation of numbers, using switches or levers which can adopt one of only two positions (on/off).

In the binary system the positions to the left of the point represent units, twos, fours, eights, etc., and to the right of the point represent halves, quarters, eighths, etc.

16	8	4	2	1	·	$\frac{1}{2}$	$\frac{1}{4}$	$\frac{1}{8}$	$\frac{1}{16}$	
1	0	1	1	0	·	1	0	0	1	(1.1)

This number represents one of the sixteens, no eights, one of the fours and so on, and this number 10110.1001 in binary notation can be shown to be the same as 22·5625 in decimal notation:

Binary $10110 \cdot 1001 = 16 + 4 + 2 + \frac{1}{2} + \frac{1}{16}$

Decimal $16 + 4 + 2 + 0 \cdot 5 + \cdot 0625 = 22 \cdot 5625$

Note that this is purely a different notation for the same number. The number given in (1.1) could be represented by a set of nine switches in which *off* corresponds to 0 and *on* corresponds to 1:

on	off	on	on	off	on	off	off	on
1	0	1	1	0 ·	1	0	0	1

Modern electronics can alter switches hundreds of millions of times a second and can thus perform very fast handling of numbers in the binary notation.

There is a duality of ideas in the mathematics of numbers, and just as we can represent a number by a pattern of symbols so we can represent a pattern of symbols by a number. Consider, for example, coding of treatment schemes for carcinoma patients, where we wish the treatment received to be represented by a simple number in order to facilitate indexing or computer processing. For simplicity we will assume that the patient may receive any combination of three treatments: radiotherapy, surgery, and chemotherapy. The possible combinations have been set out in Table 1.1, using a 1 to represent a treatment which was given, and a 0, one which was not. The resulting sequences of 0's and 1's can be interpreted as numbers in the binary notation, and their decimal equivalents give a simple coding scheme:

Table 1.1

	Radio-therapy	Surgery	Chemo-therapy	Decimal equivalent
No treatment	0	0	0	0
Chemotherapy	0	0	1	1
Surgery only	0	1	0	2
Surgery and chemotherapy	0	1	1	3
Radiotherapy only	1	0	0	4
Radiotherapy and chemotherapy	1	0	1	5
Radiotherapy and surgery	1	1	0	6
Radiotherapy, surgery and chemotherapy	1	1	1	7

This provides a good example of the way in which numbers may be used in problems which do not involve measurement or counting, though in this case the processes of arithmetic would be meaningless.

The number base may be chosen to suit the problem. Bases 8 (*octal*) and 16 (*hexadecimal*) are often chosen as a compromise between the mechanical convenience of binary and the notational inconvenience of a long string of zeroes and ones. If the number base is greater than 10 then further symbols beyond the ordinary decimal digits are needed and there is no general agreement on the ones to be used, though often the letters A, B, etc., are used to continue the symbol sequence. A great puzzle is the eventual domination of a notation to base 10 in our numbering system, for its only practical advantage is the correspondence with the number of fingers and thumbs on our hands. Base 8, which could have arisen from use of our fingers only, may well have been more useful, and the bases of 12 and 16 in the vanishing English measuring systems have a number of useful features.

Number notation is always assumed to be in base 10, unless otherwise stated, but the absence of any symbols **8** or **9** on a computer print-out may indicate that octal is being used, and a string of ones and zeroes usually indicates binary notation. But not always so; to provide light-hearted relaxation for mathematically-minded friends, ask them to complete the missing number in the sequence

$$101, \quad ?, \quad 1010, \quad 1111$$

The answer is 202, the series representing the numbers 10, 20, 30, 40, in the number base 3, but by showing them a part of the series which uses only ones and zeroes you have deliberately given them a false clue and they will almost certainly try to use the binary notation, base 2, to solve the puzzle. We will repeatedly return to this need for clues in interpreting mathematical notation.

1.2.2   Floating point notation

Floating point notation is an alternative notation for numbers, which is useful for representing a very wide range of values in a limited number of digit positions. In this notation the value is represented in two parts: the first part is a number with the point just before the left-most non-zero digit, and the second part is the number of places to the left or the right that the point must be moved to produce the desired value. If the point is to be moved to the right, the second part is an ordinary counting number, and zeroes are filled in on the right of the first part if necessary; for example

$$\cdot 1234 \quad 6 \text{ is equivalent to} \quad 123400 \cdot 0$$

If the point is to be moved to the left, the second part has a '−' symbol in front of it, and zeroes are filled in to the left of the first part, for example

$$\cdot 1234 \quad -3 \text{ is equivalent to} \quad \cdot 0001234$$

To avoid confusion with a simple subtraction sum the second part of the floating point number is often preceded by a symbol such as 'E'; for example

·1234 E2 is equivalent to 12·34

·5678 E−9 is equivalent to ·0000000005678

The floating point representation can be applied in any number base notation. It is particularly useful for automatic computations where only a fixed number of symbol positions can be allocated to a number no matter what its size, and for printing numbers in regular columns when the range of values is not known in advance.

1.2.3 Negative numbers

When we represent measures by a number it is usual to have both a scale and an origin or zero point. Thus 3°C is 3° *above* freezing and we use −3°C to represent 3° *below* freezing. Negative numbers simplify the handling of many concepts; for example a measured decrease can be regarded as a negative increase. In many physical phenomena it is possible to use these negative numbers in exactly the same formulae as with positive numbers and provided certain rules given in Section 1.3.6 are observed, the correct answer will result.

The value of a number with its sign ignored is called its *absolute value*, *modulus* or *numerical value* and the symbol | | is sometimes used for this. For example | −3 | is the same as | 3 | and is the positive number 3.

On desk calculators and within digital computers negative numbers are sometimes held in a *complement notation*. This notation is in effect the result of subtracting the modulus of the negative number from a number which is one greater than the largest number the machine can hold; its main advantage is that the complement numbers can be automatically handled by the same mechanisms which deal with positive numbers. To obtain this notation, start from the extreme left of the machine register holding the negative number and replace each digit (including leading zeroes) by its difference from 9 (or one less than the number base) until you reach the last non-zero digit, which is replaced by its difference from 10 (or the number base); the remaining zeroes may be left as zeroes, e.g.

−·0081730 is represented as 99 . . . 9·9918270

The number of leading 9's depends on the size of the register holding the numbers. The process is reversible by exactly the same rule.

1.3   Representation of arithmetic operations

1.3.1   Multiplication

The operation of multiplication is one of the most frequent in mathematical work. However, the main symbols for multiplication, '.' and '×', have become confused with other uses for the same symbols, and in recent years mathematical programming languages have been using the symbol '∗' to indicate multiplication. In these languages this symbol *must always* be used whenever the process of multiplication is indicated. *In this book we too will use an asterisk (∗) to indicate multiplication*, when we feel that this will help in clarifying the text.

1.3.2   Indices and roots

1.3.2.1   Indices

There is a special notation for repeated multiplication of a number by itself, namely, to place the number of repetitions as a superscript just above and to the right of the number; for example

$$2 * 2 * 2 \quad \text{is represented as} \quad 2^3$$

These superscripts are called *exponents, powers* or *indices* and are normally printed as shown, i.e. in slightly smaller type to the number being multiplied. However, superscripts are often used in a somewhat different fashion, e.g. in Section 1.6 and Section 9.3.2, and one has to rely on the context to decide between the different possibilities. The use of superscripts can be very inconvenient with digital computers, and the symbols $\uparrow$ or $* *$ are sometimes used in such circumstances to indicate repeated multiplication; for example:

(i) $2 \uparrow 3$ is the same as 2^3 which is the same as $2 * 2 * 2$ which is the same as 8.

(ii) $3 * * 2$ is the same as 3^2 which is the same as $3 * 3$ which is the same as 9.

(N.B. 2^1 is the same as 2).

The symbol $=$ is usually used as a shorthand for 'is the same as' or 'equal to'; thus $2^3 = 8$, $3^2 = 9$, $6 + 7 = 13$, etc.

Multiplying a number by itself is often referred to as *squaring* it, and a further multiplication as *cubing* it; thus 3^2 is 'three squared' and 2^3 is 'two cubed'. Also, we would call 9 $(=3^2)$ the *square* of 3, and 8 $(=2^3)$ the *cube* of 2.

Powers higher than 3 are referred to as the fourth power, fifth power, etc. Thus 2^5 $(=32)$ is the fifth power of 2.

1.3.2.2 Square roots

The *square root* of any given number is the quantity which when multiplied by itself results in the original number; thus 3 is the square root of 9. The process of finding the square root of a number is often referred to as *extracting* the square root, and is denoted by the symbol $\sqrt{\ }$.

> Examples:
> (i) $3^2 = 3 * 3 = 9$, and so $\sqrt{9}$ is 3.
> (ii) $2^2 = 2 * 2 = 4$, and so $\sqrt{4}$ is 2.

1.3.2.3 Cube and other roots

The process and notation of the square root can be generalized. For instance, $2^3 = 2 * 2 * 2 = 8$.
Thus three 2's multiplied together give 8, and we write $2 = \sqrt[3]{8}$.
The symbol $\sqrt[3]{\ }$ is known as the *cube* root.
Similarly

$$2^4 = 2 * 2 * 2 * 2$$
$$= 16$$

and we write

$$2 = \sqrt[4]{16}, \quad \text{the } \textit{fourth root} \text{ of } 16.$$

A somewhat more convenient notation for roots in which for example the cube root of 8 is represented by $8^{1/3}$ is discussed in Section 4.1.6.

1.3.3 Brackets

Brackets (and)—also called parentheses—have an important role in grouping operations together. The rule is that all items between a matching pair of brackets are performed before any operation outside them; for example:

$$(3+2)^2 = 5^2 = 25$$

whereas $3 + 2^2 = 3 + 4 = 7$

Brackets can be *nested* inside each other to indicate the order in which a computation is to be performed, the innermost pairs of bracketed expressions being evaluated first.

Example:

$$(8+(3+2)^2) * 4 = (8+5^2) * 4 = (8+25) * 4 = 33 * 4 = 132$$

The mathematician often uses a variety of bracket shapes to help him distinguish matching pairs of brackets (this facility is not available on computers); e.g. the last computation might have been written as

$$\{8+(3+2)^2\} * 4$$

1.3.4   Division

The symbol ÷ for division has largely been replaced by the symbol /. For example, 4/2 is four divided by two, or 1/3 is one divided by three and is an alternative representation of the fraction $\frac{1}{3}$. The / is the symbol for division in mathematical programming languages where the position-dependent symbols such as

$$\frac{5+3}{4}$$

which represents eight divided by four, would be written

(5+3)/4.

It is important to realize that *division by zero is not allowed* in mathematical operations, as it leads to inconsistencies and any process involving such a division will not be correct. The concept of *infinity* with which division by zero is sometimes associated is considered in Section 1.7.1 and in Chapter 5.

1.3.5   Order of operations

An arithmetic calculation normally proceeds in the following order:

(i) Evaluation of all operations of raising to a power.
(ii) All multiplications or divisions, and lastly
(iii) All additions and subtractions.

$3 * 2^2 - 5$ is evaluated in the order:

evaluate 2^2: $3 * 4 - 5$
evaluate multiplication: $12 - 5$
evaluate subtraction: 7

Contents of brackets are evaluated separately and then treated as a single number.

The division symbol / can give rise to ambiguity—for example $4/2 * 2$ could be interpreted as either $4/(2 * 2) = 1$ or as $(4/2) * 2 = 4$. Brackets resolve ambiguities and should always be used if one is in any doubt about the meaning of an arithmetic expression.

1.3.6   Handling negative numbers

We give here the rules for handling negative numbers; these may of course be already familiar to the reader from school mathematics.

(i) Adding a negative number is the same as subtracting the absolute value:

$$6 + (-3) = 6 - 3 = 3$$

(ii) Subtracting a negative number is the same as adding the absolute value:

$$6 - (-3) = 6 + 3 = 9$$

(iii) Multiplying two negative numbers together gives a positive answer:

$$(-6) * (-3) = +(6 * 3) = 18$$

(iv) Multiplying a positive number and a negative number gives a negative answer:

$$(-6) * 3 = -(6 * 3) = -18$$

(v) Dividing a negative number by a negative number gives a positive answer:

$$(-6)/(-3) = 6/3 = 2$$

(vi) Dividing a positive number by a negative number or vice versa gives a negative answer:

$$-6/3 = -(6/3) = -2$$
$$6/(-3) = -(6/3) = -2$$

As a guide we can say 'two negatives give a positive' in the situations just described.

1.3.7   Negative square roots and square roots of negative quantities

The fact that the multiplication together of either two positive numbers or two negative numbers results in a positive answer implies that the product of any number with itself must be positive. This means that no negative number can have an ordinary number as a square root, and any positive number has *two* square roots, equal in absolute value but opposite in sign.

Thus,

the square root of 9 is either $+3$ or -3, a statement which is written $\sqrt{9} = \pm 3$, the sign $\pm$ meaning '+ or −'.

Similarly

$\sqrt{16} = \pm 4$.

Normally, however, *it is the positive square root which is meant when we refer to* $\sqrt{}$.

We said above that no negative number could have an *ordinary* number as a square root. The term 'ordinary' was used because mathematicians have enlarged the concept of numbers to include entities some of which—the so-called *imaginary numbers* or *imaginaries*—behave as though they were the square roots of negative numbers. Such entities are called *complex numbers*. Ordinary numbers are sometimes referred to as belonging to the *real* number system, to distinguish them from the complex numbers and in particular from the imaginary numbers.

1.4   Accuracy

The representation of the 'counting' numbers 1, 2, 3, . . ., etc., presents no problems, but fractions can lead to difficulty. For example, it is impossible to represent the number $\frac{1}{3}$ exactly in the normal decimal notation. We can show that $\frac{1}{3}$ lies between 0·33 and 0·34, or, more accurately, between 0·3333 and 0·3334, or more accurately still, between 0·333333 and 0·333334, and so on. In other words we can represent $\frac{1}{3}$ to some preset accuracy only. If we use number base 2, the fraction $\frac{1}{10}$ cannot be expressed exactly, so that a number such as 4·1 when entered into a digital computer may be treated as a slightly smaller or slightly larger number. In addition to the fractions, there are measures which cannot be represented exactly in *any* integer number base. Two examples of these are the ratio of the circumference of a circle to its diameter and the ratio of the diagonal of a square to its side. As such numbers cannot be written exactly, they are occasionally given special symbols—e.g. the ratio of the circumference of a circle to its diameter is called π and is approximately 3·1416. The ratio of the diagonal of a square to its side can be shown to be equal to the square root of 2 (approximately 1·4142), for which we use the normal $\sqrt{}$ symbol, thus: $\sqrt{2}$.

In theoretical mathematics it is important to distinguish between these numbers, which are called *irrational numbers*—e.g. π, $\sqrt{2}$, and numbers which can be represented as integers or fractions, e.g. $\frac{22}{7}$ or 3·14, which are called *rational numbers*. In practice, however, we must always handle both types to an acceptable accuracy.

1.4.1 Representation to a desired accuracy

Numbers may be represented to an absolute accuracy; for example, the figures for π and $\sqrt{2}$ just given are within ·00005 of any more accurate representation. This is known as accurate to four *decimal places*. Alternatively we may consider the accuracy relative to the number itself and give only a number of *significant figures*, that is, digits counted from the left-most non-zero digit (cf. floating point notation Section 1.2.2). Five figure accuracy would normally represent the numbers to within 0·5 in 10000:

3·141593	as	3·1416
·00314593	as	·0031416
3141593	as	3141600

In representing a number to a limited accuracy we normally replace the number by one with acceptable accuracy closest to it; this is called *rounding off*. For example

12·4551 to four significant figures is 12·46

12·45499 to four significant figures is 12·45 (but is 12·4550

to four decimal places)

12·4550 is ambiguous to four significant figures, and various schemes exist which produce either 12·46 or 12·45.

Some electronic computers and most mechanical calculators do not round-off but just ignore the irrelevant digits. This is called *truncation*. It is in general more inaccurate than rounding-off—e.g. 2·9 *truncates* to 2, to the nearest integer, whereas it *rounds-off* to 3, which is a better approximation. (In view of this inaccuracy, it is worth bearing in mind that one of the leading mathematical programming languages (Fortran IV) always truncates the fractional part of any number when converting its representation from 'floating point' to 'integer'.)

The truncated value of a negative number is generally taken to be $-($the truncated value of its modulus); thus $-2·9$ truncates to $-(2·9 \text{ truncated}) = -2$.

The reader will no doubt have noticed a slight reservation in our definition of the truncation value of a negative number: 'is generally taken to be' implies that there is a certain amount of divergence on the matter, and indeed there is.

Occasionally one meets a form of truncation, especially with regard to dropping the fractional part of a number, which leads to a different result with negative numbers to that occurring with the definition given above. This form defines the truncation of a number as *the greatest number of acceptable accuracy not bigger than the original number.* Thus 2·96 truncates on this definition to 2·9, to one decimal place, and to 2 to the nearest integer. The result is thus as before —for *positive* numbers. For *negative* numbers, however, this alternative form produces a value 1 less than that produced by the standard definition—thus −2·9 'truncates' to −3.

One must always check, therefore, as to which definition is being used if truncation occurs—especially with computer programs.

1.4.2   *Accuracy during arithmetic*†

In general it is best to carry as many significant figures as you conveniently can and to round-off, not truncate. As a rough guide we can say that in the *addition* of two numbers we may have an error of up to 1 in the least significant digit. In *multiplication* or *division* we may have an error of up to five in the least significant digit. *Subtraction* is more complicated and we can lose all the significant digits; for example

$$3\cdot141593 - 3\cdot140000 = \cdot001593$$

but working with three significant digits gives

$$3\cdot14 - 3\cdot14 = 0$$

In a large number of successive arithmetic operations these errors can easily

---

† Some people would say that what we are talking about here is not *accuracy* but *precision.* There is continual argument over the exact meaning of these two terms, and it does not help a confused situation that they are often used interchangeably—even in Abramowitz & Stegun (1965) we find: '. . . linear interpolation will yield four- or five-figure accuracy, which suffices in most physical applications. Users requiring higher precision in their interpolates may . . .' To avoid involving the reader—and ourselves—in this argument we have used the term 'accuracy' throughout this section.

If we *were* asked to distinguish between the two concepts, we would say that *precision* really applies to *measurement,* and is governed by the size of the units used to make the measurement—we can be more precise with a balance weighing in milligrams than with one weighing in grams. *Accuracy,* however, is a question of how close we are to the 'true' value when we make our measurements. A measurement given as 21·014 g is very precise, but as an estimate of a weight whose true value is 22·0 g, it is very inaccurate. Thus precision does not necessarily imply accuracy, on these definitions, but accuracy would normally imply precision.

build up to be of practical importance; the topic is covered in more detail in books on numerical analysis. Wherever possible, new calculation techniques should be checked with known values or compared with experimental results.

1.5   Representing variable quantities

Nearly all mathematical work is concerned with the handling of quantities whose values can vary. As an example: there are various standards for the normal or ideal levels of basal metabolism. One of these, the Harris–Benedict standard, can be computed from the following formulae (in these formulae the letter C represents the ideal calorie consumption in kilocalories per 24 hours, W represents the weight in kilograms, H the height in centimetres and A represents the age in years):

Ideal metabolic rate:

Men: $C = 66 \cdot 473 + 13 \cdot 751 * W + 5 \cdot 0033 * H - 6 \cdot 7550 * A$

Women: $C = 655 \cdot 095 + 9 \cdot 563 * W + 1 \cdot 8496 * H - 4 \cdot 6756 * A$

These formulae give a simple computing rule that is meant to be applicable to various individuals, and so we substitute the actual values of weight, height and age in place of the letters to obtain the calculation. One of the authors has weight 72 kg, height 174 cm, and is aged 37 years, so we should replace W by 72, H by 174 and A by 37 giving his ideal basal metabolism as

$$C = 66 \cdot 473 + 13 \cdot 751 * 72 + 5 \cdot 0033 * 174 - 6 \cdot 7550 * 37$$

$$= 1677 \cdot 2 \text{ kcal per 24 hr.}$$

We have quite simply taken the letters W, H and A to represent the numerical values. In a computer program to evaluate this formula, the computer would have to allocate one of its number stores to each of the letters and would use the number stored in that store at the appropriate point in the calculation. The symbol need not be confined to being a single letter; another formula of a similar type, designed to give ideal weight in kilograms from height and average chest measurements in centimetres, is

$$\text{WEIGHT} = \frac{\text{HEIGHT} * \text{CHEST}}{240} \qquad (1.2)$$

In this formula we may regard the *words* HEIGHT, CHEST and WEIGHT as the representative symbols. In practice this system would probably be best for the simple formulae above, but in more complex problems which repeatedly use the same quantity, the use of words is very cumbersome and one tends to use single letters, resorting to the greek and gothic alphabets when the latin one is exhausted.

Representing arithmetic or other procedures in this symbolic manner is generally known as *algebraic notation*.

1.6   Choice of symbols

In choosing single letter symbols, we sacrifice the descriptive properties of the fuller word or phrase, for a quick and concise method of writing down computing rules. We attempt to overcome this deficiency in description by choosing the letter according to certain conventions, e.g. w or m for weight. It is customary to choose letters towards the end of the alphabet for quantities whose values are expected to vary between each application of the formula in which they occur, such quantities being called *variables*, and letters at the beginning of the alphabet for quantities whose values are not expected to change between applications of the formula—these quantities are called *constants*. It is customary to use i, j and k for counting in a repetitive process, to use n for the total number of repetitions, to use δ or ϵ for very small quantities, to use d, δ or Δ together with another letter for small changes, and to use greek letters—particularly θ and ϕ—for angles. However, each subject has its own conventions, often based on the initial letters of measurements being represented (see British Standard No. 1990); in medical work these conventions are not well established but the subject is endowed with an abundance of short three or four letter symbols, such as PCV (packed cell volume), Hb (haemoglobin), PCO_2 (carbon dioxide pressure), FEV (forced expiratory volume), which will do almost as well as a one letter symbol. People often employ 'hats', e.g. $\hat{x}$, or primes, e.g. x', or create their own composite arrangements of superscripts and suffices, for example, the use of $R_{f/b}^0$ to represent the 'ratio of free to bound hormone at zero concentration'. In further work in this book we consider general computing and mathematical rules, that is, we follow through the outcome of various operations quite independently of the numbers or types of measurements which will eventually be involved in a practical application. For such work symbolic representation is essential and this is the most important use of algebraic notation. In practice the mathematician relies to some extent on clues in the formulae for the interpretation of symbols. He expects x^2 to be the value of a variable x multiplied by itself, just as 3^2 represents $3 * 3$, and so symbols such as $R_{f/b}^0$ can cause confusion to someone unfamiliar with the context of the work. It is a mass of these complex and often personal symbols which scares the reader of a mathematical text and drives the printer to despair, but it is not necessary for this to happen if certain points are kept in mind.

1.7   Writing and reading algebraic formulae

The process of writing and manipulating symbols in formulae is surprisingly simple, far easier in fact than attempting to read through someone else's work. The first rule is to *choose simple but meaningful symbols*. If your work is to be arranged for a computer program then at the present time they will only accept letters from the latin alphabet, or combinations of letters such as PCV or HEIGHT, and will not be able to handle hats, primes, strange suffices or superscripts. Greek letters can still be used, though in the computer program they would be spelt out in full, e.g. DELTA for δ.

Always prepare a list of the symbols you use, what they stand for *and the units* in which they are measured. It is best to keep this list separately, though new symbols can be noted just before or after they are first used. When publishing mathematical work it is considerably easier for the reader if a complete list of symbols is included in the text as a separate item, *before* the formulae.

Reading someone else's mathematical formulations can be very much more difficult, but we give one or two suggestions for coping.

(i) Look around the formula to see whether the symbols are defined in a neighbouring paragraph. Some of the symbols may represent procedural rules rather than simple numbers, or the writer may be relying on some convention—such as that t represents time. The symbols are frequently defined *after* the formula in which they are used.

(ii) Is the formula just a rule for computation? If so it could be accepted and ignored till the computation is actually required. The computation would then be a simple substitution of the measures in the prescribed places.

(iii) Is the formula just a notational convenience (or inconvenience) and never used again? If so, it can be ignored.

(iv) It often helps in examining the meaning and implications of a formula to see the effect of increasing or decreasing variables, or to look into the effect when some variables are very large or very small.

(v) Are there groups of symbols that always seem to go together? If so can you think of a physical meaning for them, for example, if mass and volume only occur in the combination (mass/volume) then concentration is relevant. It often helps to follow the formula through in terms of the mass, length, and time units of the variables.

(vi) Remember that you are unlikely to be able to read and understand a line of algebraic notation at the same speed as a line of ordinary text—after all the writer resorted to algebraic notation because the ordinary text would be too long and cumbersome to record, and it therefore represents a condensation of thought, something which one would expect to take longer to unravel.

1.7.1   Some algebraic symbols

We have already made use of various symbols in this text to represent, e.g. the operations of arithmetic or the idea of equality between quantities or expressions. Other symbols which are simple shorthand notations for such ideas as 'greater than', 'approximately equal to', etc., are given in Table 1.2. For convenience, we repeat here some symbols which we have already used.

Table 1.2

Symbol	Meaning
$=$	'Equals', 'is equal to', or 'becomes equal to' or 'takes on the value of'.
$\doteqdot, \simeq, \simeq$	'Is approximately equal to' or 'becomes approximately equal to', or 'takes on a value approximately equal to'—the level of approximation must be taken from the context.
$>$	'Is greater than': the wide side of the symbol is nearest the larger number (e.g. $4 > 2$).
$<$	'Is less than': the narrow side of the symbol is nearest the smaller number.
$\geqslant$	'Greater than or equal to'.
$\leqslant$	'Less than or equal to'.
$\ngtr$	'Not greater than'.
$\nless$	'Not less than'.
$\neq$	'Not equal to'.
$\pm$	'Positive or, alternatively, negative'. This represents two operations and will produce two answers. E.g. $3 \pm 1 = 2$ and 4.
$\ldots$	'Continue these operations or numbers in a similar fashion'. E.g. $2 + 4 + 6 + \ldots + 20$ means $2 + 4 + 6 + 8 + 10 + 12 + 14 + 16 + 18 + 20$.
$\propto$	'Is proportional to' or 'varies as'. If $a \propto b$ where a and b are variables, then we can write $a = K * b$, where we will need additional information to determine the value of K.
$:$	'Is to' or 'the ratio of'. E.g. $a : b = 6$ means that a is 6 times as big as b.
∞	'Infinity'. This symbol means 'greater than any imaginable value'—*it is not itself a value*. The symbol $-\infty$ means 'numerically greater than any imaginable number, but negative in sign'.

1.7.2   The Σ and $\prod$ notations

Another useful symbol is Σ meaning 'the sum of'. It is used to indicate a repetitive addition, and is always associated with an *index of summation* which increases by 1 as we go from term to term. There is also a starting and finishing value for the index which are written below and above the Σ. For example

$$\sum_{i=2}^{6} x^i \quad \text{is the same as} \quad x^2 + x^3 + x^4 + x^5 + x^6 \quad \text{(powers of } x\text{)}$$

while $\quad \sum_{j=0}^{4} a_j \quad$ means $\quad a_0 + a_1 + a_2 + a_3 + a_4$

where the index of summation is simply a subscript and is used to denote the values of separate variables a_0, a_1, a_2, a_3 and a_4 which have some common property enabling them to be regarded as a group. Often the limits of the index of summation are omitted if they are considered to be obvious from the context.

This notation is particularly important in statistical work, for many of the operations in such work consist of adding together all the observations; for example the arithmetic mean of n observations $x_1, x_2, \ldots x_n$

is $\quad \dfrac{\sum_{i=1}^{n} x_i}{n}$

and their standard deviation can be computed as

$$\sqrt{\left[\frac{\sum x^2}{n} - \left(\frac{\sum x}{n}\right)^2\right]}$$

Notice that in the last expression all reference to the index has been omitted and is assumed from the context, for Σ implies a summation and the only numbers to sum are x_1, x_2, etc.

A similar type of notation is used for repetitive multiplication, using the symbol $\prod$. E.g.

$$\prod_{i=1}^{5} a_i = a_1 * a_2 * a_3 * a_4 * a_5$$

1.8   Arithmetic manipulation in algebraic notation

If we wish to study and resolve a number of arithmetic relationships, we will often have to do this before we have actual values to work with, or perhaps we may wish the answers to be applicable to many different measurements. We therefore have to follow through the processes of arithmetic using algebraic symbols for the variables and constants.

The manipulation of algebraic symbols follows exactly the process of arithmetic given in Section 1.3. However, in arithmetic we reduce the contents of brackets to single numbers before proceeding with the next stage of the calculation, but in algebraic work we do not know the values to substitute for our numbers so we cannot condense them into a single number. It is convenient to remember a few simple rules and two further definitions:

1.8.1   *Terms and expressions*

Symbols that are bound together as powers or by multiplication or by division (not subtraction or addition) are considered as single *terms*, for example

$$x^2 + \frac{x * y}{5} - y^2 + x$$

has four *terms* x^2, $\frac{x * y}{5}$, $-y^2$, and x

The sign of the term is usually associated with it.

A collection of terms separated by $+$ and $-$ signs is called an *expression*. An expression is in effect a sequence of mathematical operations.

1.8.2   *Manipulation of bracketed expressions*

(i) A bracketed expression *multiplied* by a single symbol or number is equivalent to multiplying all the terms in the bracket by the symbol or number:

$$a * (x * y + z) = a * x * y + a * z$$
$$a * (x * y - z) = a * x * y - a * z$$
$$-a * (x * y - z) = -a * x * y + a * z$$

A similar rule applies for *division* by a single symbol or number, e.g.:

$$\frac{(x * y + z)}{a} = \frac{x * y}{a} + \frac{z}{a}$$

Sometimes the resulting expression can be simplified:

$$\frac{(a * y + z * a^2)}{a} = \frac{a * y}{a} + \frac{z * a^2}{a} = y + z * a$$

(ii) When multiplying two bracketed expressions together the result is equivalent to pairing all the terms from the first bracket with all the terms in the second bracket in all possible ways:

$$(a+b+c) * (x+y) = a * x + a * y + b * x + b * y + c * x + c * y$$
$$(a+b-c) * (x-y) = a * x - a * y + b * x - b * y - c * x + c * y$$
$$(x-y) * (x+y) = x^2 + x * y - y * x - y^2 = x^2 - y^2$$

When multiplying three bracketed expressions together we take all possible *triples* of terms one from each bracket:

$$(a+b) * (c+d) * (e+f) = a * c * e + a * c * f + b * c * e + b * c * f$$
$$+ a * d * e + a * d * f + b * d * e + b * d * f$$

Sometimes addition of like terms simplifies the result, e.g.

$$(a+b) * (a+b) = a^2 + a * b + a * b + b^2$$
$$= a^2 + 2 * a * b + b^2$$

These rules can be extended up to any number of bracketed expressions. There is *no equivalent rule for division.* Some common bracketed expressions are given in the Appendix.

It must be noted that there is a widespread convention in mathematics of suppressing the multiplication sign, it being understood that the juxtaposition of two sets of symbols, each set representing a value, *implies* multiplication. This frequently leads to difficulty for the non-mathematician, who is generally unfamiliar with the clues indicating the process of multiplication. One advantage of the use of single letters for variables is that the multiplication sign can be omitted without introducing too much ambiguity; for example (1.2) could be written

$$W = HC/240$$

with a reasonably obvious interpretation.

In this book, we will also use this convention of dropping the multiplication sign ($*$) where it is felt that the reader will not be confused by this; e.g. an expression such as $4 * a * b + 3 * c$, where a, b and c are known to be single symbol variables, will be written as $4ab + 3c$ in the usual way. Where it is felt, however, that dropping the sign might cause difficulties for the reader, it will be retained, even though a mathematician would probably not do so.

.8.3   *Algebraic fractions*

Algebraic 'fractions' are handled by the rules of arithmetic also; the only difference is that we cannot condense down our results as with numbers. For instance, division by a fraction is equivalent to multiplication by its reciprocal†:

$$x \left/ \frac{b}{a} \right. = x * \frac{a}{b}$$

Addition and subtraction of algebraic fractions is carried out by expressing them in terms of the same common denominator;

$$\frac{p-2}{a+3} + \frac{q}{x+y} = \frac{(x+y)*(p-2)}{(x+y)*(a+3)} + \frac{(a+3)*q}{(a+3)*(x+y)}$$

$$= \frac{(x+y)*(p-2)+(a+3)*q}{(x+y)*(a+3)}$$

(we use here the facts that (a) a fraction can have its numerator and denominator multiplied or divided by the same quantity without altering the value of the fraction, and (b) fractions with the same denominator can be added by adding their numerators and keeping the common denominator).

1.8.4   Manipulation of equalities

The same quantity or expression may be added to the expressions on both sides of an = sign without destroying the relationship; similarly an expression may be subtracted from or multiply or divide the two sides of the equality without destroying it.

Example:

If $\dfrac{x-a}{b} + 2 = \dfrac{y-a}{b} + 1$

then multiplying each side of the relationship by b gives

$$x - a + 2 * b = y - a + b$$

and subtracting b and adding a to both sides of this gives

$$x + b = y \tag{1.3}$$

These formulae are three different ways of expressing the same relationship.

A quantity can be transferred from one side of an equality to the other provided its sign is changed. For instance, in (1.3) above, we can transfer the quantity b to the left-hand side of the equality and write

$$x = y - b$$

---

† The *reciprocal* of a is $1/a$. The *numerator* of a fraction a/b is the expression a, the *denominator* is the expression b.

There is one exception to the rule given at the beginning of this section: division by *zero*, or by any expression whose value has become zero as a result of special values being given to the variables, is forbidden. If $x=y$, we cannot write

$$\frac{x}{a} = \frac{y}{a}$$

if a is zero,

or

$$\frac{x}{a-6} = \frac{y}{a-6}$$

if $a=6$.

1.8.5   *Manipulation of inequalities*

There are rules for handling the transfer of quantities across inequalities as well as equalities, but the situation is more complicated. It is possible to add the same value to both sides of an inequality without altering its validity, or to subtract it:

Examples:

(a) If $x>y$, then $x+a>y+a$

(b) If $\frac{x}{a}-6<p$, then $\frac{x}{a}-2<p+4$ (add 4 to both sides)

Multiplication or division, however can *reverse* the inequality:

Examples:

(a) If $x>y$ then, $kx>ky$ if k is positive (i.e. $k>0$)

$kx<ky$ if k is negative (i.e. $k<0$)

(and similarly for division)

(b) If $a-6\leqslant b+2$, then $6-a\geqslant -(b+2)$

(multiplying across by -1)

There is also a reversal if *reciprocation* takes place; if, e.g.

$$x=y, \quad \text{then} \quad \frac{1}{x}=\frac{1}{y}$$

but if $x>y$,   then $\dfrac{1}{x}<\dfrac{1}{y}$

B

The rules above will be applicable to any numbers we substitute for the symbols a, x, b, y, etc. The validity of the rules can easily be demonstrated by substituting numbers for the symbols. Although we check the rules by seeing that they work for numbers, the mathematician accepts these rules of algebra as basic, and checks that his numbers satisfy them; for example, he will *define* the numbers 0 and 1 as values which satisfy the relations

$$a + 0 = a \quad \text{and} \quad a * 1 = a$$

These ideas are very important to pure mathematics but need not concern us here.

1.9   Simplifying algebraic expressions

In rule (ii) Section (1.8.2), we see that a long series of multiplications and additions (the right-hand side of the = sign) can be replaced by a comparatively simple product (the left-hand side of the = sign). We often find ourselves trying to derive an expression similar to the one on the left-hand side from a long and complicated expression similar to the right-hand side. To do this we work from clues in the formulae, and it helps to know a large number of complicated expressions and their simple forms.

The presence of these simple forms may become clearer if we use a new symbol for an expression that repeats itself, or look for common divisors in fractional expressions. Remember that *it may not be possible to simplify an expression and it may not be necessary*. A modern digital computer is as happy calculating with a complex expression as with a simplified one, and simplification is usually only needed to help with further algebraic manipulation, to satisfy an aesthetic need for neat presentation, or, when using a digital computer, to shorten computation time or save storage space.

At times it will seem that mathematical proof and manipulation is produced by magic out of a hat, but the professional mathematician has had great experience in simplifying expressions and processes. One advantage of practical applications is that we often have good experimental evidence for the desired answer before we start, and then we look several moves ahead and ask ourselves 'will this substitution lead to a form that could be reduced to the form I desire?' Unfortunately, only continual practice will improve one's facility, and the medical worker may have insufficient opportunity for doing this.

1.10   Equations

An *equation* is a statement to the effect that two mathematical expressions are equal or equivalent. If for example we take v as the volume and p as the pressure of a perfect gas, then Boyle's law states that $p * v$ has a constant value. If we denote the constant by c then the law can be stated as the *equation*

$$p * v = c$$

We may perform any operation (apart from division by zero) on both sides of this or any other equation without destroying the equality (cf. Section 1.8.4). For instance, let us divide both sides by v; this gives us

$$p = \frac{c}{v}$$

which is a means of calculating p if we know c and v.

Examples of equations:

(i) $(x+7)+(3 * x-4)=4 * x+3$

(ii) $4 * x+7=5 * x$

(iii) $a^x+b^x=c$

(iv) $R=\dfrac{\pi * r^4 * p}{8 * \eta * l}$ (Poiseuille's Law†)

In some cases, an equation is true for all values of the variables—for instance example (i) above is true for any value of x. Such equations are called *identities* and the expressions are said to be *identically equal*. The usual situation, however, is that the relationship is true only for certain values of the variable or variables in the expression; the associated problem is then to find these values, called the *roots* of the equation. They are said to *satisfy* the equation, and finding the roots is called *solving the equation*. The symbol $\equiv$ is sometimes used to indicate an identity instead of the $=$ sign; thus (i) above would be written:

$$(x+7)+(3 * x-4)\equiv 4 * x+3.$$

Examples (i) and (ii) above are examples of single variable equations. The first example is true for any value of x (i.e. it is an identity) and the second is true for $x=7$ (this answer is obtained by transferring the term $4 * x$ from the left-hand side of the equation to the right-hand side, changing its sign in the

---

† This law applies to the flow of a viscous fluid in a rigid capillary tube. r=radius of the capillary, l=length of capillary, p=pressure difference between ends, η=coefficient of viscosity, R=volume rate of flow.

process (see Section 1.8.4), which gives us $7=5*x-4*x$, i.e. $7=x$). The third example may or may not be a single variable equation, depending on which of a, b, c, and x is regarded as unknown. If a, b, and x are known, then c can be calculated; if a, b, and c are known, then it is not immediately obvious how the value of x is to be found, but the relationship is still a single variable equation. If a and b are unknown, however, then we have a two-variable equation. In such a case, a and b cannot be properly determined if there is only one equation connecting them, since any value we may care to assign to one of the unknowns leads to a different value for the other.

Even in a single variable equation, however, there may be more than one possible value satisfying the equation. For example,

$$x^2-3*x-4=0$$

is satisfied by both $x=4$ and $x=-1$, since

$$4^2-3*4-4=0$$

and $$(-1)^2-3*(-1)-4=0$$

In practice we would refer to the physical situation being represented by such mathematical expressions in order to resolve which values should be used.

Equations are handled to some extent by *transforming* them, both by use of the rules in Section 1.8 to simplify expressions through collecting related terms together on one side or other of the equation and also sometimes by substituting other mathematical expressions for some of the variables.

1.10.1   Simultaneous equations

In Poiseuille's Law given above we have five variables (R, r, p, l and η) and *one* equation, so we must measure, or have knowledge of, the values of any four of the variables in order to be able to use the equation to calculate the other one. In general if we have n variables and one equation we must know $n-1$ of the variables to use the equation to calculate the remaining one. If we have n variables and r equations (i.e. r relationships between them) we can generally reduce this to one equation between $n-r+1$ variables, and so we must know $n-r$ of the variables and use the reduced equation to calculate the remaining one. If we have n unknown variables and we wish to deduce the value of all of them we will have to establish n equations to achieve this. Such a system of equations would be known as a system of n *simultaneous equations*.

An important condition underlying the previous statements as to the number of equations needed to deduce the values of the variables is that the equations must be *independent*, i.e. it must not be possible to obtain any one of the equations by algebraic manipulation of the others, as such an equation does not supply any extra information.

For example:

$$x+y-z=1$$
$$2x+3y-2z=2$$
$$x+2y-z=1$$

are three simultaneous equations for three unknown variables, but the system is not in fact properly solvable; the third equation is simply the result of subtracting the first equation from the second; it adds no new information and the equations are not independent.

1.10.2   *Quadratic equations*

A very important form of equation which can be solved by mathematical manipulation is the *quadratic* equation

$$a * x^2 + b * x + c = 0 \tag{1.4}$$

where x is the unknown variable, a, b, and c being supposed known. Two values of x satisfy this equation; these are

$$x_1 = \frac{-b + \sqrt{(b^2 - 4 * a * c)}}{2 * a} \tag{1.5a}$$

and

$$x_2 = \frac{-b - \sqrt{(b^2 - 4 * a * c)}}{2 * a} \tag{1.5b}$$

x_1 and x_2 are therefore the roots of the quadratic equation (1.4).

The quantity $b^2 - 4 * a * c$ is called the *discriminant* of the quadratic and its value determines the nature of the roots. If $b^2 - 4 * a * c$ is positive, i.e. greater than zero, then x_1 differs from x_2 and there are two distinct roots; if $b^2 - 4 * a * c = 0$ then $x_1 = x_2 = -b/(2 * a)$ and the two roots fuse into a single value; this is known as a case of *equal* or *repeated* roots. If $b^2 - 4 * a * c$ is negative then $\sqrt{(b^2 - 4 * a * c)}$ will not exist in the ordinary or 'real' number system (Section 1.3.7) and the equation is said to have *no real roots*.

Examples:

(i) $2 * x^2 + 5 * x + 3 = 0$ has two (real) roots.
For relating this to (1.4) above, we have:
$a = 2, \ b = 5, \ c = 3$

whence

$b^2 - 4 * a * c = 1$

and therefore the roots are

$$x = \frac{-5 \pm \sqrt{1}}{2 * 2}, \quad \text{i.e. } x_1 = -1 \text{ and } x_2 = -1 \cdot 5.$$

(ii) $x^2 - 6 * x + 9 = 0$ has the repeated root $x = 3$.

(iii) $x^2 + 2 * x + 7 = 0$ has no real roots.

1.11   An example of algebraic manipulation

This example is taken from the work of Ekins *et al* (1969) on the theoretical behaviour of a mixture of a physiologic compound and a specific binding reagent. This forms the basis of 'saturation assay', a technique particularly useful in measuring very small hormone concentrations. The simplest system comprises the reaction of a binding protein and a univalent hormone. The reaction is governed by the Law of Mass Action and will result in some molecules of hormone and binding protein being bound together and others remaining free in the mixture, until a steady equilibrium is reached; all measures are taken at equilibrium. The symbols used are given in Table 1.3.

Table 1.3

P:	the concentration of free hormone (moles/litre)
Q:	the concentration of free binding protein (moles/litre)
B:	the concentration of bound hormone and binding protein (moles/litre)
p:	the total concentration of hormone (moles/litre)
q:	the total concentration of binding protein (moles/litre)
K:	the equilibrium constant of the reaction (litres/mole)
R:	ratio of B/P (dimensionless)

From the definitions in Table 1.3.

$$p = P + B \tag{1.6}$$

$$q = Q + B \tag{1.7}$$

The assay technique is to separate the bound and free hormone and measure the ratio of bound to free hormone

$$R = \frac{B}{P} \tag{1.8}$$

It was desired to examine the effect on the measure R of changing the total concentrations of hormone and binding protein, p and q and the equilibrium constant K. This means that we must find *four* relationships between the variables, viz. three to substitute the variables P, Q, and B, which are not wanted, and one to provide the required relation between R, p, q, and K. We have only three— (1.6), (1.7) and (1.8) and so we *must* get a further new relationship to solve the problem. This is provided by the Law of Mass Action, which can be expressed as:

$$K * P * Q = B \tag{1.9}$$

We may now proceed to eliminate P, Q and B, and this can be done in a variety of ways. Equation (1.8) gives a very simple substitution for B, namely $B = R * P$, and we will replace B by this in *all* the other equations:

from (1.9), $K * P * Q = R * P$ (1.10)

from (1.6), $p = P + R * P$ (1.11)

from (1.7), $q = Q + R * P$ (1.12)

Equations (1.10) and (1.11) simplify to

$$K * Q = R \tag{1.13}$$

$$p = P * (1 + R) \tag{1.14}$$

It is no use returning to any of the equations (1.6) to (1.9) as they will only re-introduce B. We proceed with (1.12), (1.13) and (1.14).

Equation (1.14) gives a substitution for P, namely

$$P = \frac{p}{1 + R}$$

and (1.13) gives a substitution for Q:

$$Q = \frac{R}{K}$$

Applying both these in equation (1.12) gives

$$q = \frac{R}{K} + \frac{R * p}{1 + R} \tag{1.15}$$

(1.15) is an expression of the desired relationship between R, p, q and K in the form of a computing rule for evaluating q from values of R, p and K. The same relationship can be expressed in other ways; for example:

$$p = \frac{1+R}{R} * \left(q - \frac{R}{K}\right) \tag{1.16}$$

which is obtained from (1.15) by bringing R/K over to the right-hand side of the equation (thus changing the sign) and then multiplying the equation across by $(1+R)/R$.

The equation was in fact used by Ekins in the form (1.16) to compute the numerical relationships between p and R; p was computed for various values of R at set values of K and q.

Equation (1.15) can also be expressed as

$$\frac{K*p}{1+R} = \frac{K*q}{R} - 1 \tag{1.17}$$

This gives a further idea of some of the processes involved. For instance the relationship (1.17) depends on $K*p$ and $K*q$ (note also how the units—moles and litres—always come out correctly in all the equations). As there are no negative concentrations in the assay the left-hand side must be positive and so on the right-hand side we must have $K*q/R > 1$, that is R must always be less than $K*q$.

On the other hand, to obtain a solution of R from equation (1.15) is not straightforward, and indeed no amount of multiplying or dividing, adding or subtracting with the equations (1.6) to (1.9) will produce a simple algebraic expression enabling R to be computed directly in terms of K, p and q.

However, if we multiply both sides of equation (1.15) by $K*(1+R)$, we obtain

$$K*(1+R)*q = R*(1+R) + R*K*p$$

which by similar manoeuvres to those already illustrated can be written as

$$R^2 + (1 + K*p - K*q)*R - K*q = 0 \tag{1.18}$$

Because this equation contains a term in R^2 as well as R, we see that (1.18) is a *quadratic* equation (cf. Section 1.10.2) in the variable R. Now the equation

$$a*x^2 + b*x + c = 0 \tag{1.4}$$

was shown earlier to have two solutions

$$x_1 = \frac{-b + \sqrt{(b^2 - 4ac)}}{2a} \tag{1.5a}$$

$$x_2 = \frac{-b - \sqrt{(b^2 - 4ac)}}{2a} \tag{1.5b}$$

Comparing (1.18) with (1.4), we see that R takes the role of x, the variable whose value is being sought, while the quantities a, b, and c are matched by 1, $(1+K*p-K*q)$ and $-K*q$ respectively. Substituting these for a, b and c in (1.5a) and (1.5b), we obtain two alternative expressions for R:

$$R = \frac{-(1+K*p-K*q)+\sqrt{[(1+K*p-K*q)^2+4*K*q]}}{2} \quad (1.19a)$$

and

$$R = \frac{-(1+K*p-K*q)-\sqrt{[(1+K*p-K*q)^2+4*K*q]}}{2} \quad (1.19b)$$

The question arises, are both these alternatives valid expressions for R in terms of K, p and q? And if not, which one do we use? To see how questions like this are answered in practice, let us consider the case when both $K*p$ and $K*q$ are known and equal to, say, 13 and 12 respectively. Then the two alternative expressions for R give

$$R = \frac{-(1+13-12)+\sqrt{[(1+13-12)^2+4*12]}}{2} = -1+\sqrt{13} = 2 \cdot 61$$

and

$$R = \frac{-(1+13-12)-\sqrt{[(1+13-12)^2+4*12]}}{2} = -1-\sqrt{13} = -4 \cdot 61$$

We have two *mathematically* possible answers; however, the physical situation excludes a negative answer for R, and so we can expect a value of $R=2\cdot61$ in the situation $K*p=13$, $K*q=12$.

As it happens, in this particular example it can be shown that any answer arising from (1.19a) will be positive for physically feasible values of $K*p$ and $K*q$, and any answer from (1.19b) will be negative, so the formula (1.19a) is the one to use at all times.

Note that (1.19a) is a long and cumbersome expression. We would probably use it only for numerical work, and there is no notational advantage in using it rather than continuing to use R to represent the measured ratio of B/P.

Chapter 2
Graphs

2.1   Introduction

Graphs are a common and familiar method of data presentation. However, there are various terms and definitions associated with them, and also some points of technique worth keeping in mind when drawing them; for the benefit of those readers who have either forgotten these details or to whom they are unfamiliar to start with, we briefly review the subject in this chapter.

2.2   Definitions

2.2.1   Axes

The system in most common use is called the *rectangular Cartesian* system, after Rene Descartes (1596–1650). It consists of two lines, called the *axes of reference* (or simply the axes), which intersect at right angles in a point called the *origin*. Such a configuration is sometimes called a *frame of reference*. Axes not at right angles to each other are called *oblique Cartesian axes*, but are hardly ever used. We will deal exclusively with rectangular Cartesian axes.

Each axis has some quantity associated with it in any particular application, and the axis is named after this quantity. For instance in graphing the results of a follow-up study subsequent to operation or treatment, we might have the horizontal axis as the time axis and the vertical axis representing the number or percentage of survivors. Formally, however, the horizontal axis is known as the *x-axis*, and the vertical one as the *y-axis*. The usual practice is that positive values of x are measured off on the x-axis from zero at the origin and increasing as we move to the right along the x-axis, while negative x values are measured from the origin decreasing as we move to the left along the x-axis. Correspondingly, positive values of y are measured upwards from zero at the origin and negative values downwards (Fig 2.1).

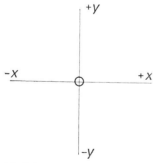

Fig 2.1

There is, however, another axis sign convention possible, shown in Fig 2.2.

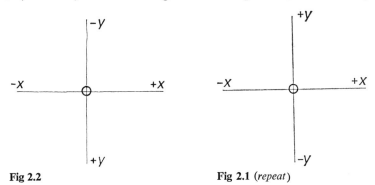

Fig 2.2   Fig 2.1 (repeat)

We see that in this system the axes have a different relationship to those of the system in Fig 2.1; also we find that no matter how we move the two systems around in the plane, they cannot be brought into coincidence with the signs of all their directions overlapping. They are irreconcilable systems, which bear the same relationship to each other as do right-handed and left-handed gloves.

The system in Fig 2.1 is called a *right-handed system* and that in Fig 2.2 a *left-handed system*. There are various rules for distinguishing them, rules which involve rotation of the axes in the plane. We will simply content ourselves with saying that any axis system which can be made to coincide in all respects with that in Fig 2.1 is a right-handed set of axes, and any system with a similar relation to the set in Fig 2.2 is a left-handed set.

Right-handed systems are sometimes referred to as having *even parity*, and left-handed systems as having *odd parity*. The right-handed system is the one normally used, but left-handed systems occasionally occur—for instance in certain radiotherapy calculations. It is often important to distinguish between the two types, because in some mathematical formulae arising out of the use of

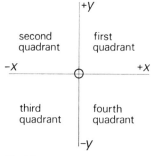

Fig 2.3

graphs positive signs are changed to negative signs, and vice versa, if we use left-handed axes instead of right-handed ones.

Whatever system we use, we see that the axes divide the space in which they lie into four sections or *quadrants*. These are numbered as follows: the area bounded by the lines where both *x* and *y* are *positive* is called *the first quadrant*; that where *x* is negative and *y* positive is called the *second quadrant*; where both are negative is the *third quadrant*, and where *x* is positive and *y* negative is the *fourth quadrant* (Fig. 2.3).

2.2.2   Co-ordinates

Each pair of values (x, y) is used to define a point in the plane of the axes, by measuring off the specified number of units in the *x*-direction and then moving the required number of units in the *y*-direction. E.g. if $x=4$ and $y=3$ we have:

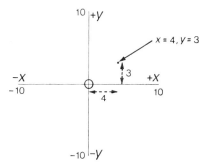

Fig 2.4

In this example, *x* and *y* are both positive, but negative values are handled similarly:

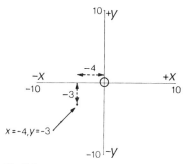

Fig 2.5

When a point is associated with a pair of numbers in this way, they are called the *co-ordinates* (also written *coordinates*) of the point. The x-value is called the *abscissa*, and the y-value *the ordinate*.

The standard notation for a point specified by co-ordinates is to refer to it as the pair: (abscissa, ordinate). Thus, for instance, the point corresponding to $x=4$, $y=3$ would be referred to as 'the point (4,3)'; similarly, the point $x=-2$, $y=1$ would be the point $(-2,1)$.

(Query: What are the co-ordinates of the origin? Answer: (0,0)).

2.3   Points and curves

Plotting a graph is a standard scientific activity. However, whenever we plot a graph, especially as a result of experimental work, it is as well to realize what we are really doing. This is the marking off of a series of points in the plane, which then appear to highlight a curve. By drawing the curve so defined, we then hope to obtain values for the coordinates of points not yet observed directly. We are assuming, in fact, that if we had been able to measure other—or all—the values between or even beyond the actual measured values, the results would have ended up on the same curve as that on which the existing points seem to lie. Now normally this is a reasonable assumption to make in practice; occasionally, however, things can go wrong and an illustration will be given in Chapter 3 of a situation which is not as straightforward as it looks at first sight.

2.4   Drawing graphs

Few graphs are straight; they usually curve, bend or twist, though it is sometimes possible to 'transform' the data so as to end up with a straight-line graph (see Chapter 3). Not everybody, however, has the ability to draw a good 'freehand' graph through a set of points, and this is perhaps the reason why we see so many graphs made up of straight-line segments, in spite of the possible disadvantages of this practice (Section 2.4.3). It is surprising that instruments for drawing curved graphs do not appear to be used as commonly in medicine as in, say, engineering, though medical work makes just as much use of graphs as does any other discipline. But then it must be admitted that even undergraduate mathematicians are not in general initiated into the mysteries of actually drawing properly the curves which so freely decorate their textbooks and notes.

There are two types of instrument for drawing smooth curves through sets of points: the *french curve* and the *spline*.

2.4.1   *French curves*

French curves come in sets, though they can be bought individually. Each one is a piece of transparent plastic with curved internal and external edges.

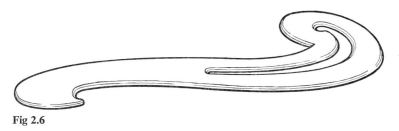

Fig 2.6

They are used as a straight-edge would be used, by being laid on the paper so that the points lie on one of the curved edges:

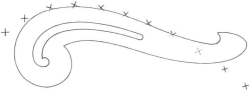

Fig 2.7

It usually happens that only some of the points to be joined lie on a single edge of the curve. In that case, different edges are used in succession to form a linked series of curves. However, there is a right way and a wrong way to do this; when following on from one curve to another, make sure that the final part of the first curve lies along the initial part of the second one, otherwise a smooth final result will not be obtained (Fig. 2.8).

If possible, successive sections should have at least two data points in common.

2.4.2   *Splines*

These are pieces of flexible wood, perspex or plastic-covered metal, which can be bent into curved shapes to follow the trend of points, and then used by running a pencil along them. The plastic-covered metal ones are easiest to use, as they retain the shape into which they are bent, whereas the perspex or wood splines have to be held in shape by weights. However, it is not always possible to re-straighten the plastic/metal type of spline, especially if it has been sharply

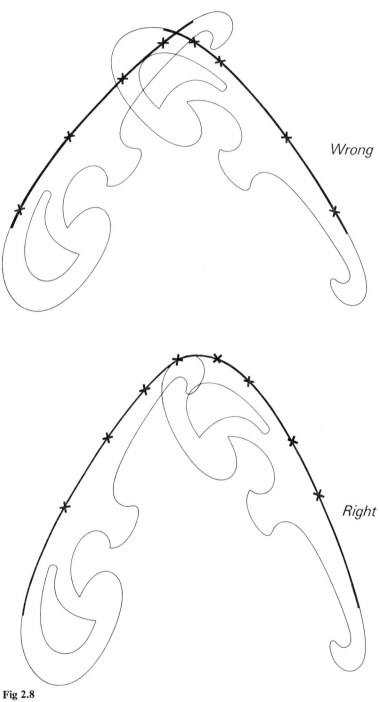

Wrong

Right

Fig 2.8

bent; after a while it develops 'kinks', which can cause difficulties. In any case, splines are not suitable, in general, for drawing sharply turning curves; french curves are best for this.

2.4.3   Presentation

It is surprising how often graphs are badly presented. A well-drawn graph should indicate the point positions without ambiguity, and the scales should be clearly marked along the axes. In many diagrams, especially those which contain more than one graph for comparison purposes, the point positions are frequently 'indicated' by solid triangles, squares or circles, and only a few scale points indicated on the axes. These circumstances make the actual values used to plot it almost impossible to retrieve from the graph, and since they are usually not tabulated, one is really left with less information than the experimenter had available to present. Admittedly, since proofs are made by logic, not by pretty pictures, graphs should not be used to *prove* anything, but simply to display information, indicate trends and suggest overall behaviour of the system being observed. But by the same token, then, graphs should not be the only presentation of the results if quantitative deductions are being made.

A bad practice is to clutter up the picture with large numbers of graphs for comparison purposes—there are too many examples in the literature where the result resembles a bird's nest. It is better to group the graphs onto separate diagrams or boil them down to averages and standard deviations. And if you have a standard deviation or estimate of experimental error for your points, it is a good idea to show this on the graph:

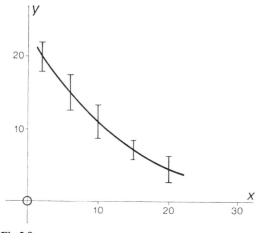

Fig 2.9

Another common practice which one often sees in medical journals is to draw the graph of a set of points by joining successive points with straight-line segments. In doing this, it should be borne in mind that the estimate of a value of y for a value of x lying between two known values is then based solely on the two points at the beginning and end of the line segment joining them, and we lose any information about the shape of the curve between those two points which is contributed by the other points:

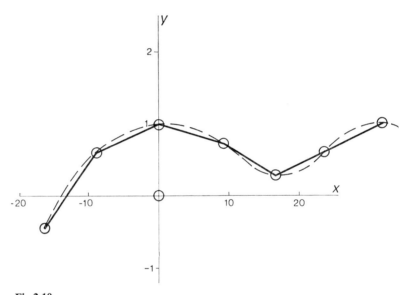

Fig 2.10

Also, this procedure makes no allowance for experimental and observer error in measuring and plotting the points—it may be that the 'best' curve to draw through the points does not actually pass through all or even any of them (Fig. 2.11).

This particular topic will be dealt with in Chapter 11.

It sometimes happens that the values being recorded on a graph do not allow the origin to be conveniently included in the drawing, in which case the values for one or both axes start at non-zero values (Fig. 2.12).

However, where possible the origin should be included in a graph, otherwise it is very easy to distort and exaggerate the shape of the graph and the effects of changes in y due to changes in x (Fig. 2.13). (This technique is sometimes used deliberately; for instance, if these had been graphs of death rate against amount of smoking, Fig 2.13a would probably be far more effective as anti-smoking propaganda than Fig 2.13b!)

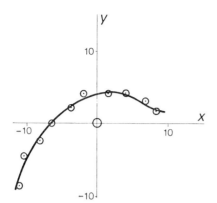

Fig 2.11

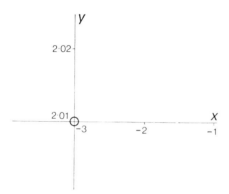

Fig 2.12

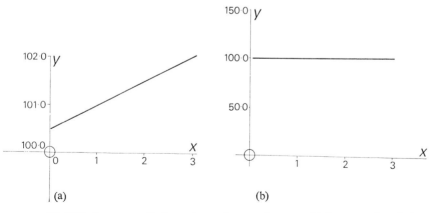

Fig 2.13. An apparently large change in y as x increases (a) is seen to be relatively small, in fact (b).

Sometimes, the axis is 'broken' to show the origin:

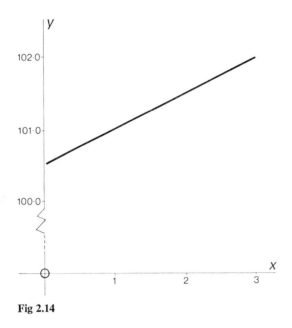

Fig 2.14

Candidly, this does not seem to us to help very much; it might be better to include along with the actual graph a scaled-down version including the origin. But as we said earlier, a graph is not a logical argument, merely an indication of behaviour.

Chapter 3
Functions

3.1   Introduction

Mathematics deals with *relationships*. Almost invariably, mathematical investigations are concerned with the way in which changes in the value or behaviour of some entity or other lead to corresponding changes in a related item or items. In practical terms, this means that mathematics is a natural approach to the handling of cause and effect, and for attempting to define the relationship between the two—it is for this reason that mathematics has been so successful a tool in scientific work. For instance, we might be concerned with the way the rate of salt excretion from the body alters as a result of changes in ambient temperature, or attempting to relate the rate at which cells are disrupted by irradiation to various incident dosage levels. Situations such as these lend themselves to a mathematical approach.

In order to be able to handle relationships mathematically, we need first some definitions to help give precision to our statements.

3.2   Variables and constants

We have already met in Chapter 1 the concepts of a variable and of a constant. A *variable* is simply a quantity which may take different values, i.e. *vary* in value. A *constant*, on the other hand, has a fixed value. Both the names arise naturally from their definitions. The diameter of the pupil of the eye is a variable—its size for any individual depends on the amount of light falling on the eye. The ratio of the circumference of a circle to its diameter is a constant = 3·1416 (approximately); for all circles, big or small, the ratio is constant or unchanging. This is an example of a pure numerical constant. We can also have physical, biological or chemical constants, for example the melting point of a metal at a given atmospheric pressure or the molecular weight of a specific compound. Experimentally determined constants, however, always have an uncertainty due to experimental error, but are regarded as 'constants' within this limitation.

3.3   Functions

If two variables are related by the fact that the value to be given to one of them can be determined only when the value of the other is known, the first variable is said to be a *function* of the second. Referring to the examples in Sections 3.1 and 3.2 above: the salt excretion rate is a function of the ambient temperature, other factors being fixed; the cell disruption rate is a function of the incident radiation dosage, and the pupil diameter is a function of the incident light.

3.4   Independent and dependent variables

Following on from the idea of a functional relationship between two variables, it is apparent that a series of values of one of them will set up a series of corresponding values of the other; in a sense, we can say that the second variable *depends* on the first, since the value of the first variable has to be given before we can determine the value of the second variable. For example, two variables, x and y, may be related as in Table 3.1.

Table 3.1

x	y
1	2
2	4
2·5	5
7	14
20	40

It will be easily seen that y is twice x (or x is half of y); but to use the functional relation between them, we may have to decide which of them is to have its value determined by the other. If x is to be allowed to vary in order to determine y, then we will be considering y as a function of x; whereas if y is the variable whose value will point to that of x, we will be regarding x as a function of y.

In order to make quite clear the direction of the relationship, special terms are used to describe the variables. The one whose value determines that of the other is called the *independent* variable, while the variable whose value is so determined is called the *dependent* variable. If y is a function of x, x is the independent variable and y the dependent variable; but if we turn the relationship inside-out and wish to regard x as a function of y, we are then giving y the role of independent variable and making x the dependent variable.

Thus, for example, if we are investigating the way in which height varies with age, then age will be the independent variable and height the dependent one. In mathematics, we are free to choose whichever variable we like as the independent variable and develop our argument from that standpoint; in practice however, we frequently have very little choice in the matter—for example, any relationship involving *time* will almost inevitably have it as the independent variable, if only because time moves on whether we like it or not.

3.5   Functions in theory and practice

Functional relationships between variables can be studied either experimentally or theoretically. Although much of what follows holds for both approaches, the underlying assumption of this chapter will be that we are dealing with *theoretical* relationships. The main difference between the two viewpoints is that experimental studies are limited in the range and scope of values studied; in theoretical work this is not the case. With experimental work, either the independent variable is given a limited set of distinct (or *discrete*) values and the values of the dependent variable recorded, or else the observations are restricted to a range of values. For example, we may be recording serum globulins (the dependent variable) in a patient or animal every half-hour (time, the independent variable) over a period of 24 hr; this will give us forty-nine (not forty-eight!) pairs of discrete readings. Or we may make a continuous EEG or ECG recording over a period of time. With theoretical relationships, on the other hand, we assume that the law relating our variables is known completely, and that for *any* value we may care to give the independent variable, it is possible to compute *or otherwise define* the value of the dependent variable. (We will see later (Section 3.6.2) why the italicized words have been included.)

3.6   Function definition

3.6.1   *Functional expressions*

If y is given as a function of x, this means that x's value has to be manipulated or used in some way in order to obtain the value of y. Quite often, the way in which x is to be handled in order to obtain y will be defined as a sequence of mathematical operations on x. But we have already seen (Section 1.8.1) that the medium for denoting sequences of operations on a variable is the *mathematical expression*—e.g. $x^2 + 2x - 7$ means 'square x, add the result to twice x, and then subtract 7'. So, for example, if y is obtained from x by, say, squaring x and adding 3 to the result, then we are forming $x^2 + 3$, and y will have the value of that expression for any given value of x. It would be a logical step in such a case to write

$$y = x^2 + 3$$

and this is in fact the most common way of expressing known functional relationships, the term 'function' being applied both to the dependent variable and to the equivalent expression in the independent variable. Thus we can talk of the function

$$y = x^2 + 3$$

or the function $\left.\begin{array}{l}\\ \\ \\ \\ \\ \\ \\ \\ \end{array}\right\}$ y as a function of x

$$y = (x^3 + a)/(x - 1)$$

or $z = w^3 - \dfrac{7 \cdot 4}{w} + b^2$ z as a function of w

(where a and b are constants).

Such expressions may be short and simple, or quite extended and complex. They may even involve other functions: e.g.

$$y = \sqrt{x} - 7x^2$$

which includes the 'square root' function. In such definitions, the dependent variable is on the left-hand side of the '=' sign, and the mathematical expression involving the independent variable is on the right-hand side.

3.6.2   Other means of function definition

Not all functions, however, are or can be defined by simple sequences of operations. For example, the 'square root' function which occurred above has no simple equivalent expression; $\sqrt{x}$ is defined as the (positive) quantity whose square is equal to x, which although a perfectly valid definition, gives no indication as to how x is to be obtained. The reader will probably be inclined to comment—with justice—that such theoretical definitions are all very well, but if no method of computing the function is included in its definition, what is one to do when faced with clothing these concepts with actual numbers? He or she might even argue that such functions contradicted the fundamental definition of a function, in that given x, we are not in a position to compute $\sqrt{x}$ as a result of its definition.

To this we would reply that there is no reason why we should not define a function by its properties rather than by directions for its computation, always keeping in mind, however, that the definition has to lead us to a means of computing the function should we require this. And in fact this is how most mathematical functions have been developed; the need for each one has arisen out of some situation whose solution demanded a function with particular properties, and having defined it by these properties, the mathematician has then had to devise means of computing the function, based on its definition. In other words, functions have been defined—usually—by their 'function', i.e. by their behaviour and by what they are supposed to do. To this extent, we suggest that the term 'function' in mathematics may not be as dissimilar from its use in medical applications, e.g. physiology, as some writers have thought.

In fact, we see now that there are two ways of dealing with functions. The first way is to define a computational scheme—i.e. a mathematical expression—and deduce the properties of the function from this; the second—and the one which occurs most frequently in practice—is to define the function by its properties and deduce a computational scheme from these properties.

Both these methods of definition are valid, and in developing the topic, we will use them as and when we need them.

3.7   Functions as graphs

In the previous chapter we discussed the use of graphs in presenting experimental data. We now apply the idea of a graph to the handling of functions.

It is easy to see how graphical ideas can be adapted to presenting functions. We have an independent variable and a dependent one; if we assign the x-axis to the independent variable, and the y-axis to the dependent one, then each pair of values will define a point. Take for example the function $y = x^2 + 3$:

x	y
-2	7
-1	4
0	3
1	4
2	7
3	12

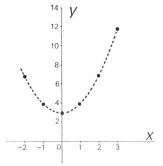

Fig 3.1

As with experimental data, the points can be joined up by a curve, shown by the broken line in Fig 3.1. But unlike experimental data, the value of *y* is supposed to be known for *all* values of *x*, and therefore we can in theory accurately plot the curve for any range of values of *x*.

However, even without the infilling curve, the scattered and relatively sparse set of points plotted above gives us something of the 'feel' of the function. We see for example that as *x* 'moves along the *x*-axis' (i.e. takes a succession of values) from negative to positive values, *y* drops in value and then rises again; in particular, the lowest value it attains in the range of *x* being studied seems to be 3. Information of this kind is frequently of more use than the calculation of specific values—and often is not very obvious from the form or definition of the function. Admittedly, in the example given, it is not difficult to see, both from the table of values and from the observation that x^2 is $\geqslant 0$ for all and any *x* and therefore $x^2+3 \geqslant 3$ for all *x*, that the value of *y* never falls below 3, and that *y* falls to 3 in value and then rises again. But deducing the behaviour of a function from its mathematical form alone can sometimes present difficulties, and a graph can be of great value in indicating the overall nature of such a function. The study of the techniques for sketching the graphs of functions without having to work out the co-ordinates of a large number of points is known as *curve-tracing* (see Section 8.10.3 for further discussion of this topic).

It is as well, however, to state here and now that the reading of the values of unplotted points from a graph through those already plotted can be an extremely deceptive activity, and care is always necessary. Take for example the following:

Table 3.2

x	*y*
−3	5·4
−2	2·67
−1	1
0	0
1	0·33
2	1·6
3	3·86

which plot as Fig 3.2

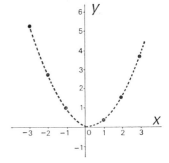

Fig 3.2

The curve looks quite reasonable, with y always positive, and in particular the value of y for $x = -0.4$, say, appears to be about 0.25. However, the function being plotted, and whose values at unit intervals are given in Table 3.2, is in fact

$$y = \frac{x^3}{2x+1}$$

which really looks like this:

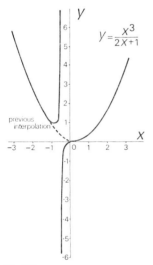

Fig 3.3

and for $x = -0.4$ the value of y is actually negative $= -0.32!$ This is because the function changes very rapidly between $x = -1$ and $x = 0$. The moral is that in experimental work, a graph is a guess at what is happening between known values, and must be considered as nothing better than that, while in theoretical work, a graph should not be plotted without a thorough mathematical investigation of the function concerned. For this, the theories of *limits* (Chapter 5) and of the *differential calculus* (Chapter 9) are usually needed.

The above example was one of *interpolation*, i.e. estimation of unknown values *within* the range of observed values. Even more care is needed in *extrapolation*, i.e. estimating (=guessing, often enough) values outside the range plotted. Considerations of this kind are of importance when extrapolating from observed data in order to estimate a threshold—for example, when estimating minimum permitted radiation dose.

3.8   Units

When dealing with functions, the values of the variables are usually treated as though they were pure numbers, without physical dimensions. The theory of functions does not concern itself with the units in which the measurements may be made, even though in applications of the theory, the variables may correspond to actual physical quantities. Function theory deals solely with numerical magnitudes and changes in numerical magnitudes; the units in which variables may be measured—feet, ohms, grams/c.c., etc—do not enter into the discussion or affect the conclusions.

3.9   Implicit and explicit functions

Sometimes a function relation between two variables is given as an equation which has not actually been solved for the dependent variable; for example

$$y - 4x^3 + x = 0 \tag{3.1}$$

defines a relation between x and y but does not express y directly as a function of x—which we would need to do if we wished to plot y against x. To get this into the form we have been using up to now, we would have to bring all the terms in x to the right hand side of the '=' sign:

$$y = 4x^3 - x \tag{3.2}$$

When, as in (3.2), y is defined directly in terms of x, y is said to be an *explicit* function of x; but where the relationship is not defined explicitly, as in (3.1), y is said to be an *implicit* function of x. We could also say, of course, that (3.1) defines x as an implicit function of y, but since the equation (3.1) contains a term in x^3 as well as x, the conversion to an explicit form is then more difficult, though it can be done.

We see that sometimes the distinction between implicit and explicit forms may be trivial, as above with y defined as a function of x. Often, however, the manipulation may be difficult or even impossible. In general, implicit relationships are more awkward to handle than explicit ones, but they have their uses, and it is sometimes possible—and more convenient—to deduce the properties of an implicitly defined dependent variable without having to manipulate it into an explicit form.

3.10   Some specific types of functions: linear, polynomial and rational forms

We now discuss some functions of relatively simple type which are nevertheless of considerable use and importance.

3.10.1   Linear functions

The simplest functional relation between two variables is the straight equality

$$y = x \tag{3.3}$$

where x is the independent variable. This means that for any given value of x, y takes the same value. If $x = 6$, so does y; if x becomes $-72 \cdot 14$, y does also. The meaning of (3.3) above is that y is equal to x *for each and every value of x*. If we plot pairs of values from (3.3), they appear to be on a straight line through the origin,

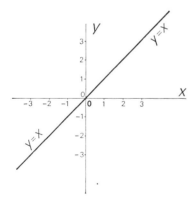

Fig 3.4

and indeed this is the case; the graph of $y = x$ is in fact a straight line through the origin.

The function $y = x$ is a member of a class of functions all of which have straight-line graphs, and which are for this reason known as *linear functions*.

Slightly more complicated examples are

$$y = x + 1 \tag{3.4}$$

$$y = 3 - 7 \cdot 18x \tag{3.5}$$

$$2y = x\sqrt{2} - 8 \cdot 511 \tag{3.6}$$

$$-\frac{y}{\sqrt{3}} + 2x - 1 \cdot 8 = 0 \tag{3.7}$$

The common property of the terms in these functions is that they contain only x's and y's; there are no products or quotients of x and y, nor higher powers of these variables. In each case, if we plot the graphs, we find we can draw a straight line through the points plotted (Figs 3.5 and 3.6).

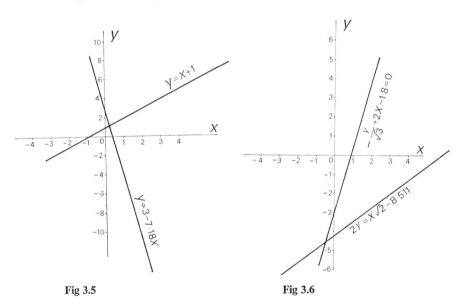

Fig 3.5   Fig 3.6

3.10.2   The general linear function

The most general linear function is of the implicit form

$$ly + mx + n = 0 \tag{3.8}$$

i.e. $$ly = -mx - n \tag{3.9}$$

where l, m and n are constants. However, if $l \neq 0$, this can be expressed explicitly as

$$y = -\frac{m}{l}x - \frac{n}{l} \tag{3.10}$$

or $y = ax + b$ (3.11)

where we have put a for $-m/l$ and b for $-n/l$. This form (3.11) is a commonly used one; in it, the quantity multiplying x—i.e. the constant a—is called the *slope*.

Examples (3.4) to (3.7) above can all be obtained by giving special values to the constants a and b or l, m and n. For instance, if $a=1$ and $b=1$ in (3.11), we get $y=x+1$, which is example (3.4); if we put $a=-7{\cdot}18$, $b=3$ in (3.11), we obtain $y=-7{\cdot}18x+3$, which is example (3.5). Similarly, in (3.8), $l=2$, $m=-\sqrt{2}$, $n=8{\cdot}511$ gives us example (3.6), while $l=-1/\sqrt{3}$, $m=2$, $n=-1{\cdot}8$ gives us example (3.7).

It is possible to prove that the graph of (3.8) is a straight line for any values of l, m and n, though we will not give the proof here.

3.10.3   Properties of linear functions

Linear functions have a number of useful properties. In the first place, they are mathematically simple and easy to handle, since they involve only the first powers of the variables, and not higher powers or other functions. Secondly, if it is known that two variables have a linear relation, then since a straight line is fixed once two points on it have been determined, we need only plot two points on the graph and then obtain the whole graph by drawing a line with a straight-edge through the two points. The two easiest points to obtain are normally those in which the straight line cuts the axes. If $y=ax+b$, it can be shown that these are the points $(0, b)$ and $(-b/a, 0)$:

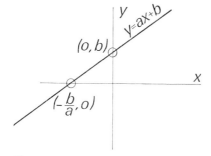

Fig 3.7

For instance, if $y = 3x - 12$, then we are taking $a = 3$ and $b = -12$, and the graph of this function is the straight line through the points $(0, -12)$ and $(4, 0)$:

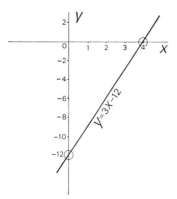

Fig 3.8

As with everything else, commonsense must be used when drawing straight line graphs by this method. If the two points of intersection with the axes are rather close together, then a slight error in ruling the short line between them will be steadily magnified into a large one as the line length is increased:

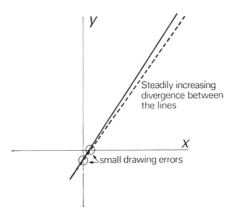

Steadily increasing divergence between the lines

small drawing errors

Fig 3.9

To guard against this, additional points should be plotted. It is a good idea in any case to check a line graph drawn through two points by making sure that a third point some distance away has co-ordinates satisfying the defining function.

A further important characteristic of linear functions is the simple way in which changes in the value of the independent variable bring about changes in the value of the dependent variable. Consider the linear function

$$y = 6x + 3 \qquad (3.12)$$

for example. For the set of values

$$x = -4, \ -2, \ 0, \ 2, \ 4, \ 6$$

we obtain

$$y = -21, \ -9, \ 3, \ 15, \ 27, \ 39$$

(E.g.   if $x = 2$, then $y = 6 * 2 + 3 = 15$.)

Notice that the values of y change by a constant amount ($+12$) as x changes by a constant amount ($+2$). Furthermore, the ratio of the change in y to the change in $x = 12/2 = 6$, which is the value of the multiplier of x in (3.12). This is an example of a property of linear functions, which in algebraic terms can be stated as follows: if $y = ax + b$, and x_1, x_2 are two values of x corresponding to values y_1, y_2 of y, then the change $(x_2 - x_1)$ in x is related to the corresponding change $(y_2 - y_1)$ in y by the relation

$$(y_2 - y_1) = a(x_2 - x_1)$$

i.e. $\dfrac{y_2 - y_1}{x_2 - x_1} = a.$

In other words, if y is linearly related to x, then changes in y are proportional to changes in x.

3.10.4   Non-linear functions

The linear relationships (3.8) and (3.11) contain no powers, functions, quotients, or products of either variable; terms such as x^3, $\sqrt{y}$, xy do not appear. Any functional relation containing such quantities will not be of the form (3.8) and is therefore said to be *non-linear*. The graph of such a function is not a straight line. For example

$$y = \pm \sqrt{x}$$

$$y = 3x^3 + x - 1$$

$$p = (q + 7)/(q + 2) \qquad (3.13)$$

are non-linear functions. This is true even of (3.13), which does not apparently

c

contain any powers or products, but is nevertheless not expressible in the form
(3.8). In fact, if we multiply across by $q+2$, we obtain $pq+2p=q+7$, again a
non-linear function. Other examples of such functions are, e.g.

$$y^2 = x^2 + a^2 \tag{3.14}$$

$$y^2 - 3x + y = 0 \tag{3.15}$$

$$p - q - \frac{3}{q} = 7 \tag{3.16}$$

As an example of the varied forms which the graphs of non-linear functions can
take, we illustrate those of $y = \pm \sqrt{x}$ and $y = 3x^3 + x - 1$:

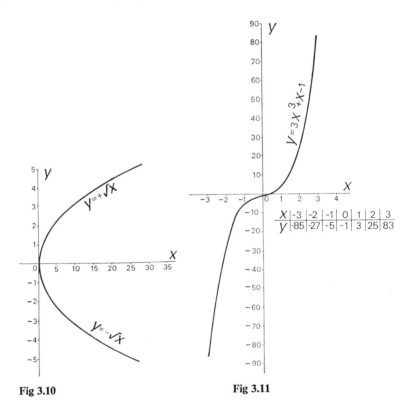

Fig 3.10   Fig 3.11

N.B. An expression containing a variable x solely in the form $ax+b$, where
a and b do not involve x, is said to be *linear in x*; thus (3.15) is linear in x but
non-linear in y.

3.10.5   Transformations

Although the relation between two variables may be non-linear, it may be possible to *transform* it into a linear form by introducing subsidiary variables. This is often done in order to take advantage of the simplicity of linear functions.

Consider for example the implicit form

$$\sqrt{\tau} = k_0 + k_1\sqrt{\gamma} \tag{3.17}$$

used by Schmid-Schonbein *et al* (1968) in a discussion of the mechanics of blood-flow. In (3.17), τ is the shear stress of the blood and γ the shear rate; k_1 and k_2 are constants (or more correctly, *parameters*: see section 3.11. The relation is non-linear; however, if we introduce two new variables, u and v say, defined by

$$u = \sqrt{\tau}$$

$$v = \sqrt{\gamma}$$

we obtain

$$u = k_0 + k_1v \tag{3.18}$$

which expresses u as a linear function of v, i.e. expresses $\sqrt{\tau}$ as a linear function of $\sqrt{\gamma}$. So by working with $\sqrt{\tau}$ and $\sqrt{\gamma}$ rather than τ and γ, we can handle the problem with a linear function and simplify the mathematics, returning if necessary to τ and γ at the end of the analysis.

3.10.6   Multiple-valued functions

An examination of the graph of $y = \pm\sqrt{x}$ (Fig 3.10) shows that it is different from the functions we have illustrated so far, in that any given value of x gives rise to two different values of y, equal in magnitude but opposite in sign. If $x = 9$, then both $+3$ and -3 can be taken as the value of $\pm\sqrt{x}$, since each squared gives 9. This is an example of a *multiple-valued function*—to a given value of the independent variable there corresponds more than one value of the dependent variable. Note that this is not the same situation as having different values of the independent variable giving rise to the same value of the dependent variable, which is the case with, e.g., $y = 3x^2 - x - 7$ ($y = -5$ for $x = -\frac{2}{3}$ and for $x = 1$). This is still an ordinary *single-valued* function of x; for any particular value of x there is but one value of y.

3.10.7   *Functions undefined over a region*

The reader will see also that there are no points on the graph of $y = \pm \sqrt{x}$ for negative values of x. This is because the square of either a positive or a negative quantity is always positive, and hence in the ordinary number system, there is no number which can act as the square root of a negative quantity. We say, therefore, that $y = \pm \sqrt{x}$ is *not defined* for $x < 0$. In this example, the region of non-definition is the whole of the negative x-axis, but it is possible to have a function which is not defined over a finite section of the x-axis, e.g. $x^2 - y^2 = 1$
i.e. $y = \pm \sqrt{(x^2 - 1)}$:

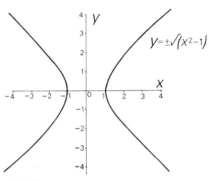

Fig 3.12

Or again, it is possible to have a function which is defined *only* over a finite part of the x-axis, e.g. $x^2 + y^2 = 1$ (i.e. $y = \pm \sqrt{[1 - x^2]}$):

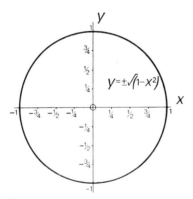

Fig 3.13

Functions of this kind represent something of an enlargement of the idea of a function which has been building up in previous sections. It is now clear that there may be values of the independent variable for which it is not possible to find a value of the dependent variable. Until now, our examples have always implied that any value of the one would give rise to a corresponding value of the other, although the definition given in Section 3.3 does not actually say this, and in fact was worded so as to allow for the possibility of being unable to give a value to the dependent variable.

3.10.8   Polynomials

An expression of the form

$$a_0 + a_1 x + a_2 x^2 + a_3 x^3 + \ldots + a_n x^n$$

i.e. $$a_0 + \sum_{i=1}^{n} a_i x^i$$

where $a_0, a_1, a_2, a_3, \ldots a_n$ are constants

is called a *polynomial* in x, and if

$$y = a_0 + \sum_{i=1}^{n} a_i x^i \tag{3.19}$$

y is said to be a *polynomial function* of x. The constants $a_1, a_2, \ldots a_n$ are called the *coefficients* of the powers of x; the constant a_0 is called the *absolute term*. The constant n is called the *order* or *degree* of the polynomial (both terms are in common use).

    Examples:

(i) $3 + 4x + 7x^2 - 3 \cdot 2x^3 + 0 \cdot 01x^4$

(a *fourth-order* polynomial in x; the absolute term is 3. The coefficient of x is 4, of x^2 is 7, of x^3 is $-3 \cdot 2$ and of x^4 is $0 \cdot 01$).

(ii) $-1 + 5w^2 - 0 \cdot 1w^4 + 2w^6$

(a sixth-order polynomial in w, the coefficients of the odd powers of w being all zero).

If $n = 1$ in (3.19), we have y as a linear function of x; if $n = 2$, y is said to be a *quadratic* function of x; if $n = 3$, y is called a *cubic* function of x; $n = 4$ results in a *quartic* or *biquadratic* function; $n = 5$ gives a *quintic* function; and so on.

(We suppose that $n=7$ gives a *septic* function, which is a nice coincidence in a medical context!)

One reason for the importance of polynomials is that they are easily-computed expressions which can be used to *approximate* the values of functions of more complicated form; for example if x lies between ± 1, it can be shown that

$$\sqrt{(1+x)}$$

has very nearly the same value as

$$1+\tfrac{1}{2}x-\tfrac{1}{8}x^2+\tfrac{1}{16}x^3.$$

Table 3.3 $\sqrt{(1+x)}$ and $1+\tfrac{1}{2}x-\tfrac{1}{8}x^2+\tfrac{1}{16}x^3$

x	$-0\cdot9$	$-0\cdot5$	$-0\cdot3$	$-0\cdot1$	$0\cdot0$	$0\cdot1$	$0\cdot3$	$0\cdot5$	$0\cdot9$
$\sqrt{(1+x)}$	0·3162	0·7071	0·8367	0·9487	1·0	1·0488	1·1402	1·2247	1·3784
$1+\tfrac{1}{2}x-\tfrac{1}{8}x^2+\tfrac{1}{16}x^3$	0·4148	0·7109	0·8376	0·9487	1·0	1·0488	1·1405	1·2266	1·3944

The approximation is best for positive or small negative values of x (the problem of approximation is dealt with in Chapters 10 and 11). Since computing the values of polynomials is comparatively simple on a desk calculator or an electronic computer, we have therefore the means at hand to compute the values of functions which have not been defined by a simple mathematical expression.

3.10.8.1 Computation of polynomials by 'nesting'

It was stated in the previous paragraph that polynomials are 'easily computed' expressions. However, anyone faced with computing the value of, e.g.

$$16x^8-3\cdot4x^7+4\cdot01x^6-7x^5+0\cdot5x^4-2\cdot11x^3-7x^2+3\cdot1x-5 \qquad (3.20)$$

for, say $x=2\cdot1$, might be forgiven for wondering whether 'easily-computed' was quite the phrase to use. As written, the computation requires thirty-six multiplications and eight additions or subtractions; even if advantage is taken of the fact that $x^3=x^2*x$, $x^4=x^3*x$, etc., this still leaves fifteen multiplications and eight additions or subtractions. Either way, at the very least a desk calculator would be needed, but even so the computation would be laborious and prone to error. A computer program could be written to do the work, of course, but the time and effort involved might not be felt to be worth it for a 'one-off' calculation, and in any case there is a more efficient method for carrying out the calculation, which we will now discuss.

This method, known as 'nesting', saves multiplication and thus reduces the risk of accumulating round-off errors, and it also enables the complete calculation to be carried out on a desk calculator without pencil-and-paper copying of intermediate results. Alternatively, it leads to a computer program of maximum efficiency.

Consider the polynomial

$$f = cx^2 + bx + a.$$

In this form, computing f for any value of x takes at least three multiplications and two additions: we must form x^2, $c * x^2$ and $b * x$, which gives the three multiplications, and then use two additions to add cx^2, bx and a. However, we can write

$$f = cx^2 + bx + a$$

as

$$f = (cx + b) * x + a.$$

In this form only two multiplications are needed: $c * x$ and $(cx + b) * x$, but still two additions: $cx + b$, and $(cx + b)x + a$.

This alternative form of f can be computed in two main steps:

Form

$$g = c * x + b$$

$$f = g * x + a \qquad (= (cx + b) * x + a)$$

If there is a term in x^3, say

$$f = dx^3 + cx^2 + bx + a$$

then the same technique can be used on this. As written, this would take at least five multiplications: x^2, x^3 $(= x^2 * x)$, dx^3, cx^2 and bx, and three additions: $dx^3 + cx^2$, $(dx^3 + cx^2) + bx$, $(dx^3 + cx^2 + bx) + a$. Applying our previous approach, we write

$$f = ((dx + c) * x + b) * x + a.$$

or in steps,

$$h = dx + c$$

$$g = hx + b \qquad = (dx + c) * x + b$$

$$f = gx + a \qquad = ((dx + c) * x + b) * x + a$$

which requires three multiplications and three additions, a saving of two multiplications.

Notice that each step consists of the same pair of operations: multiply the previous answer by x and add a coefficient. The highest coefficient of x is used as the 'previous answer' to begin with, and we carry on down the list of coefficients in order of decreasing powers of x. A little experimentation shows that the method extends to polynomials of any order.

Our polynomial (3.20) would be represented as

$$(((((((16x-3\cdot4)x+4\cdot01)x-7)x+0\cdot5)x-2\cdot11)x-7)x+3\cdot1)x-5 \qquad (3.21)$$

which looks rather fearsome, but whose evaluation can be handled in single steps as with the simpler forms already discussed. In this form, eight multiplications and eight additions suffice to calculate the expression for any value of x, a considerable saving in effort.

The form of (3.21) is the characteristic one of a 'nested' polynomial; bracketed expressions are 'nested' within one another, rather like those children's box toys where each box contains within itself a smaller box.

In addition to the saving of effort, 'nesting' a polynomial is easier and safer to carry out on a desk calculator than the more obvious method, since the computation can be kept entirely on the machine; after each step the answer is transferred to the keyboard in preparation for the next step and no other copying operation is needed. Indeed, if the machine has an automatic transfer from accumulator to keyboard, then the whole process is completely mechanical (though round-off will still have to be carried out by the operator).

Applying this to (3.21) for $x=2\cdot1$, the steps are, assuming a desk calculator is being used:

(1) Enter the value $x=2\cdot1$ in the multiplier register and lock it there.
(2) Enter 16 (the coefficient of x^8) on the keyboard.
(3) Form $16 * 2\cdot1$.
(4) Add $-3\cdot4$ (the coefficient of x^7) to the answer.
(5) Transfer the result to the keyboard (or copy it to the keyboard if there is no transfer mechanism).
(6) Multiply by $2\cdot1$.
(7) Add $4\cdot01$ (the coefficient of x^6) to the result, etc., etc.

Steps (5), (6) and (7) are repeated, substituting the various coefficients in turn, until the process terminates with the addition of the absolute term, -5.

Care must be taken to use a machine with a large enough keyboard and registers, of course. The nesting method can be easily adapted as an algorithm for a computer program, and it is not difficult to write the program so that *any* polynomial can be computed, given the degree, the coefficients and the value of the independent variable.

The method also serves to illustrate a point of frequent occurrence in practical computation, namely, that particular mathematical forms may be algebraically cumbersome, but arithmetically easy, and vice versa. For algebraic work, the form (3.20) is more compact, but for arithmetic calculation the form (3.21) is preferable.

3.10.9   *Rational functions*

If

$$y = \frac{a_0 + a_1 x + a_2 x^2 + \ldots + a_n x^n}{b_0 + b_1 x + b_2 x^2 + \ldots + b_m x^m}$$

where n, m and a_0, $a_1 \ldots a_n$, b_0, $b_1 \ldots b_m$ are constants, then y is said to be a *rational function* of x. We see that a rational function is the quotient of two polynomials.

Note that if $b_1 = b_2 = b_3 = \ldots = b_m = 0$ (i.e. all the coefficients of the denominator are zero), then a rational function degenerates into a polynomial; if $a_2 = a_3 = a_4 = \ldots = a_n = 0$ as well, the polynomial becomes a linear function; and if $a_1 = 0$ as well, the linear function degenerates into a constant.

Examples:

$$w = \frac{a}{b+z}$$

$$y = \frac{x^3}{2x+1}$$

which we met with earlier,

$$p = \frac{-1 + 3 \cdot 2q - 17 \cdot 8q^2}{2 - 8 \cdot 001q + 0 \cdot 023q^2}$$

The graphs of such functions are variegated and not classifiable; as an example, we give the graph of $y = \dfrac{1-x}{1+x}$:

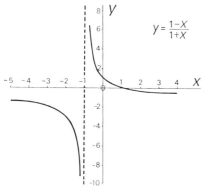

Fig 3.14

At $x = -1$, $y = 1/0$, i.e. becomes undefined, since division by zero is forbidden (Section 1.3.4). The graph has two branches, separated by a vertical line through $x = -1$. (In terms of *limits* (Chapter 5) $\lim_{x \to -1} y = \pm\infty$, the sign depending on the direction from which $x = -1$ is approached.)

Along with polynomials, rational functions are very useful in approximating to other functions.

3.11   Parameters

It often happens that a quantity which could vary or be varied in a given situation is constrained to hold a fixed value—for example, the temperature in a constant temperature bath or a particular value set for a variable resistance. These values then define the particular system in which some other variable operates—e.g. we may be observing mass action transfers at fixed temperatures or electrical outputs from a network with fixed values of resistance, etc. Or take as a further example the Schmid-Schonbein relation already referred to (Section 3.10.5):

$$\sqrt{\tau} = k_0 + k_1\sqrt{\gamma}$$

The relationship of interest is that between τ and γ, but the exact nature of this will depend on the values of k_0 and k_1. For instance, the ratio of change in $\sqrt{\tau}$ to change in $\sqrt{\gamma}$ is equal to k_1 (Section 3.10.3). Once k_0 and k_1 have been fixed, however, they define the detail of the system within which τ and γ can change. Different values of k_0 and k_1 define different systems for the relationship between τ and γ.

Such 'variable constants' are called *parameters*. They are quantities capable of having different values but which hold a fixed value in order to define a particular case of a general relationship.

3.12   General notation

So far, we have discussed only particular functions. Sometimes, however, we need a notation for indicating a function without necessarily giving its exact mathematical form.

The symbol

$$f(x)$$

(spoken as 'f of x')
is used to denote a function of x where the form of the function may or may not

need to be specified. The quantity in the parentheses ( )—here x—is called the *argument* of the function. If we need to distinguish between different functions in a discussion, we can use subscripts:

$$f_1(x), \quad f_2(x)$$

or some other letter instead of f:

$$g(x), \quad F(x), \quad \phi(x), \quad \lambda(x).$$

In such a situation, if y is the dependent variable, we write

$$y = f(x) \quad (\text{or } y = g(x), \text{ etc.}).$$

Sometimes, in order to cut down the number of symbols, the notation

$$y = y(x)$$

or $\qquad \lambda = \lambda(t)$

is used, meaning 'y is a function of x', or 'λ is a function of t'. However, novices are advised to avoid this economy until they feel confident of their ability to manipulate symbols.

3.13   Functional form and change of variable

The definition of a function sets up a relationship which is one of *form*, unaffected by the choice of symbols or values. So for example, if

$$f(x) = 4x^2 - 2x + 7 \tag{3.22}$$

then $\qquad f(t) = 4t^2 - 2t + 7$

and $\qquad f(3) = 4 * 3^2 - 2 * 3 + 7 = 37 \tag{3.23}$

Furthermore, with the same definition of $f(x)$

$$f(x+1) = 4 * (x+1)^2 - 2 * (x+1) + 7 \tag{3.24}$$

i.e. reduced to its simplest terms, $f(x+1) = 4x^2 + 6x + 9$

and $\qquad f(x+a) = 4 * (x+a)^2 - 2 * (x+a) + 7 \tag{3.25}$

i.e. $\qquad f(x+a) = 4x^2 + 6ax + 4a^2 - 2a + 7.$

Note that if we substitute $a = 1$ in (3.25), we obtain (3.24), and that if $x = 0$,

$f(x+a) = f(a) = 4a^2 - 2a + 7$. More complex examples are:

$$f\left(\frac{1}{x}\right) = \frac{4}{x^2} - \frac{2}{x} + 7 \tag{3.26}$$

and $$f\left(\frac{x+1}{x+2}\right) = 4 * \left(\frac{x+1}{x+2}\right)^2 - 2 * \left(\frac{x+1}{x+2}\right) + 7 \tag{3.27}$$

where again $f(x)$ is defined by (3.22).
Again, if

$$g(x) = \sqrt{(x-1)} \tag{3.28}$$

then $$g(z + \tfrac{1}{2}) = \sqrt{[(z + \tfrac{1}{2}) - 1]} = \sqrt{(z - \tfrac{1}{2})} \tag{3.29}$$

and $$g(\sqrt{z}) = \sqrt{(\sqrt{z} - 1)} \tag{3.30}$$

Examples (3.22)–(3.30) show that basically it is the form of the function which matters, not the argument. A conclusion deduced about

$$g(x) \text{ for } x = a$$

will also be true of

$$g(\sqrt{z}) \text{ for } \sqrt{z} = a.$$

So if $g(1) = 5$,

then $$g\left(\frac{2x+1}{x+3}\right) = 5 \text{ for } \left(\frac{2x+1}{x+3}\right) = 1$$

i.e.   for $x = 2$.

The reader will probably have noticed that there is a possibility of a notational ambiguity between $f(x+1)$ meaning 'the function f with $(x+1)$ as argument' and $f(x+1)$ meaning $f * (x+1)$. In practice, this rarely leads to difficulty since it is the first interpretation which is usually intended and in any case the interpretation should be easily deducible from the context. Where it is not, whoever wrote the text is guilty of very bad notation.

3.14   Roots of a function; roots of an equation

If a function is zero for some finite value or values of the independent variable, such values are called the *roots* of the function. Symbolically, any value k for which

$$f(k) = 0$$

is a root of $f(x)$. It is also common usage to speak of the *roots of the equation*

$f(x)=0$, and k would be referred to as a root of this equation if $f(k)=0$. Another way of referring to the situation would be to say that k *satisfies* the equation $f(x)=0$ if $f(k)=0$. The process of finding the roots of an equation is called *solving the equation* (cf. Section 1.10).

Examples:

(i) $x=3$ is a root of $f(x)=2x^3-5x^2-9$
    since $f(3)=2*3^3-5*3^2-9=0$

(ii) $x=2$ is a root of $\sqrt{(x^2-4)}=0$
     So is $x=-2$.

Some functions do not have any roots at all—for example the function $1/x$. Other functions have innumerable roots—this is much more common a situation than having no roots. The functions of trigonometry (Chapter 6) are examples of such functions.

Finding the roots of functions or equations constitutes a major part of practical mathematics; we normally wish to find values of the independent variable for which our dependent variable will satisfy given conditions and this in general leads to a question of locating roots. Different types of equation demand different techniques for finding roots, though *formal*—i.e. algebraic manipulative—methods for finding roots are not very numerous, and functions do not occur very often for which it is possible to deduce general formulae for finding the roots. By far the most common approach to solving the equations met with in practice is to use *numerical* or *approximation* methods; some details of these are given in Chapter 11.

N.B. If we plot the graph of $y=f(x)$, the roots of $f(x)=0$ are the x-values of the points where the graph crosses the x-axis. This is the basis of many techniques for finding roots.

3.15   Functions of more than one variable

In many physical situations, the simple functional dependence with which we have been dealing up until now is inadequate. Frequently our observations depend on more than one variable—there may be many variables, all varying independently of one another and all contributing to the changes in the observed variable. For example, if we have solute diffusing through a volume, the concentration at any point depends not only on the time at which the measurement is made, but also on the position of the point of measurement within the volume. Or again, in radiation dosimetry the dose accumulating at a given point in the patient depends on the time since the implant and the distance of the point from the implant.

We are led, therefore, to an extension of the single variable functional dependence represented by $y=f(x)$. It would appear that a (dependent) variable —e.g. concentration or radiation dose—can depend on more than one independent variable—e.g. on distance and time. The mathematical notation for such dependence is a straightforward extension of the single independent variable case: if y is a variable whose value depends on the values of two independent variables—x and t, say—then we write

$$y=f(x, t)$$

or $$y=y(x, t)$$

The implication here is that a change in y can result from changes in x alone, changes in t alone, or changes in both x and t.

The notation extends easily to functions of more than two variables; e.g. $z=f(x, y, t)$ expresses the fact that z is a function of the three variables x, y and t.

Examples:

(i) $z=x^2+y^2-6x$

expresses z as a function of the variables x and y.

(ii) $w=xyz$

is a function of the three variables x, y and z

$$\text{(iii)} \quad R_{b/t}=\frac{q}{\dfrac{p}{1+R_{b/t}}+\dfrac{1}{K}} \tag{3.32}$$

used by Ekins, Newman & O'Riordan (1968) in a paper on radioimmunoassay. Here q, p and K are the independent variables, $R_{b/t}$ the dependent variable. Because $R_{b/t}$ appears on both sides of (3.32), it is therefore defined *implicitly* as a function of q, p and K (cf. Section 3.9).

3.15.1   *Multivariable graphs*

Representation of a function of two variables by a graph is achieved by various extensions of the procedure for a single variable. What is frequently done with e.g.

$$y=f(x, t)$$

is to choose one of the independent variables—t, say—and then plot y as a function of t for a series of steps in value of x, each x-value resulting in a different graph of y against t, and the complete ensemble of curves being plotted on the same sheet of graph paper. A typical example is the following based on data in a paper by Mori (1969) on the antigenic structure of human gonado-trophins.

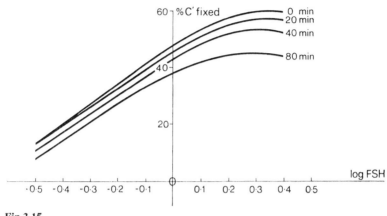

Fig 3.15

Here we have plotted the percentage of complement fixed, C', as a function of the *logarithm*† of the concentration of FSH (follicle stimulating hormone) for various periods of incubation with neuraminidase plus β-glucosidase.

The technique cannot be extended very easily to functions of more than two variables; the best that can be done in such cases is to repeatedly plot the dependent variable as a function of one of the independent variables, for various fixed values of the other variables. An example is Fig 3.16, taken from the paper by Ekins, Newman & O'Riordan (1968) mentioned earlier.

Here $R_{b/t}$ is plotted as a function of p for a series of values of q, and fixed K.

A problem arising with such representations is that of interpolating for values of that independent variable which is represented only for certain fixed values. For example in Fig 3.16, we have values of $R_{b/t}$ against p for $q=1\cdot0$ and $q=0\cdot375$; how do we find values of $R_{b/t}$ for $q=0\cdot6$ say?

One way to tackle this is to find points between the two curves for $q=1\cdot0$ and $q=0\cdot375$ whose vertical distance from one or other of these curves is in a suitable proportion to the corresponding vertical distance between the curves.

† Section 4.3.

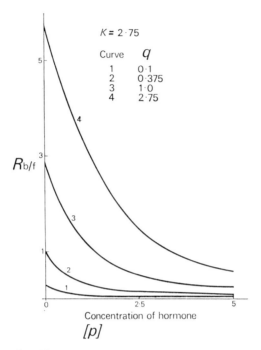

Fig 3.16

E.g. in Fig 3.17, if A is a point on the $q=0.6$ curve, then

$$\frac{BA}{BC} = \frac{0.6-0.375}{1.0-0.375};$$

since BC can be measured, BA is known and therefore A can be plotted for the value of p at the vertical line BC.

Repetition of this process for various values of p gives the graph for $q=0.6$.

This is not always satisfactory, since the variation between curves may not be properly represented by a proportion. In such cases, more complicated methods of interpolation are needed.

An alternative method of presentation which can sometimes be used is the *carpet graph*. This method involves little more effort than is needed for the previous technique described, and interpolation is much easier. The family of curves is plotted as before, but for each curve the origin of the coordinate system is moved horizontally by an amount proportional to the change in the value of the stepping variable. The result is as though each curve had been plotted on a separate sheet of graph paper and the sheaf shuffled sideways—e.g. if we replot

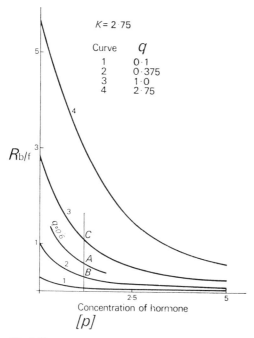

Fig 3.17

Fig 3.15 in this way, shifting the origin one unit to the right for a change of 20 min in incubation time, we have:

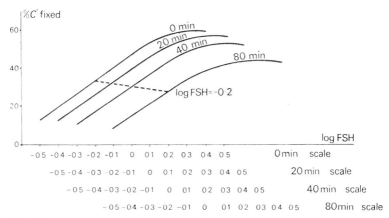

Fig 3.18

Using these scales, the value of C' for a particular log FSH value is marked on each curve, and joining these points gives a curve of constant log FSH value

(Fig 3.18). Repeating this for various log FSH values gives the characteristic carpet:

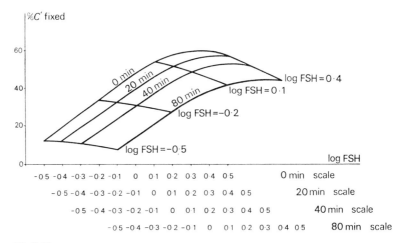

Fig 3.19

Interpolation is straightforward. Suppose, for example, that we wish to obtain the value of C for log FSH $= -0.3$ and incubation time $= 60$ min. We first plot the curve of log FSH $= -0.3$, by marking off this point on each curve of constant incubation time (remembering that each curve has a different origin of co-ordinates). We then use the fact that on any curve of fixed log FSH, the point of its intersection with the 60 min incubation time curve must lie a *horizontal* distance of 1 unit to the right of its intersection with the 40 min incubation time curve, since the time curves are displaced one unit to the right for every 20 min increase in incubation time. Applying this reasoning to the newly-plotted log FSH $= -0.3$ curve gives us the 60 min incubation time point on it.

Repeating this procedure with all our constant log FSH curves gives the 60 min incubation time curve itself (Fig. 3.20).

For fuller discussion of the technique of carpet graphs see Ellis (1955).

Another method for representing functions of two variables graphically is to plot pairs of values of the *independent* variables against one another for a *fixed* value of the *dependent* variable, repeating the process for different values of the dependent variable. The result will be a set of *contours* each of constant dependent variable value; they are exactly analogous to contour lines of height on a map, taking height as the dependent variable and the map grid co-ordinates as the independent variables. (This type of presentation is the standard method for representing two-dimensional dose distributions in radiotherapy.)

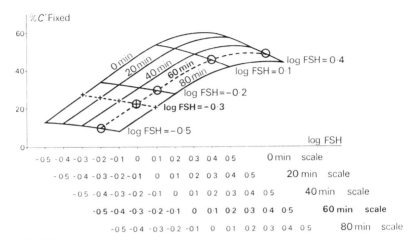

Fig 3.20

A technique used occasionally in the past, but which the advent of computers has made more accessible, is to take advantage of the fact that functions of two variables can be represented as surfaces in three-dimensional space (see Chapter 8). This is an extension of the ordinary graph, which represents a function of one variable as a curve in two-dimensional space. Computers can be made to display such surfaces on cathode ray oscilloscopes, either as perspective drawings, isometric charts or as stereoscopic pairs; they can also plot these drawings by being programmed to drive a mechanical graph-plotter. Such techniques are mainly used at present to give an overall picture of the behaviour of the function rather than as a means of deriving actual readings, but there is no reason why they should not be used for the latter purpose—certainly the programming techniques exist for enabling this to be done.

Chapter 4
Indices, The Binomial Theorem and Logarithms

4.1   Powers and indices

Previous chapters have made use of the idea of a *power* of a constant or of a variable, for example

$7^3 = 7 * 7 * 7$, the third power (or 'cube') of 7

$b^5 = b * b * b * b * b$, the fifth power of b.

Each of the superscripts 3 and 5 in these examples is known as the *index* or *exponent* of the corresponding power.

We can also have a power of a function, e.g.

$$\left(1 + x^5 - \frac{1}{x}\right)^3 = \left(1 + x^5 - \frac{1}{x}\right) * \left(1 + x^5 - \frac{1}{x}\right) * \left(1 + x^5 - \frac{1}{x}\right)$$

the third power ('cube') of $(1 + x^5 - 1/x)$, or more generally

$$[f(x)]^m = \overbrace{f(x) * f(x) * \ldots * f(x)}^{m \text{ factors}}$$

where m is a positive integer, being the index of the mth power of $f(x)$.

The properties of indices and powers as defined in this way are a part of school mathematics; for completeness and also for the sake of readers who may have forgotten this theory, we give first some basic results. The point of doing so is that we will then develop some consequences and extensions of these ideas which will prove to be of great practical importance. Although we will work almost entirely in terms of powers of a single variable our results will clearly be true for powers of functions also.

4.1.1   *Rules for multiplication and division of powers*

(1) If m and n are two positive integers then for any a:

$$a^m * a^n = a^{(m+n)}, \text{ usually written } a^{m+n} \tag{4.1}$$

In words: to *multiply powers of the same quantity, add the indices.* This is proved by considering the number of a's in the product of a^m and a^n.

The fact that in these particular circumstances the operation of *multiplication* is replaced by one of *addition* has important practical applications, as we shall see.

Examples:

(i) $2^7 * 2^4 = 2^{7+4} = 2^{11}$

(ii) $\left(x - \frac{1}{y} + 3\right)^3 * \left(x - \frac{1}{y} + 3\right)^5 = \left(x - \frac{1}{y} + 3\right)^8$

(2) Repeated application of (4.1) proves the following result (all indices being positive integer quantities):

$$a^m * a^n * a^l * a^t \ldots a^s = a^{m+n+l+t+\cdots+s} \tag{4.2}$$

Examples:

(i) $2^3 * 2^5 * 2^6 * 2^4 * 2^2 = 2^{3+5+6+4+2} = 2^{20} \ (=1{,}048{,}576)$

and if we work out the values of 2^3, 2^5, 2^6, 2^4 and 2^2 and multiply them together, their product is found to be also 1,048,576, as the result (4.2) demands.

(ii) $(ax^2 - bx + 7) * (ax^2 - bx + 7)^4 * (ax^2 - bx + 7)^3 = (ax^2 - bx + 7)^8$

It is important to remember that powers of different quantities or expressions cannot be compounded together in this way—only like terms can be so treated. For example

$$4^5 * 3^7 * 5^6 * 4^3$$

can be simplified only to the extent of compounding the powers of 4:

$$4^5 * 3^7 * 5^6 * 4^3 = 4^{5+3} * 3^7 * 5^6$$

$$= 4^8 * 3^7 * 5^6$$

Again, as a further example:

$$(a+b)^3 * (x-y)^2 * (a+b)^8 * (x-y)^4 = (a+b)^{11} * (x-y)^6$$

(3) If m and n are any two positive integers, then for any a:

$$(a^m)^n = (a^n)^m = a^{m*n} \tag{4.3}$$

In words: *raising of a power to a power multiplies the indices.*
As with (4.1) this is proved by considering the number of factors on each side of the equation.

Examples:

(i) $(2^5)^7 = 2^{35} = (2^7)^5$

(ii) $\left(\left(2x+\dfrac{1}{y}\right)^3\right)^4 = \left(2x+\dfrac{1}{y}\right)^{12}$

The relation (4.3) can sometimes be used to simplify expressions, e.g.

$$(x^2 - 2xy + y^2)^3 = ((x-y)^2)^3 = (x-y)^6$$

(4) The rule (4.3) can be generalized as follows:

$$(\ldots((a^m)^n)\ldots)^k = a^{m*n*\cdots*k} \tag{4.4}$$

Examples:

(i) $(4^3)^2 = ((2^2)^3)^2 = 2^{12} \ (=4096)$

(ii) $(((x-y)^3)^7)^2 = (x-y)^{42}$

(iii) $((((p-a)^3)^b)^b) = (p-a)^{3b^2}$

(5) If a and b are any two numbers, and m is a positive integer, then

$$(a * b)^m = a^m * b^m \tag{4.5}$$

In words: *the power of a product equals the product of the powers.*
The proof follows from the definition of a power and by counting terms on each side of (4.5).

Examples:

(i) $(3 * 4)^5 = 3^5 * 4^5 \ (= 3^5 * 2^{10})$

(ii) $((x * y)^m)^n = (x^m y^m)^n = x^{mn} y^{mn} = (x * y)^{mn}$

(6) Relation (4.5) is easily extended to more than two variables:

$$(p * q * r * \ldots * z)^s = p^s * q^s * r^s * \ldots * z^s \tag{4.6}$$

Examples:

(i) $(30)^5 = (3 * 2 * 5)^4 = 3^4 * 2^4 * 5^4$

(ii) $(p * q * r)^7 = p^7 * q^7 * r^7$

(iii) $(x^2 - y^2)^2 \ (x+y)^2 = \{(x+y) \ (x-y)\}^2 \ (x+y)^2 = (x+y)^4 \ (x-y)^2$

(7) If m and n are positive integer quantities, and m is $> n$ then

$$a^m / a^n = a^{m-n} \tag{4.7}$$

In words: *To divide powers of the same quantity, subtract the index of the divisor from the index of the dividend†.*

This result is proved in the usual way, by counting factors on each side of the equation. The fact that division can be replaced by a subtraction has important practical consequences.

Examples:

(i) $2^{17}/2^8 = 2^{17-8} = 2^9$

(numerical check: $2^{17} = 131,072$; $2^8 = 256$; $2^{17}/2^8 = 131,072/256 = 512$; $2^9 = 512$).

---

† *Divisor:* the quantity dividing.   *Dividend:* the quantity being divided.

(ii) $(x-y)^8/(x-y)^3=(x-y)^5$

(iii) $(a^m/a^n) * a^l = a^{m-n+l}$

(iv) $\left(\dfrac{x^m}{x^n}\right)^3 = \dfrac{(x^m)^3}{(x^n)^3} = \dfrac{x^{3m}}{x^{3n}}$

$= x^{3m-3n} = x^{3(m-n)} = (x^{m-n})^3$

4.1.2   The use of tables of powers

So far we have simply stated the rules for manipulation of powers. We now consider some applications. Consider a list of powers of some number—for ease of arithmetic, let us use 2, though our discussion will be valid for any number.

Table 4.1 Powers of 2

Index	n	1	2	3	4	5	6	7	8	9	10	11	12
Power	2^n	2	4	8	16	32	64	128	256	512	1024	2048	4096

With such a table, multiplication of powers of 2 is easy. To find the value of say, 16 * 256, we take the index 4—corresponding to 16, add it to the index 8 —corresponding to 256, and look up the value of the power of 2 corresponding to the sum of the two indices; this procedure is simply making use of the relation (4.1). Thus we have $4+8=12$; this corresponds to $2^4 * 2^8 = 2^{12}$, by our law (4.1), and $2^{12}=4096$, from the table. Thus we can carry out the multiplication: 16 * 256 = 4096 by looking up the powers representing 16 and 256, and then looking up the number corresponding to their sum.

A table such as Table 4.1 above will therefore enable us to replace multiplication of numbers which are powers of 2 by the simpler process of addition. Obviously similar tables for other numbers will enable other powers to be multiplied in the same manner.

Division is similarly carried out by subtraction:

$$512=2^9$$
$$64=2^6$$
$$512/64=2^9/2^6=2^{9-6}=2^3=8$$

However, as it stands, this procedure is very limited in scope—it is very uncommon to find that the numbers we need to multiply and divide are exact powers.

4.1.3   Extension of the idea of a power

The preceding discussion raises the question: is it possible to extend the idea of a power to include in Table 4.1 numbers which are not integral powers of 2? If we could 'fill the gaps' in this table, so that there was a value of n corresponding to 3, 5, 6, 7, 9, , , .. etc., this would enable a much wider variety of arithmetic to be carried out, and would open up the possibility of replacing *any* multiplication by a simple addition in conjunction with the use of a table.

Graphically the idea seems feasible. If we plot 2^n against n from Table 4.1 we have Fig. 4.1. These points seem to highlight a curve (Fig. 4.2).

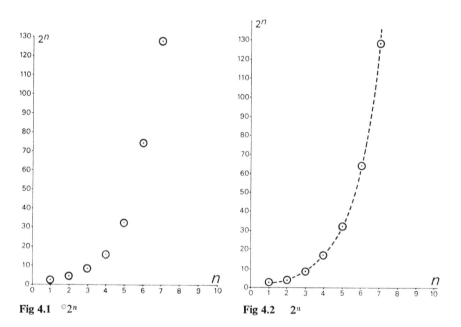

Fig 4.1 $\circ 2^n$ Fig 4.2 2^n

Now we can read values off this curve. For instance if the curve is drawn fairly accurately, the value 5 on the 2^n-axis seems to correspond to a value of $n = 2 \cdot 3$. Purely symbolically, we seem to be saying that

$$2^{2 \cdot 3} = 5 \qquad \text{(Fig. 4.3)}.$$

Similarly the value 7 on the 2^n-axis corresponds to $n=2\cdot8$. Suppose we now read off the 2^n-value corresponding to $n=2\cdot3+2\cdot8$, i.e. $n=5\cdot1$. It is *35*, the *product* of 5 and 7. In other words, values read off our curve appear to behave in exactly the same way as powers of 2 read from Table 4.1.

We see, therefore, that to *multiply* two numbers together, we read off the

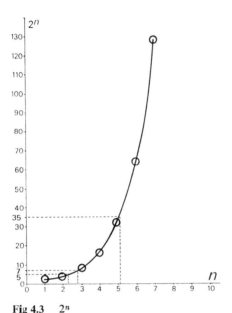

Fig 4.3 2^n

values of n along the x-axis which correspond to the two numbers along the y-axis, *add* the two n-values together, and then read off our answer. Division is similarly carried out by using subtraction instead of addition.

Clearly if we can find a logical extension of the idea of an index, such that any number can be expressed as a power of some quantity or other, we will have a means whereby multiplication and division can be transformed into addition and subtraction. As we develop our subject, it will become apparent that as well as being an arithmetic convenience, this can be a very useful tool from both an algebraic and a graphical point of view.

4.1.4 *Non-positive integer powers*

Our approach is by a process of generalization which is very characteristic of mathematics and the mathematical way of thinking.

Up until now a^n has been defined, for any a, solely for n a positive integer; from this definition we derived the rules for multiplication and division given in the previous sections. Now suppose for the moment that we were to drop some of the restrictions on the values of the indices in these rules—e.g. the apparently incontrovertible ones that indices must be greater than zero, or must be integers; could we still attach meaning to the resultant expressions if we continue to require them to obey the rules? In other words, having used a restricted set of values to define a set of rules, can we enlarge our concepts by making the *rules* our starting point and relaxing some of the original restrictions?

The basic criteria for this approach are that the results must be *consistent*, i.e. lead to no contradictions, and also include the cases which originally led to the rules. The value of this kind of generalization is that it almost invariably leads to new concepts and reveals underlying connections between topics which beforehand had been regarded as separate entities. We will also see in this particular instance that the new concept arising from our process is the *logarithm* (although it must be admitted that the discovery of logarithms originally came about in a different way).

4.1.4.1 Negative indices

Consider the rule (4.7):

$$a^m / a^n = a^{m-n}$$

for $m > n$.

Let us now relax the restriction that m must be greater than n, and see where the application of (4.7) will now lead us.

First, a numerical example. Let $m = 3$, $n = 4$. Then our rule (4.7) would have us say that

$$a^3 / a^4 = a^{3-4} = a^{-1}$$

But $\quad a^3 / a^4 = \dfrac{1}{a}$

Thus we are led to an *interpretation* of a^{-1}, namely that

$$a^{-1} = \frac{1}{a} \tag{4.8}$$

and if we now take this as a *definition* of a^{-1}, we can test whether the criteria stated above are satisfied, namely does such a definition lead to contradiction and do the consequences of it include all the familiar rules and behaviour for positive indices?

We find that the new definition fits in very well with our rules so far. For example, we would now have

$$a^m * a^{-1} = a^{m-1}$$

which is true, because

$$a^m * a^{-1} = a^m * \frac{1}{a} = a^{m-1}$$

Again, (4.7) would give us

$$a^m / a^{-1} = a^{m-(-1)} = a^{m+1}$$

This is quite consistent:

$$a^m / a^{-1} = a^m \Big/ \left(\frac{1}{a}\right) = a^m * a = a^{m+1}$$

The result

$$a^{-1} = \frac{1}{a}$$

generalizes without difficulty to the following:

$$a^{-m} = \frac{1}{a^m} \tag{4.9}$$

Examples:

(i) $3^{-2} = \dfrac{1}{3^2} = \dfrac{1}{9}$

(ii) $x^m * x^{-n} = x^{m-n}$

(iii) $3^{-4} * 3^{-2} = 3^{-6}$

(iv) $(a^{-5})^2 = a^{-10}$

(v) $(b^{-5})^{-3} = b^{-5*(-3)} = b^{15}$

(vi) $(7^{-m})^n = 7^{-mn} = (7^{-n})^m = (7^n)^{-m} = (7^m)^{-n}$

Notice that we are now restricted a little as to the possible values a can have in an expression such as a^{-2} or a^{-n} generally: we now have to say that a^{-n} *is defined only for non-zero a*. This is, of course, because 0^{-n} would equal $1/0^n$, which is not allowed (cf. Section 1.3.4).

4.1.4.2   The index zero

We have now given a meaning to a^m, where m is a positive or negative integer. We can also give it a meaning for $m=0$, as follows:
We have

$$a^n/a^n = 1$$

for any values of x and $n \neq 0$ (n integral). But

$$a^n/a^n = a^{n-n} = a^0$$

Hence for *any non-zero* value of a, we can *define*

$$a^0 = 1 \tag{4.10}$$

Examples

(i) $6^0 = 1$

(ii) $(\tfrac{1}{4})^0 = 1$

(iii) $\left(bc - af + \dfrac{1}{3w}\right)^0 = 1$

Note that

$$1 = 1^0 = 2^0 = 3^0 = \ldots$$

We see, therefore, that in order to be able to use the a^0 notation, we have to add a rider that $a^0 = b^0$ *does not prove that* $a = b$.

(To avoid a similar kind of inconsistency, it is necessary also to rule that $1^m = 1^n$ *does not prove that* $m = n$.)

4.1.5   *The graph of* 2^n

We can now fill in further points on our graph of 2^n, namely values for $n=0$, -1, -2, -3, ... corresponding to $2^0 = 1$, $2^{-1} = 0 \cdot 5$, $2^{-2} = 0 \cdot 25$, $2^{-3} = 0 \cdot 125$, etc. (see Fig. 4.4).

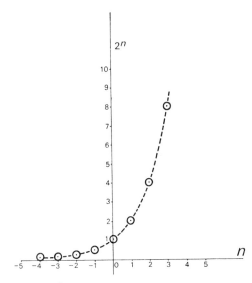

Fig 4.4 2^n

4.1.6   *Fractional indices*

By keeping the rules of manipulation, but relaxing some of the basic premises which led to them, we have given a meaning to a^n, where n is now a positive or negative integer, or zero, and where the only restriction on a is that it cannot be zero unless n is positive. The logical next step is: can we enlarge the concept to give a meaning to a^n when n is a fraction?

Normally, n is used in mathematics as a symbol for an integer value; to show that we are now investigating non-integral indices, we will continue the discussion in terms of a^x, x being generally accepted as a symbol which can take any value.

4.1.6.1   The index $\frac{1}{2}$

Consider the symbol:

$$a^{1/2}$$

and play the game according to the rules. Then

$$a^{1/2} * a^{1/2} = a^{1/2+1/2} = a^1 = a$$

This is equivalent to saying that $a^{1/2}$ is a quantity whose product with itself is equal to a; by definition, therefore, it must be the *square root* of a, i.e.

$$a^{1/2} = \pm \sqrt{a}$$

To avoid ambiguities, the standard definition of $a^{1/2}$ is that it represents the *positive* square root.

Numerical examples:

$$9^{1/2} = 3, \quad 64^{1/2} = 8, \quad 1^{1/2} = 1$$

$$2^{1/2} = 1 \cdot 414 \ldots$$

We see immediately that $a^{1/2}$ is not defined by this procedure for negative a. This new definition does not violate any of our previous rules. For example

$$(a^6)^{1/2} = a^{6*1/2} = a^3, \quad \text{which is correct:} \quad a^3 * a^3 = a^6.$$

Negative fractional indices can be treated in the same way as negative integer indices:

$$b^{-1/2} = \frac{1}{b^{1/2}} = (b^{-1})^{1/2} = (b^{1/2})^{-1}$$

$$16^{-1/2} = \frac{1}{16^{1/2}} = \frac{1}{4}$$

$$3^{-1/2} = \frac{1}{1 \cdot 732 \ldots}$$

In short, our new definition of $a^{1/2}$ fits in perfectly satisfactorily with our previous ideas, but with the new restriction that a cannot be negative. This new extension of the idea of an index thus brings square roots within the scope of this notation.

4.1.6.2   The index $\dfrac{1}{n}$

We have—if we use the normal rules—

$$a^{1/3} * a^{1/3} * a^{1/3} = a^{1/3+1/3+1/3} = a$$

which would seem to define $a^{1/3}$ as the cube root of a: $\sqrt[3]{a}$. There is no ambiguity of sign here, since $\sqrt[3]{a}$ has the same sign as a. Generally,

$$\overbrace{a^{1/n} * a^{1/n} * \ldots * a^{1/n}}^{n \text{ factors}} = a^{\overbrace{(1/n)+(1/n)+\cdots+(1/n)}^{n \text{ factors}}}$$

$$= a^{n*1/n}$$

$$= a$$

Hence we can define:

$$a^{1/n} = \sqrt[n]{a} \tag{4.11}$$

i.e. $a^{1/n} = $ *the nth root of a*

valid for all positive, negative or zero values of a if n is odd, but only for non-negative values of a if n is even. It takes the sign of a where the value of a is within this range of validity. If a is negative, then

$$a^{1/n} (n \text{ odd}) = -(|a|)^{1/n}$$

Examples:

(i) $32^{1/5} = \sqrt[5]{32} = 2 \quad (=(2^5)^{1/5})$

(ii) $(-32)^{1/5} = (-2^5)^{1/5} = -(2^5)^{1/5} = -2$

(iii) $(x^2 + 2xy + y^2)^{1/2} = ((x+y)^2)^{1/2} = (x+y)$

4.1.6.3   The index $a^{m/n}$

It is very easy now to give a meaning to $a^{m/n}$, m and n integral. We define:

$$a^{m/n} = (a^{1/n})^m = (a^m)^{1/n} \tag{4.12}$$

i.e. $a^{m/n}$ is *(the nth root of a)^m or equivalently, the nth root of a^m.*

Again, we must place some restrictions on a. If when m/n has been reduced to its lowest terms, n is even, a cannot be negative; if m/n is negative, a cannot be zero.

Examples:

(i) $4^{3/2} = (4^{1/2})^3 = 2^3 = 8$

$= (4^3)^{1/2} = 64^{1/2}$

(ii) $(-32)^{-7/5} = (-2^5)^{-7/5} = ((-2^5)^{1/5})^{-7}$

$= (-2)^{-7}$

$= \dfrac{1}{(-2)^7}$

$= -\dfrac{1}{128}$

The new definition enables us to give a formal meaning to mixed decimal indices; for instance:

$$3^{4\cdot71} = {}^{3471}/{}_{100}$$

$$= {}^{100}\sqrt{3^{471}}$$

though in practice such values would be calculated using logarithms (Section 4.3) and in terms of comparative size we would tend to think of $3^{4\cdot71}$ as a quantity somewhere between 3^4 and 3^5 in value rather than as ${}^{100}\sqrt{3^{471}}$.

4.1.6.4   Use of fractional indices

Fractional indices are sometimes met with in dealing with interrelations between surface area and volume, or surface area and weight. A well-known example is the empirical formula due to DuBois & DuBois (1916), relating body surface area (S) to weight (W) and height (H):

$$S = 71\cdot84 \; W^{0\cdot425}H^{0\cdot725} \tag{4.13}$$

(S in cm^2, W in kg, H in cm).

Again it is known that with similar shapes of different sizes, the surface area increases as the *square* of the linear dimensions and the volume as the *cube* of the linear dimensions (Maynard Smith, 1968). Thus, for example, with two solids of similar shape one of which is three times the size of the other, the bigger solid has 9 ($=3^2$) times the surface area and 27 ($=3^3$) times the volume of the smaller solid. This has been put to use in deducing the volumes of body organs from observations of surface area and conversely (Fischer & Wolff, 1964) through the relationships

$$\text{volume} \propto (\text{surface area})^{3/2}$$

and conversely

$$\text{surface area} \propto (\text{volume})^{2/3}$$

(these are deduced from the facts that volume $\propto$ (linear measurement)^3 and surface area $\propto$ (linear measurement)^2).

The proportionality constant for any application has to be obtained experimentally by observations on a series of specimens of the organ involved.

4.1.7   *The generalization of 2^n*

We now appear to be in a position to fill in our graph of 2^n for all rational values of n, though it should be noted that all our definitions so far are purely formal ones, in that we have given no procedures for calculating the values of our fractional powers. For this we need logarithms (Section 4.3).

D

4.1.8   The function a^x

In the preceding sections, we have in fact been discussing the *function* a^x, which we have been able to define always for positive a, sometimes for negative a, and only for rational x. At this point, the further theoretical development of the meaning of a^x becomes difficult. Indeed for a fully satisfactory theory, a new type of number concept is needed—the so-called *complex number* (Chapters 1 and 7)—and a new starting point also. Modern mathematical theory bases the concepts of powers and logarithms (Section 4.3) on the differential and integral calculus (Chapter 9), but this point of view required considerable mathematical hindsight to develop, and we have yet to discuss the techniques which are needed for this approach.

The difficulties are due to the problem which arises at this point, of defining a^x for x irrational—e.g. $3^{\sqrt{2}}$ or e^π. However, in practical work, we always work with rational numbers (usually in decimal form), either *per se* or as approximations to irrationals. If we need the value of $\sqrt{2}$, for instance, we write it as $1 \cdot 41$ or $1 \cdot 414$ or $1 \cdot 4142 \ldots$ etc., according to the degree of accuracy required, and hence $3^{\sqrt{2}}$ is $3^{1 \cdot 41}$, or $3^{1 \cdot 414}$, etc., depending on the required accuracy.

4.2   The Binomial Theorem

4.2.1   The theorem for positive integer indices

An algebraic result of widespread application arises out of the properties of powers of a *sum or difference* of two quantities.

Consider the expression $(a+x)^2$. If we write this as $(a+x) * (a+x)$ and multiply out all the terms, we obtain

$$(a+x)^2 = a^2 + 2ax + x^2$$

A similar operation with $(a+x)^3$ yields

$$(a+x)^3 = a^3 + 3a^2x + 3ax^2 + x^2$$

and with $(a+x)^4$,

$$(a+x)^4 = a^4 + 4a^3x + 6a^2x^2 + 4ax^3 + x^4.$$

It will be seen that there is a certain discipline in the formation of the terms of these expressions. In the first place, the coefficients of the various powers in any expression seem to rise and fall in a symmetrical way as we take the terms in turn—for $(a+x)^2$ they are 1, 2, 1; for $(a+x)^3$ they are 1, 3, 3, 1, and for $(a+x)^4$ the sequence of coefficients is 1, 4, 6, 4, 1. Again, each term involves powers of a and/or x and the sum of the indices of the powers in any term is constant for any particular expression, equalling the index of the power of $(a+x)$. For example, in the case of $(a+x)^4$ the sum of the indices in any given term on the right-hand side of the relationship equals 4 while for $(a+x)^3$ it equals 3. In addition the powers increase or decrease in a uniform way.

It will probably come as no surprise to the reader, therefore, to be told that there is an underlying reason for these relationships, and they that are all particular instances of a general theorem, known as the *Binomial Theorem* or *Binomial Expansion* (any expression of the form $a+x$ is referred to as a *binomial expression*). This is stated as follows:

$$(a+x)^n = a^n + \frac{n}{1} a^{n-1}x + \frac{n(n-1)}{2*1} a^{n-2}x^2 + \frac{n(n-1)(n-2)}{3*2*1} a^{n-3}x^3$$

$$+ \frac{n(n-1)(n-2)(n-3)}{4*3*2*1} a^{n-4}x^4 + \ldots + x^n \qquad (4.14)$$

where n *is a positive integer.* If we substitute $n=2$, or 3, or 4 into (4.14) the particular results for $(a+x)^2$, $(a+x)^3$ and $(a+x)^4$ are obtained as above.

The coefficients of the powers of a and x in (4.14) are of a very special kind. The coefficient of $a^{n-r}x^r$ for any $r \leqslant n$ is

$$\frac{n(n-1)(n-2)(n-3)\ldots(n-r+1)}{r(r-1)(r-2)(r-3)\ldots 3*2*1} \qquad (4.15)$$

and is usually denoted by

$$^nC_r$$

or

$$\binom{n}{r}$$

—both notations are in common use.

Examples:

(i) $^6C_4 = \dfrac{6*5*4*3}{4*3*2*1} = 15$

(there are always as many factors in the numerator of ^nC_r as in the denominator).

(ii) $^nC_n = 1$ for any positive integer n.

(iii) $^nC_1 = n$ for any positive integer n.

(iv) $(2+0.5)^4 = 2^4 + 4*2^3*0.5 + \dfrac{4*3}{2*1}*2^2*(0.5)^2$

$$+ \frac{4*3*2}{3*2*1}*2*(0.5)^3 + \frac{4*3*2*1}{4*3*2*1}*(0.5)^4$$

The Binomial Expansion is sometimes useful for approximating powers of numbers close to integers. For example,

$$(2 \cdot 001)^{10} = (2 + 0 \cdot 001)^{10}$$

$$= 2^{10} + 10 * 2^9 * 0 \cdot 001 + \frac{10 * 9}{2} * 2^8 * (0 \cdot 001)^2$$

$$+ \text{terms in } (0 \cdot 001)^3, (0 \cdot 001)^4, \dots \text{ etc.}$$

$$\doteqdot 2^{10} + 5 \cdot 12 + 0 \cdot 01$$

$$= 1029 \cdot 13$$

Care must always be taken in such cases to check that the discarded terms can be safely neglected.

The Binomial Theorem takes a special form in the case where one of the binomial terms—say a—is equal to 1:

$$(1+x)^n = 1 + {}^nC_1 x + {}^nC_2 x^2 + {}^nC_3 x^3 \dots + x^n \qquad (4.16)$$

4.2.1   Extension of the Binomial Theorem to non-integer indices

We know that $(a+x)^p$ can be given a meaning for any value of the index p, subject to conditions on the value of $(a+x)$. We have also seen that for positive integer values of p, the function $(a+x)^p$ has the expansion (4.14). It is perhaps natural, therefore, to wonder whether some form of expansion exists for $(a+x)^p$ when p is not a positive integer.

It was shown by Newton and others that *if p is any number whatsoever* then

$$(1+x)^p = 1 + px + \frac{p(p-1)}{2*1} x^2 + \frac{p(p-1)(p-2)}{3*2*1} x^3 + \frac{p(p-1)(p-2(p-3)}{4*3*2*1} x^4$$

$$+ \dots \quad (4.17)$$

provided that $|x| < 1$.

The point about the series (4.17) is that it does not terminate unless p is a positive integer, $=n$, say, when all terms after x^p vanish because they contain the factor $p-n$ ($=0$) in the numerator of the coefficients. In this case (4.17) becomes the binomial expansion (4.16).

The sum of terms on the right-hand side of (4.17) is an example of an *infinite series*. The idea that an unlimited number of terms can add up to a finite amount is at first sight a strange one, but it is a fact of mathematical life that this is sometimes the case (this topic is dealt with in more detail in Chapter 10).

Some special cases of the expansion (4.17) are given in the Appendix, page 392.

The result (4.17) enables us to expand $(a+x)^p$ for any p. We use the fact that

$$(a+x)=a\left(1+\frac{x}{a}\right)=x\left(1+\frac{a}{x}\right),$$

and write

$$(a+x)^p=a^p\left(1+\frac{x}{a}\right)^p \quad \text{if} \quad |x|<|a|$$

or
$$=x^p\left(1+\frac{a}{x}\right)^p \quad \text{if} \quad |x|>|a|$$

then expand the binomial expression using (4.17).

The Binomial Theorem gives us a useful approximation for $(1+x)^p$ when x is small; if we can neglect the terms in x^2, x^3 etc., then we have

$$(1+x)^p \doteqdot 1+px$$

as a linear approximation. If we must include the term in x^2 as well, then

$$(1+x)^p \doteqdot 1+px+\frac{p(p-1)\,x^2}{2},$$

a quadratic approximation.

4.2.2   Applications of the Binomial Theorem

The Binomial Theorem is used extensively in mathematics and statistics. In mathematics it is an indispensable tool in such areas as the development of formulae in the *differential calculus* (Chapter 9), in the theory of *limits* (Chapter 5) and in obtaining methods for approximating and calculating mathematical functions. In statistics it is the basis of the *binomial distribution*, used to determine the probabilities of the observed proportions of dichotomous events such as patterns of Mendelian inheritance, incidence of complications after treatment, etc.

4.2.3   Note on the Binomial Coefficients

The quantity

$$^nC_r=\frac{n(n-1)(n-2)\ldots(n-r+1)}{r(r-1)(r-2)\ldots 3*2*1},$$

and also its numerator and denominator, all occur on their own account in many mathematical applications. It can be shown that ^nC_r is equal to *the number of distinct selections* (also called *combinations*) *which can be made by taking r objects at a time from a group of n different objects*. This is a function which arises in the mathematical theory of permutations and combinations, and there is a logical reason for such a quantity making its appearance in the Binomial Expansion, but we will not develop this topic here; the reader is referred to texts on algebra such as Green (1968).

The denominator of ^nC_r is the product of all the integers from r to 1 inclusive, and is known as *factorial r*, written

$$r!$$

or $\lfloor r$

If $r=6$, for example, then

$$6! = 6 * 5 * 4 * 3 * 2 * 1$$

$$= 720$$

The value of $r!$ increases rapidly with r (see Appendix, p. 392). We see that $r!$ is defined only for r an integer >0, but although one would not expect 0! to be defined, there are various reasons for formally defining its value as being 1.

The numerator of ^nC_r is usually denoted by ^nP_r; thus

$$^nP_r = n(n-1)(n-2)(n-3) \ldots (n-r+1).$$

It can be shown that this is *the number of permutations* (also called *arrangements*) *of n objects taken r at a time*. The difference between this and a combination or selection is that the order in which the objects are chosen is ignored in a combination but important in a permutation.

Examples:

(i) $^5P_4 = 5 * 4 * 3 * 2 = 120$

(ii) $^nP_1 = n$

(iii) $^nP_n = n!$

(iv) $^nC_r = {}^nP_r/(r!)$

$$= \frac{n!}{r!(n-r)!}$$ (a useful alternative to (4.15) as an expression for ^nC_r)

4.3   Logarithms (or 'logs')

We have seen how multiplication and division can be reduced to addition and subtraction by expressing the quantities concerned as powers of some number or other. In our development, we used powers of 2—or as it is sometimes expressed, we used 2 as a *base*. However, any positive number could have been used, and we will see both in this chapter and later on (Chapter 9) that other bases are to be preferred.

One thing we have not done is to show how to calculate these powers; we have not shown how to find, for example, the power of 10 which is equal to $16 \cdot 2$. Fortunately, we do not need to get involved in this question; tables of powers, specially constructed for this very purpose, have been in existence for well over three centuries. They have been known as *logarithms*.

The original computational methods used to obtain them were extremely laborious—it was all pencil-and-paper work (or perhaps more accurately quill-and-paper work), as there were no mechanical calculating aids. Modern tables are produced with aid of digital computers, and use more sophisticated methods than were available to the old arithmeticians, but the old tables, with errors eliminated over a long period of time, are still completely adequate, and formed the basis of all such tables until comparatively recently.

4.3.1   Definitions of logarithms and antilogarithms

If $y = a^x$, then x is defined as *the logarithm of y to the base a*.
     This is written:

$$x = \log_a (y). \tag{4.18}$$

In this definition, *a must be positive. So must y*—we will see later (Section 4.3.3.) why this should be.

With regard to the use of brackets in the form $\log_a (y)$, it is usually the practice to omit the brackets if y is a number or a single algebraic variable, and write: $\log_a y$. Where y is in fact an arithmetic or algebraic expression, the brackets are retained, though sometimes one meets with e.g.

$$\log_a \frac{3+4y}{1+y}$$

where $\log_a \left(\frac{3+4y}{1+y} \right)$

is meant. Since both representations are met with in practice, we will ourselves sometimes use brackets and sometimes omit them (where this will not lead to ambiguity) in order to accustom the reader to both notations.

We see that Table 4.1 is a table of logarithms, to the base 2, of the numbers 2, 4, 8, 16, ... For example, since $2^7 = 128$, this gives us $\log_2 128 = 7$. The base 1 is clearly trivial, since $1^x = 1$, for all x, and we therefore do not consider it.

There is a converse definition to (4.18), namely, that if $x = \log_a y$, then y is said to *be the antilogarithm of x to the base a*, and written

$$y = \text{antilog}_a x \ (=a^x) \tag{4.19}$$

Before looking into the question of the best base to use, we will derive some results which are true for any base. They will be concerned entirely with logarithms, since the main activity with antilogarithms is to read them out of the tables, whereas logarithms usually involve some manipulations.

4.3.2   Logarithms of products, quotients and powers

We quote the following rules without proof; the proofs follow straightforwardly from the definition of a logarithm and by the use of the theory of indices:

(a)   *The logarithm of a product = the sum of the logarithms of the factors*

In symbols: $\log_a (x * y) = \log_a x + \log_a y$

(b)   *The logarithm of a quotient = the logarithm of the dividend minus the logarithm of the divisor.*

In symbols: $\log_a (x/y) = \log_a x - \log_a y$

(c)   *The logarithm of the power of a quantity = the index of the power multiplied by the logarithm of the quantity.*

Symbolically: $\log_a x^s = s * \log_a x$

There is a deduction which follows from the last result, namely:

(d) $x^s = a^{s * \log_a x}$

a rather bizarre proposition which is nevertheless sometimes useful. It enables any power of any positive variable (here x) to be expressed as a power of any other positive variable (here a).

In (a)–(d) above, the quantities a, x and y are all positive. The quantity s in rules (c) and (d) can be positive or negative, or zero.

Examples:

(i) $\log_7 15 = \log_7 5 + \log_7 3$ (Rule (a))

(ii) $\log_9 0 \cdot 7 = \log_9 (7/10) = \log_9 7 - \log_9 10$ (Rule (b))

(iii) $\log_2 [(x+y)^3] = 3 * \log_2 (x+y)$ (Rule (c))

(iv) $\log_{10} \sqrt{7} = \frac{1}{2} \log_{10} 7$ (because $(7 = 7^{1/2})$ (Rule (c))

(v) $0 \cdot 7^{10} = 4^{10 * \log_4 0 \cdot 7}$ (Rule (d))

(vii) Show that if

$$E_h(v) = E_0 + 30 \cdot 7 \log \frac{P_v}{L_v}$$

and

$$E_h(a) = E_0 + 30 \cdot 7 \log \frac{P_a}{L_a}$$

then

$$E_h(v) - E_h(a) = 30 \cdot 7 \log \frac{L_a P_v}{L_v P_a} \quad \text{(Hlavova \textit{et al}, (1968))}$$

We have: $E_h(v) - E_h(a) = \left(E_0 + 30 \cdot 7 \log \frac{P_v}{L_v} \right) - \left(E_0 + 30 \cdot 7 \log \frac{P_a}{L_a} \right)$

$$= E_0 + 30 \cdot 7 \log \frac{P_v}{L_v} - E_0 - 30 \cdot 7 \log \frac{P_a}{L_a}$$

$$= 30 \cdot 7 \left(\log \frac{P_v}{L_v} - \log \frac{P_a}{L_a} \right)$$

$$= 30 \cdot 7 \log \left(\frac{P_v}{L_v} \middle/ \frac{P_a}{L_a} \right) \qquad \text{(Rule (b))}$$

$$= 30 \cdot 7 \log \frac{L_a P_v}{L_v P_a} \quad \left(\text{since } \frac{P_v}{L_v} \middle/ \frac{P_a}{L_a} = \frac{P_v}{L_v} * \frac{L_a}{P_a} \right)$$

4.3.3   *Logarithms of negative numbers*

Since our base is always positive by definition, its powers are positive as well. It follows, therefore, that no negative number can be represented by a power of any base, and therefore that *no negative number can have a logarithm*. So, for example $\log_{10} (-4)$ does not exist in our definition of a logarithm. Similarly *the logarithm of zero does not exist* (cf. example viii of Section 5.8).

4.3.4   *Logarithms of particular values*

Since for any value of a we have $a^0 = 1$ (Section 4.1.4) this gives

$$\log_a 1 = 0 \quad \text{for any } a \qquad (4.20)$$

i.e. the logarithm of 1 to any base is zero.

Again, since

$$a = a^1,$$

we see that

$$\log_a a = 1 \qquad\qquad\qquad\qquad (4.21)$$

or in words,

for any base, the logarithm of the base itself = 1.

Thus for example:

(i) $\log_2 1 = \log_5 1 = 0$

(ii) $\log_2 2 = 1$, $\log_{10} 10 = 1$, $\log_{74.2} 74 \cdot 2 = 1$

(iii) $\log_{10} 10^n = n \log_{10} 10 = n$

(iv) $\log_a \left(\dfrac{1}{x}\right) = \log_a 1 - \log_a x$

$$= -\log_a x \qquad \text{(from (4.20))}$$

This last example is of some importance. As an illustration:

(v) $\log_{10} \dfrac{1}{1000} = -\log_{10} 1000 = -3 \log_{10} 10 = -3$

(This could also be deduced as follows:

$$\log_{10} (1/1000) = \log_{10} (10^{-3}) = -3 \log_{10} 10 = -3)$$

4.3.5   Change of base

It sometimes happens that we need the logarithm of a number to a particular base when all we have available are logarithms to some other base. The following rule enables us to use our available table to obtain the new logarithm:

The logarithm of a number to a new base = the logarithm of the number to the old base divided by the logarithm of the new base to the old base.

Symbolically:

$$\log_b x = \log_a x / \log_a b \qquad\qquad\qquad (4.22)$$

Example:

Given that

$$\log_{10} 2 = 0 \cdot 3010,$$

and $\log_{10} 3 = 0 \cdot 4771,$

then $\log_2 3 = \dfrac{0 \cdot 4771}{0 \cdot 3010} = 1 \cdot 5850$

(i.e. $3 = 2^{1 \cdot 585}$)

and generally to convert logarithms to base 10 into logarithms to base 2, we multiply base 10 logarithms by $1/0 \cdot 3010$, i.e. by $3 \cdot 3223$.

One consequence of the result (4.22) is that logarithms to different bases differ by a multiplicative factor $(= 1/\log_a b)$ which depends on the bases chosen.

4.3.6   Choice of base

Of all the possible bases for logarithms, there are two in general use to the virtual exclusion of all others. One is the base 10. The other is one which is at first sight a very strange choice: an *irrational* number, a non-terminating decimal denoted in practice by the symbol e. Its value to twelve decimal places is $2 \cdot 718281828459 \ldots$, and it and π $(= 3 \cdot 141592653590 \ldots)$ are the two most important and most widely occurring of all the mathematical constants. A mathematical definition of e is given in Chapter 5.

4.3.7   Common logarithms

Logarithms to base 10 are called *common logarithms*, and are usually written without the base being indicated. Thus

$$\log 7$$

would normally be taken to mean $\log_{10} 7$.

The use of common logarithms in aiding multiplication and division are a part of school mathematics and everyday scientific work. However, the choice of base 10 is purely as an aid in manual calculation, the base deriving its popularity from the fact that common logarithms of numbers with the same significant figures differ by an integer. The difference depends on the relative positions of the decimal point in the numbers; thus, e.g.

$$\log 3 \cdot 140 = 0 \cdot 4969$$

$$\log 314 \cdot 0 = 2 \cdot 4969$$

This results in tables of common logarithms being shorter and more convenient to handle (provided one remembers the rules!) but it should be kept in mind that the widespread use of the base 10 is not fundamental to the idea of a logarithm, nor to its application. It is quite conceivable that with the advent of the high-speed digital computer and the increasing availability of sophisticated desk calculators, the common logarithm will lose some if not all of its pre-eminence. However, that time is not yet, and for convenience we summarize now the rules for the use of common logarithms along with an exposition of one or two points which sometimes seem to cause difficulties.

4.3.8   Use of common logarithms

Our remarks in this section apply only to common logarithms. In general, the (common) logarithm of a number is not an integer, but consists of a *signed* integer *plus* a fraction (the integer part may be zero). The integer part is called the *characteristic*, and the fractional part the *mantissa*. The convenience of common logarithms is due to the fact that numbers with the same significant figures have common logarithms with the same mantissa; only their characteristics differ. For this reason, it is usual to tabulate only the *mantissae of integers*; to find the logarithm of any other number, we look up the mantissa of the integer with the same significant figures, and then determine the characteristic for our original number by the following rules:

(i) *The characteristic of the logarithm of a number >1 is one less than number of digits in the integer part of the number.*

(ii) *The characteristic of the logarithm of a fraction $= -(1+the$ number of significant zeroes in the decimal representation of the fraction).*

Examples:

(i) $\log 2 \cdot 0 = 0 \cdot 3010 \ldots$ (characteristic $=$ zero, mantissa $=$ $0 \cdot 3010$)

(ii) $\log 20 \cdot 0 = 1 \cdot 3010$ (*two* figures before the decimal point means a characteristic of *1*, mantissa as with log 2)

(iii) $\log 0 \cdot 0002 = -4 + 0 \cdot 3010$ (*three* significant zeroes means a characteristic of -4; mantissa as with log 2)

Note that the logarithm of the fraction $0 \cdot 0002$ is in fact *negative* in value

$(= -3 \cdot 6990)$; this is true of all fractions, i.e. *the logarithm of a fraction is negative*.† There are two different ways in which we can represent the logarithm of a fraction. We can either have a positive mantissa and a negative characteristic —for example $\log 0 \cdot 0002 = 0 \cdot 3010$ (the mantissa) -4 (the characteristic)—or a negative mantissa and a negative characteristic: $\log 0 \cdot 0002 = -0 \cdot 6990$ (the mantissa) -3 (the characteristic). The first way (positive mantissa) has the advantages that the mantissa is the same as that for an integer with the same significant digits as the fraction whose logarithm is being obtained, and therefore we can use directly the same table of mantissae as with numbers > 1, whereas with the second method the mantissae are negative and are different to those for numbers > 1. It is therefore universal practice to adopt the first method, and such logarithms are written in a special way to show that the characteristic is negative and the mantissa positive. This way consists of putting a *bar* over the characteristic, thus:

$$\log 0 \cdot 0002 = -4 + 0 \cdot 3010 = \bar{4} \cdot 3010$$

$$\log 0 \cdot 2 = -1 + 0 \cdot 3010 = \bar{1} \cdot 3010$$

$$\log 0 \cdot 02 = \bar{2} \cdot 3010 = -2 + \cdot 3010 = -1 \cdot 6990$$

(This is in fact a form of complement notation—cf. Section 1.2.3).

If we have a logarithm in the all-negative form we can easily convert to the standard form by the following method:

(i) Subtract 1 from the negative integer part of the logarithm and write the result as the characteristic in the 'bar' form.

(ii) Add 1 to the (negative) fractional part of the logarithm to obtain the positive mantissa.

Examples:

(i) $-0 \cdot 4259$ has integer part zero and fractional part $= -0 \cdot 4259$. Subtract 1 from the integer part, giving -1, i.e. $\bar{1}$. Add 1 to the fractional part, giving $1 - 0 \cdot 4259 = 0 \cdot 5741$. Hence $-0 \cdot 4259 = \bar{1} \cdot 5741$.

(ii) $-1 \cdot 3010 = \bar{2} \cdot 6990$, since $(-1) - 1 = -2 = \bar{2}$ and $1 - 0 \cdot 3010 = 0 \cdot 6990$

The technique depends on the fact that adding and then subtracting the same quantity from a number leaves us with the original value.

---

† This is true not only with common logarithms but for all bases > 1.

The graph of log (x) is shown in Fig 4.5.

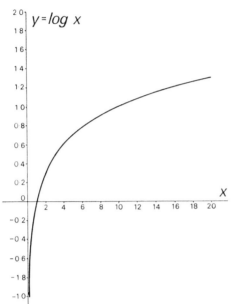

Fig 4.5 Log x.

4.3.8.1   Powers and roots using logarithms

Logarithms are very useful for dealing with powers and roots of numbers. For this purpose the rule

$$\log x^s = s * \log x \qquad\qquad (4.23)$$

is used.

The technique is to find log x, multiply it by s, and then look up the result in the table of antilogarithms. For example, to find $3^{4.1}$:

$$\log 3 = 0 \cdot 4771$$

$$\log 3^{4.1} = 4 \cdot 1 * \log 3 = 4 \cdot 1 * 0 \cdot 4771 = 1 \cdot 9561$$

Antilog $0 \cdot 9561 = 9038$. The characteristic 1 in $1 \cdot 9561$ shows us that the answer is $90 \cdot 38$.

The only point of difficulty usually encountered is with roots of fractions, due to the 'bar' notation in the characteristic.

To illustrate:

Example:

Find $(0 \cdot 117)^{1/3}$

Now $\log (0 \cdot 117)^{1/3} = \frac{1}{3} * \log 0 \cdot 117$ (cf. equation (4.23)).

From the tables, $\log 0 \cdot 117 = \overline{1} \cdot 0682$

If we divide this by 3, we get a negative fraction and also a positive one:

$\overline{1}/3 = -0 \cdot 3333$

$0 \cdot 0682/3 = 0 \cdot 0227$

This can be resolved by adding them together, result $-0 \cdot 3106$, and then converting to the standard form as shown earlier:

$-0 \cdot 3106 = \overline{1} \cdot 6894$.

From the tables, antilog $0 \cdot 6894 = 4891$. The characteristic $\overline{1}$ shows that the answer is $0 \cdot 4891$.

There is another way of dealing with the logarithms of roots of fractions, which has the advantage of shortening the arithmetic.

The technique is to subtract and add the same integer quantity to the logarithm of the fraction *before* carrying out the division which arises from the root (e.g. by 3 in the example above), subtracting from the characteristic and adding to the mantissa. The value of the logarithm will be unaltered by this. The amount to subtract and add is that which makes the resulting characteristic *the next lowest exact negative integer multiple* of the divisor. The resulting division automatically gives the correct characteristic.

With $(0 \cdot 117)^{1/3}$, we have:

$$\log (0 \cdot 117)^{1/3} = \frac{\overline{1} \cdot 0682}{3}$$

The next lowest negative integer multiple of 3 below $\overline{1}$ is $\overline{3}$, i.e. we have to subtract 2 from the existing characteristic. Hence 2 must be added to the mantissa, and we have

$$\log (0 \cdot 117)^{1/3} = \frac{(-1 - 2) + (2 + 0 \cdot 0682)}{3}$$

$$= \frac{-3 + 2 \cdot 0682}{3}$$

$$= \overline{1} \cdot 6894$$

as before.

4.3.9   Natural logarithms

Logarithms to base e are known variously as *natural* logarithms, *Naperian* logarithms or (less commonly) *hyperbolic* logarithms. They offer none of the computational conveniences of common logarithms. The choice of e as a base is due to certain properties of the function e^x. These are very relevant to *growth and decay processes* in biology and medicine, but their development in this context requires the differential and integral calculus, which we have yet to discuss (Chapter 9). The properties of e and e^x arise from its definition; however, this involves the theory of *limits* (Chapter 5), and so for the moment we will say no more about e, except to note that the symbol

$$\ln (x)$$

or simply

$$\ln x$$

is coming into increasing use as the form for $\log_e x$, and we will ourselves use this notation. The reader is warned, however, that in mathematical texts it is common to find $\log x$ used for $\log_e x$ and not for $\log_{10} x$. However, it is usually easy to see from the context which base is implied. Note that a table of e^x or e^{-x} is in fact a table of *natural antilogarithms*.

4.3.10   Conversion factors between common and natural logarithms

We saw in Section 4.3.5 that logarithms to different bases were related by a multiplicative factor. Between common logarithms and natural logarithms, the relation is:

$$\ln x = 2 \cdot 302585 * \log x$$

$$\log x = 0 \cdot 434294 * \ln x$$

The quantity $0 \cdot 434294$—i.e. the conversion factor from natural logarithms to common logarithms—is sometimes called the *Modulus* and denoted by M.

The relationship between common and natural logarithms is illustrated graphically in Fig 4.6. This is a copy of Fig 4.5, but with the addition of a scale for reading off $\ln x$ down the right hand side. The curve is the same for both $\log x$ and $\ln x$—the difference is in the vertical scales; any value on the right-hand scale is $2 \cdot 302 \ldots$ times the value represented by the corresponding point on the left-hand scale.

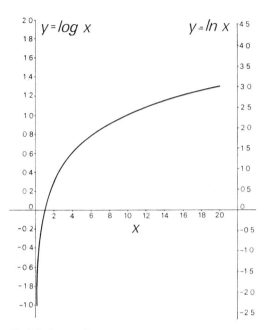

Fig 4.6 Log x, ln x.

Generally speaking, natural logarithms are met with in theoretical mathematical work and in using computers, while common logarithms are the more usual choice in manual numerical work.

N.B. Digital computer programs almost invariably give the logarithms of fractions in the all-negative form.

4.3.11   Other bases

The advent of digital computers, which unlike human beings usually count in powers of 2 rather than 10, has meant that occasionally logarithms to base 2 or base 8 ($=2^3$) are needed. Logarithms to base 2 occur also in *information theory*, an advanced mathematical theory dealing with the coding of messages and the capacities of the channels which carry them. Usually such logarithms are obtained from common logarithms by the rule given in Section 4.3.5. The base 2 is also important in calculating speeds of sorting data into order on computers.

One application where logarithms to different bases have been used has been in the manual calculation of bioassays—see for example Finney (1952). It is

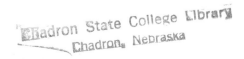

usual for assays to be evaluated in terms of the logarithms of the doses of the preparations, and if the ratio of successive doses is a constant, then using this constant (or a power of it) as a base for logarithms simplifies the arithmetic. However, the increasing use of digital computers in bioassay work is reducing the need for this technique, since to a computer a given calculation generally entails the same work whatever the values of the numbers involved.

In what follows, we will use the notation log for common logarithms, ln for natural logarithms and $\log_a$ to indicate a logarithm to any base.

4.3.12   Applications of logarithms

4.3.12.1 The scaling property of logarithms

Logarithms were originally invented in order to ease manual calculations involving multiplication and division. However, the advent of the desk calculator and the electronic computer has led to the use of tables of logarithms for this purpose becoming fairly uncommon, and the interest and utility have shifted to the properties of the logarithm considered as a *function*. From this viewpoint it is probably the most important and widely used function in medical work.

A particularly useful application for logarithms occurs where we are considering proportionality changes in a variable with a very wide numerical range. Consider for instance the death rate from infections and parasitic diseases (*International Statistical Classification* Nos. 1–138) during the period 1941–1967 (Registrar General, 1941–1967). In 1941, the crude death rate for England and Wales was 1093 deaths per million living while in 1967 the figure was eighty-two deaths per million living. In the later years reduction in the death rates of the order of 10 per million living are of interest in studying our increasing success in conquering these diseases, but in 1941 reductions of 10 per million would have been of little practical interest; at that time attention would be concentrated on reductions of the order of 100 per million living. In Fig 4.7(a) we have attempted to show these results graphically. In order to get the death rate for 1941 onto the graph we have had to set the scale so that the top of the graph reaches up to 1100 deaths per million, with the result that the continuing drop since the mid 1950's is hardly noticeable. In Fig 4.7(b) we have taken the same data, but this time we have plotted the *logarithm* (to base 10) of the death rates instead of the death rates themselves, and this curve shows the dramatic drop in the death rates from these diseases without losing the details of current changes. To make the graph easier to interpret we have included in brackets the actual death rate beside the value of the logarithm on the vertical scale.

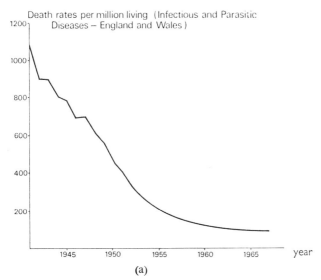

(a)

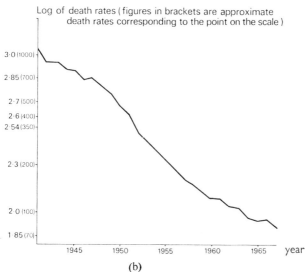

(b)

Fig 4.7   Crude death rates from infections and parasitic diseases (I.S.C. 1–138) England and Wales 1941–1967

The usefulness of the logarithm in this context arises from the fact that the proportionate change in log x relative to x increases as x becomes smaller. For example, the logarithms of numbers in the range 10 to 100 lie between 1 and 2 in value, whereas in the much larger range 1000 to 10,000 the logarithms still change by only one unit—from 3 to 4.

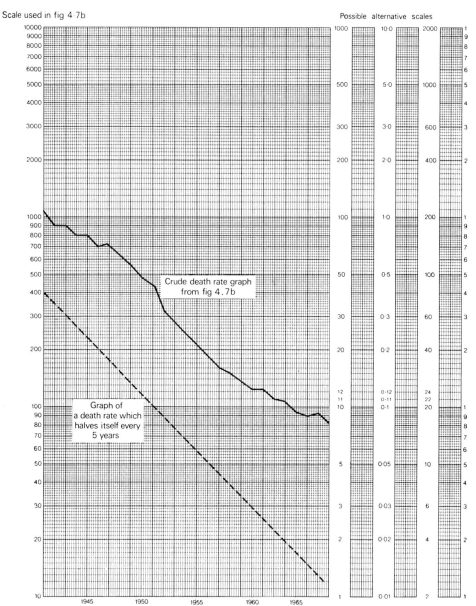

Fig 4.8   3 cycle log/linear graph paper

Another way of looking at this property is to note that a succession of values with a constant *multiplicative* factor between successive pairs will have a constant *additive* increase in their logarithms:

Examples:

(i) The common logarithms of 10, 100, 1000, 10,000, . . . are 1, 2, 3, 4, . . .

(ii) The natural logarithms of $1 \cdot 5$, 3, 6, 12, . . . are (to five decimal places) $0 \cdot 40547$, $1 \cdot 09862$, $1 \cdot 79176$, $2 \cdot 48491$, . . . with a common increase of $0 \cdot 69314$ or $0 \cdot 69315$ (the variation is due to round-off).

4.3.12.2 Logarithmic graph paper

Let us consider Fig 4.7(b) more closely. The logarithms of the death rates are noted on the *y*-axis, and beside them are given the actual death rates corresponding to the logarithmic values. But we could omit the logarithmic values, leaving only the actual values, and the graph would still be quite satisfactory for conveying the required information. Comparing the death rates written on the vertical axes of Fig 4.7(a) and 4.7(b) we see that the effect is to distort the evenly-spaced scale of Fig 4.7(a) so that in Fig 4.7(b) equal linear intervals represent a constant multiplicative increase between the values represented at the end-points—the distance from 100 to 200 is equal to the distance from 200 to 400, and also to the distance between e.g. 350 and 700, and so on. But this property of a constant *additive* increase corresponding to a constant *multiplicative* increase is the logarithmic property referred to previously, and hence the scale used in Fig 4.7(b) is referred to as a *logarithmic* scale—intervals on such a scale are proportional to the logarithms of the ratio of the numbers represented by the end-points. This property is independent of the base to which the logarithms are taken, since logarithms to different bases differ simply by a proportionality factor (Section 4.3.5).

It is clear that it should be possible to construct a special type of graph paper which instead of having regular, equally-spaced lines had a distorted and labelled scale as in Fig 4.7(b). With such graph paper it would be possible to plot graphs directly onto a logarithmic scale without ever having to refer to a table of logarithms.

As it happens, the use of logarithmic scales for plotting data is so frequent that it has been found commercially worthwhile to print this special graph paper (Fig 4.8), and it is generally available at technical stationers. Indeed, in many laboratories one is more likely to find a pad of logarithmic graph paper than the ordinary kind. The commonest type of logarithmic graph paper is scaled as in Fig 4.8, with one regular scale and one logarithmic scale, and is called variously *log/linear, semi-log, log one-way* or *log/equal divisions*.

There are also specific versions of it referred to as e.g. 'log/inch' or 'log/cm'. Another type of logarithmic graph paper has a logarithmic scale on *both* axes, and is usually referred to as *log/log* paper.

It will be seen from Fig 4.8 that the distance from 10 to 100 on the vertical scale equals the distance from 100 to 1000, which equals the distance from 1000 to 10,000. This means that the graph paper can be drawn to repeat itself in *cycles*, the intervals in the first cycle representing, say, the numbers 10 to 100, the second 100 to 1000, and so on. Or again, the first cycle could represent the interval $0 \cdot 01$ to $0 \cdot 1$ in steps of $0 \cdot 01$, when the second cycle would represent the range $0 \cdot 1$ to $1 \cdot 0$ in steps of $0 \cdot 1$, the third cycle $1 \cdot 0$ to $10 \cdot 0$ in steps of $1 \cdot 0$ and so on.

Note that *zero cannot occur on a logarithmic scale.*

Logarithmic graph paper is not base-dependent—it can be used to plot natural logarithms, for example, just as well as common logarithms, since the effect is simply to stretch the representation on the scale by a constant scale factor. In practice, however, common logarithms with a factor of 10 per cycle are used so often that the logarithmic scale usually has *each cycle* printed with the scale 1 to 10, and the actual scale used is obtained by putting the appropriate number of zeroes (with decimal point if required) before or after each scale mark. Various interpretations of the scale have been put down the right-hand side of Fig 4.8. As the logarithmic scale has an interval based on multiples, the gap between scale lines in the second cycle will represent a ten-fold increase in the numbers represented by the corresponding gap in the first cycle, etc. It is also possible to multiply the actual scale numbers by a constant (e.g. 2 on the right hand side of Fig 4.8).

The range of numbers which can be covered on a single sheet of logarithmic graph paper depends on the number of cycles provided. Figure 4.8 is an example of *3 cycle log/linear paper*.

Interpolation on a logarithmic scale for a value not already marked on it should strictly speaking be logarithmic interpolation—i.e. measuring off on the scale a length corresponding to the logarithm of the number. However, a linear interpolation is usually accurate enough (e.g. the point representing $6 \cdot 1$ can be taken to be halfway between $6 \cdot 0$ and $6 \cdot 2$).

The technique for constructing special graph papers shown in this section could be applied to any function which it is desired to plot. Logarithms are by far the most usual, but other graph papers are printed, notably 'probability paper' which is equivalent to computing the cumulative Gaussian distribution of the variable before plotting it, and is frequently used in bioassay work.

4.3.12.3 Applications in statistical analysis

(i) In the example of the study of death rates from infectious and parasitic diseases given above, one's interest is roused by a *percentage* decrease in the death rate. There are many other biological variables where we tend to be interested in changes expressed as a percentage of the value of the variable rather than as a fixed increment. In particular, in most clinical measurement techniques the accuracy is expressed as a 'percentage error', that is, we expect the difference between replicate determinations to increase proportionally to the absolute value being measured. For example in discussing precision of measurement of serum thyroxine Ekins, Williams & Ellis (1969) measured different levels of serum thyroxine and used the standard deviation as a measure of error. Three values they obtained were $50 \cdot 5$ ng†/ml, $72 \cdot 8$ ng/ml, and $122 \cdot 6$ ng/ml with standard deviations of $2 \cdot 86$ ng/ml, $3 \cdot 8$ ng/ml, and $7 \cdot 2$ ng/ml respectively, giving about a 5% error. In the statistical analysis of these results, or for presenting them graphically it is extremely inconvenient to have the actual value of the error varying. However if we work instead with the logarithms of the data, the error remains as a constant increment from the logarithm of the measured value:

$$\log (0 \cdot 05 * 50 \cdot 5) = \log (0 \cdot 05) + \log (50 \cdot 5)$$
$$\log (0 \cdot 05 * 122 \cdot 6) = \log (0 \cdot 05) + \log (122 \cdot 6)$$

(ii) Another application of the logarithm is in removing the long skew tail from the distribution of 'normal' values of many biological measurements. In general it is more convenient to handle distributions of measures which are equally spread about some central (i.e. mean) value, and it often happens that the logarithms of our observations have this property.

(iii) In studying the action of drugs we often carry out trials at doses of, for example, 10, 100 and 1000 units, in the expectation of a similar change in response for each factor of 10. Drug doses are often plotted on a logarithmic scale.

4.3.12.4 Growth and decay: exponential and power law relationships

There are many biological systems which grow or decay in a multiplicative fashion. For example, in an ideal culture a single cell will divide into 2, the 2 cells will divide into 4, the 4 into 8 and so on. After t divisions there will be 2^t cells in the culture. If n is the number of cells, then

$$n = 2^t$$

i.e. $\log n = t * \log 2$ (4.24)

---

† 1 ng = 1 nanogram = 10^{-9} gram.

A graph of $\log n$ against t should therefore be a straight line (Section 3.10.1), and indeed a plot of n against t on log/linear paper produces a straight line:

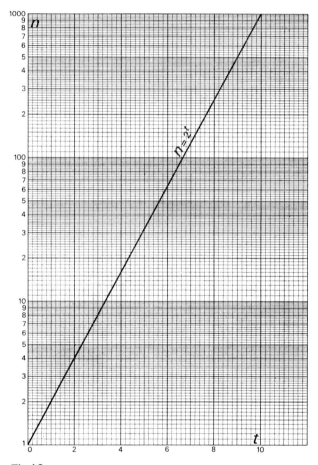

Fig 4.9

Equation (4.24) is a particular case of the relationship

$$y = Ae^{k*x} \qquad (4.25)$$

or more generally

$$y = Ap^{k*x} \qquad (4.26)$$

(the 'exponential law') which is a common and widely occurring form in biology; many growth and decay processes can be modelled by it to some extent or other.

Using natural logarithms, (4.25) becomes

$$\ln y = kx + \ln A \qquad (4.27)$$

and (4.26):

$$\ln y = (k * \ln p) * x + \ln A; \qquad (4.28)$$

a plot of such a functional relationship on log/linear paper produces a straight line.

On the other hand, the form

$$y = Ax^k \qquad (4.29)$$

(the 'power law') which is another frequent visitor to the biomathematical scene, is transformed into

$$\ln y = \ln A + k * \ln x \qquad (4.30)$$

which plots as a straight line, not on log/linear paper, but on *log/log paper*—as is the case, for example, in the following figure from a paper by Siegal & Williams (1969) on the prediction of operative survival in cirrhotic and portal hypertensive patients:

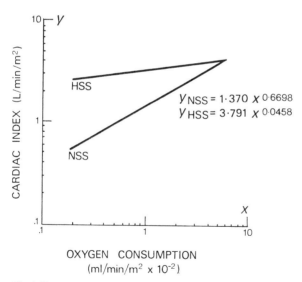

Fig 4.10

Alternatively, if plotting a set of results for y against x on log/linear paper produces a set of points which lie more or less on a straight line, then we know that—within the limits of experimental error—it is valid to postulate that the underlying relationship is of the form

$$y = Ap^{kx}$$

(p will normally be taken to be 10 or e), whereas a straight line plot on log/log paper implies a relationship

$$y = Ax^p$$

In the first type, the independent variable is the index while in the second type it is the base.

As an example of such a differentiation between possible alternative mathematical forms, we give the investigation of Berenbaum (1969) into the relationship between dose and cell survival for various alkylating and antimetabolite agents, prior to a theoretical derivation of optimum treatment schemes. Berenbaum considered the following two relationships, where F is the fraction surviving, and D the dose:

$$F = e^{-\alpha D}, \text{ which is equivalent to } \ln F = -\alpha D \tag{4.31}$$

$$F = \left(\frac{D}{D_0}\right)^{-\gamma}, \text{ equivalent to } \ln F = -\gamma (\ln D - \ln D_0) \tag{4.32}$$

If the relationship is as in (4.31) then a plot of $\ln (F)$ against D should give a straight line, while if the relationship is as in (4.32) then a plot of $\ln F$ against $\ln D$ should give a straight line. The comparison is most easily conducted using two different types of graph paper, one being log/linear with the log scale on the F axis and the linear scale on the D axis, and the other being log/log. The results for 6-mercaptopurine are given in Fig 4.11.

4.3.12.5 Half-life and decay constant

One of the commonest questions which arise with a situation modelled by

$$y(t) = Ae^{-\lambda t}$$

(λ a positive constant and t denoting time) concerns the point at which y is 50% of its starting value at $t = 0$. The corresponding value of t is called the *half-life* and often denoted by $t_{1/2}$; the constant λ is sometimes referred to as the *decay constant* or *time-constant* of the relationship. Usually we are interested in finding $t_{1/2}$, given λ, or in finding λ, given $t_{1/2}$.

We have

$$y(0) = Ae^{-\lambda * 0}$$

$$= A \tag{4.33}$$

$$y(t_{1/2}) = Ae^{-\lambda * t_{1/2}} \tag{4.34}$$

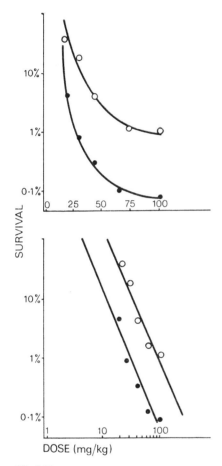

Fig 4.11

But $y(t_{1/2}) = \frac{1}{2} * y(0)$, by definition

i.e. $y(t_{1/2}) = \frac{1}{2} * A$ (from (4.33))   (4.35)

From (4.34) and (4.35), we have

$$Ae^{-\lambda * t_{1/2}} = \frac{1}{2} * A$$

and therefore

$$e^{-\lambda * t_{1/2}} = \frac{1}{2}$$

Taking natural logarithms, we obtain

$$-\lambda * t_{1/2} = \ln\left(\tfrac{1}{2}\right) = -\ln(2) \quad \text{(Section 4.3.4)}$$

i.e. $\lambda * t_{1/2} = 0 \cdot 693$

In words: Decay Constant multiplied by Half-Life $= 0 \cdot 693$ (4.36)

From this, given either $t_{1/2}$ or λ we can determine the other. Note that this result is independent of the starting value A.

A graphical method for determining the half-life is to plot two values of y against t on log/linear paper and draw a straight line through them, then read off on this graph the value of t at which y has half its initial value. (It is wise to check the accuracy of your straight line by plotting an additional point or two to make sure that they lie on the line.) From this we can then find λ through the relationship (4.36).

4.3.13   Finding the constants of a straight line log/linear plot

The relationship

Decay Constant $*$ Half-Life $= 0 \cdot 693$

enables us to calculate the decay constant where a straight line has been fitted on a log/linear plot to experimental data decreasing in value with time. However, this is not always a convenient or feasible method to use, and we give now some general formulae for finding the constants of straight line log/linear plots.

A straight line fit, with the dependent variable (y) on the log scale implies, if we use natural logarithms, that

$$\ln y = ax + b \qquad (4.37)$$

equivalent to

$$y = Be^{ax}$$

where $B = e^b$ (4.38)

While it is a and B which we usually need, it is a and b which are obtained most easily from the linear plot, with B found from b by the relationship (4.38).

The constants a and b can be obtained by considering two points on the line. If the two points are (x_1, y_1) and (x_2, y_2) then

$$a = \frac{\ln(y_1) - \ln(y_2)}{x_1 - x_2} \tag{4.39}$$

$$= \frac{\ln(y_1/y_2)}{x_1 - x_2} \tag{4.39a}$$

$$b = \frac{x_1 * \ln(y_2) - x_2 * \ln(y_1)}{x_1 - x_2} \tag{4.40}$$

and $B = e^b$ as before. This can be proved using (4.37).

Example:

Consider Fig 4.12. Taking the two points (x_1, y_1) and (x_2, y_2) as shown, we have

$$x_1 = 2 \cdot 5 \qquad y_1 = 1 \cdot 1$$
$$x_2 = 4 \cdot 0 \qquad y_2 = 0 \cdot 6 \tag{4.41}$$

Note that although y is plotted on a logarithmic scale it is the *actual values* of y_1 and y_2 which we read from the scale. The corresponding logarithms of y_1 and y_2 needed to calculate the quantities a and b have to be found from tables or by measurement with a ruler (v.i.)

From tables

$$\ln(y_1) = \ln(1 \cdot 1)$$
$$= 0 \cdot 0953$$
$$\ln(y_2) = \ln(0 \cdot 6)$$
$$= -0 \cdot 5108$$

and therefore from (4.39) and (4.41):

$$a = \frac{0 \cdot 0953 - (-0 \cdot 5108)}{2 \cdot 5 - 4 \cdot 0}$$
$$= -0 \cdot 4040$$

i.e. $a = -0 \cdot 40$ to the accuracy we can expect from the graph.

Again, from (4.40) and (4.41)

$$b = \frac{2 \cdot 5 * \ln(0 \cdot 6) - 4 \cdot 0 * \ln(1 \cdot 1)}{2 \cdot 5 - 4 \cdot 0}$$
$$= 1 \cdot 1054$$

whence $B = e^b$
$$= 3 \cdot 0$$

Thus the graph represents

$$y = 3e^{-0 \cdot 4x}$$

When calculating a, the arithmetic is simplified if y_1/y_2 is some convenient constant, especially if $x_1=0$. We then use the form (4.39a) rather than (4.39). For example, suppose $y_1/y_2=2$, and $x_1=0$, then the equation for a reduces to

$$a = -\frac{0 \cdot 693}{x_2}$$

As we saw earlier, this example has a particular application when x represents *time*; in this case x_2 is the half-life, and we have as before

$$a = -\frac{0 \cdot 693}{\text{half-life}}$$

(cf. section 4.3.12.4)

The slope a can also be found by direct measurement on the graph with a ruler, as follows: first establish a conversion factor by measuring the distance on the y-axis between any point y and the point $e * y$—e.g. between the points 1 and $2 \cdot 71$ or 10 and $27 \cdot 1$. Call this f. Then as before select two points (x_1, y_1) and (x_2, y_2) on the graph and measure the distance on the y axis between y_1 and y_2. The value of a is given by

$$a = \frac{\text{Distance between } y_1 \text{ and } y_2}{f * (x_1 - x_2)} \qquad (4.42)$$

Example:

Taking Fig 4.12 again we have:

$$f = \text{distance between 1 and } e * 1$$
$$= 3 \cdot 35 \text{ cm.}$$

Distance between y_1 and $y_2 = 2 \cdot 0$ cm.
Therefore

$$a = \frac{2 \cdot 0}{3 \cdot 35 * (2 \cdot 5 - 4 \cdot 0)} = -0 \cdot 40 \qquad (4.43)$$

as before. (Note that if y_1 is $<y_2$, then the distance between y_1 and y_2 must be taken as *negative*.)

If it is possible to read the point $x=0$ on the graph then we can also read the constant B directly off the log scale.

For at $x=0$, $y=B * e^0$, i.e. $B = $ *the value of y at x=0, i.e. the value of y where the straight line cuts the y-axis*. (cf. Section 3.10.3).

Example:

In Fig 4.12, the straight line cuts the y-axis where $y = 3 \cdot 0$. Hence $B = 3 \cdot 0$, as before

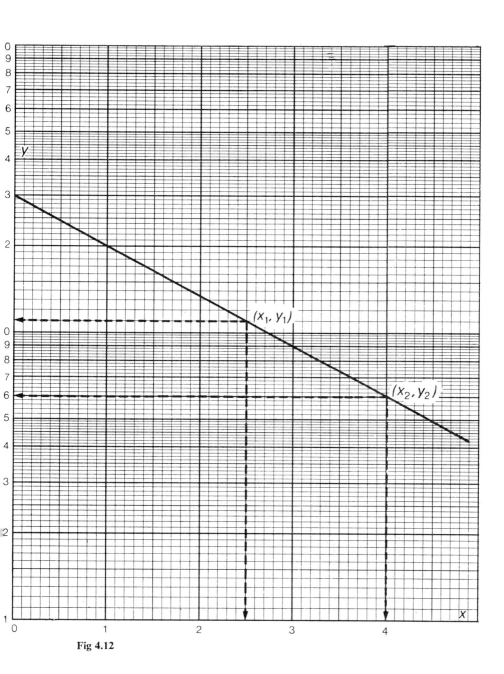

Fig 4.12

If we have found the constant a by measurement, and we cannot read the value $x=0$ off the graph, we can still find B directly by measurement from the graph, through the relationship (4.37). However, this formula is computationally sensitive to round-off inaccuracies in a, especially for large values of x. We have

$$b=\ln (y_1)-ax_1$$

or alternatively we can use

$$b=\ln (y_2)-ax_2$$

We measure off a distance whose end points are in the ratio y_1. In the Fig 4.12 this will be any distance whose end points are in the ratio $1\cdot1$, e.g. between 1 and $1\cdot1$ or between 5 and $5\cdot5$; obviously if the point 1 is on the log scale then it is easiest to measure from there. Then using our conversion factor f as before, we have

$$b=\frac{\text{Distance between the points in the ratio } y_1}{f}-ax_1 \qquad (4.44)$$

For example, in Fig 4.12, the distance between 1 and $1\cdot1$ is $0\cdot3$ cm. With $f=3\cdot35$ as before, $x_1=2\cdot5$ and $a=-0\cdot4$, we have

$$b=\frac{0\cdot3}{3\cdot35}-(-0\cdot4)*2\cdot5$$

$$=1\cdot09$$

$$B=e^{1\cdot09}=3\cdot0$$

N.B. If y is <1 the distance corresponding to it must be taken as negative. For example, if we use the value $x_2=4\cdot0$ and $y_2=0\cdot6$ in (4.44) the distance between $1\cdot0$ and $0\cdot6$ on the logarithmic scale is $1\cdot7$ cm, which we take as $-1\cdot7$ cm; this gives

$$b=\frac{-1\cdot7}{3\cdot35}-(-0\cdot4)*4=1\cdot09 \text{ as before.}$$

4.4   The role of e

The emphasis on e in the previous sections makes it perhaps appropriate to end this chapter with a few comments on this constant. It was stated earlier that the importance of e arose out of the properties of e^x, and these are undoubtedly very useful. But for any x we have

$$e^x=p^{\lambda x}$$

$$e^{kx}=p^{\lambda kx}$$

where p is any convenient alternative base, and $\lambda = \log_p e$ (see Rule (d) Section 4.3.2, putting e for x, p for a, and x or kx for s there). From this we see that all bases in power relationships are equivalent as far as mathematical manipulation is concerned—certainly e plays no special role in logarithmic plots (Section 4.3.12.2).

For example, consider the function

$$y = 3e^{-0\cdot4x} \tag{4.45}$$

of the previous section. Using base 10 rather than base e this becomes

$$y = 3 * 10^{-(0\cdot4*\log_{10}e)x}$$

i.e.
$$y = 3 * 10^{-0\cdot17x} \tag{4.46}$$

(cf. Section 4.3.10).

Both (4.45) and (4.46) are exactly equivalent and are different descriptions of the same relationship. And indeed if we work through Section 4.3.13 substituting 10 for e and using logarithms to base 10—i.e. common logarithms—rather than natural logarithms, all the formulae in that section remain valid and we obtain the result (4.46). For we have now

$$\log(y) = ax + b$$

corresponding to

$$y = B * 10^{ax}$$

where $B = 10^b$ (i.e. $B =$ antilog b).

Our formulae (4.39), (4.39a) and (4.40) then become

$$a = \frac{\log y_1 - \log y_2}{x_1 - x_2}$$

$$= \frac{\log(y_1/y_2)}{x_1 - x_2}$$

$$b = \frac{x_1 * \log(y_2) - x_2 * \log(y_1)}{x_1 - x_2}$$

and if we substitute the values of x_1, y_1, x_2 and y_2 used before, we obtain the values $a = -0\cdot18$, $B = 3\cdot0$ (compare those given in (4.46)—the difference in the values for a is due to round-off arising from a small computational difference in the third decimal place).

We would suggest therefore, that although it is an important and useful constant, the mystic aura with which e has become endowed is unjustified. Now and again one encounters a feeling in medicine and biology that life itself

E

is a manifestation of e, but the main point about e is that it is a mathematically convenient and universally accepted base for powers in which the variable is the index. It is not the be-all and end-all of such relationships, however; other bases can be and are used as needed. The important aspect of the form Be^{ax} is not the occurrence of e but the use of the variable x in the index position, as distinct from the form Bx^a, where x is the base.

Chapter 5
Limits and Continuity

5.1   Introduction

Although the essence of a function is that for any value of the independent variable, we should be able to define a value or values of the dependent variable (or at least to decide whether or not it has a value), situations frequently arise where it is not obvious from the definition of the function what this value is to be, although all the indications are that there is one.

Consider for example the function

$$y = \frac{\ln x}{2 * (x-1)} \qquad\qquad (5.1)$$

where ln x, it will be recalled from Chapter 4, is the natural logarithm of x.

We can compute y for any positive x with the exception of $x=1$; for this value of x, both numerator and denominator vanish in (5.1) and leave us with

$$y(1) = \frac{0}{0}$$

This is undefined and undefinable; no value can be given to it. However, if we calculate a succession of values of y on either side of $x=1$, we have:

Table 5.1   Values of $y = \dfrac{\ln x}{2 * (x-1)}$ near $x=1$

x	$x-1$	$\ln x$	$y = \dfrac{\ln x}{2 * (x-1)}$
1·3	0·3	0·26236	0·43727
1·2	0·2	0·18232	0·45580
1·1	0·1	0·095310	0·47655
1·05	0·05	0·048790	0·48790
1·01	0·01	0·0099503	0·49752
1·001	0·001	$0·9995 * 10^{-3}$	0·49975
1·0001	0·0001	$0·99995 * 10^{-4}$	0·49998
1	0	0	?
0·9999	−0·0001	$−0·10001 * 10^{-3}$	0·50005
0·999	−0·001	−0·0010005	0·50025
0·99	−0·01	−0·010050	0·50250
0·95	−0·05	−0·051293	0·51293
0·9	−0·1	−0·10536	0·52680
0·8	−0·2	−0·22314	0·55578
0·7	−0·3	−0·35667	0·59445

We see that the value of y seems to approach closer and closer to $0 \cdot 5$ as x gets nearer and nearer to the value 1 from either below or above $x = 1$.

It would appear, in fact, that although y cannot actually be computed for $x = 1$, it would not be altogether unreasonable to say that its value *is* $0 \cdot 5$ at $x = 1$; certainly it would appear that we can get as close as we please to the value $0 \cdot 5$ for y if we take x a sufficiently small distance from 1, and calculate accurately enough.

This concept of being able to approach as close as we please to some sort of *limiting* value for a variable without actually being able to attain that value is the basis of the mathematical theory and technique of *limits* and *limiting processes*. Examples of it occur frequently in all application of mathematics, including biology and medicine, and the theory is crucial to the differential and integral calculus (Chapter 9).

5.2   Limits

The technical phrase for the situation just described is that y *tends* to the value $0 \cdot 5$ as x *tends* to the value 1; or more briefly, that $y \rightarrow 0 \cdot 5$ as $x \rightarrow 1$. Another way of putting it is to say that the *limit* of y as x tends to 1 is $0 \cdot 5$. However, so far we have simply computed closer and closer values to the limit in this case, and we have not really defined what we mean by 'limit'. As it happens, to *prove* that the limit (insofar as we will define the term later on) is $0 \cdot 5$ in the example just given requires rather more sophisticated techniques than this chapter will develop.

5.3   Limits at infinity

5.3.1   *Transients and steady-states*

Another kind of limiting situation occurs where the independent variable is free to increase or decrease (i.e. increase negatively) to an unlimited extent. The mathematical formulation of many physical situations often consists of the sum of two functions of time, one a function which dies away with increasing time and the other a function which as time goes on approaches closer and closer to a constant value (or it may be a constant to begin with) or perhaps settles down to an oscillation of some kind. The first function is usually known as a *transient*, the second as the *steady-state* or *equilibrium state*.

For instance, consider the function

$$x(t) = \frac{1}{f+E}(f + 0 \cdot 21E - 0 \cdot 79f \exp(-(f+E)t/V)) \tag{5.2}$$

used by Wayne & Chamney (1969) in a discussion on Oxygen Tent Performance.†
E is the tent gas exchange rate, f the oxygen inflow rate, V the tent gas volume
and t the time in minutes from starting the oxygen inflow and closing the tent
(assumed to be the same). The constant $e = 2 \cdot 718281828 \ldots$ is the base of
natural logarithms (Chapter 4). E, f and V are also taken to be constants with
respect to time, though, strictly speaking, they are in fact parameters, since they
vary from tent to tent but are fixed for any particular tent. x is the oxygen
concentration v/v.

We can write the function $x(t)$ as

$$x(t) = \frac{f + 0 \cdot 21E}{f + E} - \frac{0 \cdot 79f \exp\left(-(f+E)\,t/V\right)}{f + E} \tag{5.3}$$

Now as t increases, the term $\exp(-(f+E)t/V)$ becomes smaller and smaller,
no matter what values f, E and V may have—take for example $f = 18 \cdot 0$ litres/min,
$E = 17 \cdot 0$ litres/min, $V = 145$ litres ('Trial I' of the paper):

Table 5.2   Values of $\exp(-(f+E)t/V)$ as t increases

t (min)	0	1	2	3	4	5	10	20
$\exp(-(f+E)t/V)$	1·000	0·787	0·619	0·487	0·383	0·301	0·091	0·008

From this, it is clear that as t increases, the effect of $-0 \cdot 79 f \exp\left(-(f+E)t/V\right)$
becomes less and less, and $x(t)$ comes closer and closer to the value
$(f + 0 \cdot 21E)/(f + E)$. As long as t is finite, however, the transient
$-0 \cdot 79 \exp\left(-(f+E)/t/V\right)$ will contribute some effect although completely
negligible after a while. This leaves $(f + 0 \cdot 21E)/(f + E)$ as the steady-state or
equilibrium state of $x(t)$.

Under such circumstances, we say that $x(t)$ tends to $(f + 0 \cdot 21E)/(f + E)$ as
t increases without limitation, or 'tends to infinity'. In other words the limit of
$x(t)$ as t 'tends to infinity' is $(f + 0 \cdot 21E)/(f + E)$. Infinity, as was emphasized in
Chapter 1, is not a value; it is shorthand for 'greater than any imaginable
number'.

Looked at another way, we can allow the system to approach as closely
as we please to the steady-state by waiting long enough. If we want $x(t)$ not to
differ from the steady-state by more than, say, 0·001, then we must wait until
$0 \cdot 79 f \exp\left(-(f+E)t/V\right)$ is $<0 \cdot 001$. Taking logarithms to base e, this means

---

† In Wayne & Chamney's paper, $e^{-(f+E)t/V}$ is written as $\exp(-(f+E)t/V)$; the
function e^x is often written as $\exp(x)$, for convenience in writing and printing.
See also Section 5.14.

that

$$\ln{(0 \cdot 79f)} - (f+E)t/V < \ln{(0 \cdot 001)}$$

i.e. $\ln{(0 \cdot 79f)} - \ln{(0 \cdot 001)} < (f+E)t/V$ (Section 1.8.5)

i.e. $\ln{\left(\dfrac{0 \cdot 79f}{0 \cdot 001}\right)} < (f+E)t/V$ (Section 4.3.2.)

i.e. $t > \dfrac{V}{f+E} \ln{(790f)}$ (Section 1.8.5)

Since f, E and V are supposed known, we can find the threshold value of t satisfying our requirements. With our previous values for f, E and V, this gives

$$t > 39 \cdot 84 \text{ min.}$$

In other words at about 40 min. after the start of the experiment, the concentration will not differ from the steady state by more than $0 \cdot 001$. In practice, of course, the system will have settled down to a level indistinguishable from the steady-state long before this—we will have been unable to measure the transient quite early on (in the Wayne & Chamney paper, the graph of $x(t)$ has flattened out after about 20 min.).

(The problem is a little more complicated if we require the transient to have dropped below some percentage level of the concentration, but the value of t can be found for this situation also.)

5.3.2   Infinity as a limit

Another limiting situation arises where as the independent variable approaches some finite value, the dependent variable becomes greater and greater, finally becoming infinite at the limit point. For example, if $y = 1/x^2$, then as x approaches zero y becomes greater and greater:

Table 5.3   Values of $y = 1/x^2$

x	0·5	0·1	0·01	0·001	10^{-75}	...
$y = \dfrac{1}{x^2}$	4·0	100·0	10,000·0	1,000,000	10^{+150}	...

In fact we can always find a value of x near zero such that the corresponding value of y is greater than any number we can think of, no matter how large. If we ask that y be $> 1,000,000$ then taking $x < 1/1000$ will achieve this; if we require $y > 10^{2000}$, then take $x < 10^{-1000}$.

Under such circumstances, we say that y tends to infinity as x tends to zero or $y \to \infty$ as $x \to 0$.

Finally, there is the situation where as the independent variable becomes greater and greater, so does the dependent one. An example is

$$y = x^2$$

In this case, we say that y tends to infinity as x tends to infinity, or $y \to \infty$ as $x \to \infty$. Another way of putting it is that y *tends to infinity with x*.

When dealing with infinity as a limit, one can meet limit problems in which the limit is not as easily indicated by computation as e.g. with the case of the limit for $y = \ln x / \{2 * (x - 1)\}$. Consider, for example the function

$$y = x\,e^{-x}$$
$$= x / e^x$$

As $x \to \infty$ so does e^x. The limit of y as $x \to \infty$ would appear to be ∞ / ∞, meaning 'the quotient of two numbers each greater than any imaginable number'; naturally enough, this is as undefinable as $0/0$; but whereas we could approach as closely as we pleased to $x = 1$, approaching 'infinity' is not quite so easy, though we can deal with numbers that for all practical purposes are 'close' enough:

Table 5.4   Values of $x\,e^{-x}$

x	10	100	1000	...
e^x	$2 \cdot 203 * 10^4$	$2 \cdot 688 * 10^{43}$	$1 \cdot 95 * 10^{434}$	...
$x\,e^{-x}$	$0 \cdot 454 * 10^{-3}$	$0 \cdot 372 * 10^{-41}$	$0 \cdot 51 * 10^{-431}$	...

Although it is clear that $x\,e^{-x}$ is getting rapidly smaller and smaller as x increases, to *prove* that it has zero as a limit—in the sense already discussed with other situations, namely, that by taking x large enough we can make $x\,e^{-x}$ differ from zero by as little as we like—is not straightforward. As with $\ln x / \{2 * (x - 1)\}$ rather more sophisticated mathematics are needed than are covered in this chapter. We will return in a later Section (5.7) to some other considerations raised by this example.

5.4   Formal definition of a limit

We saw earlier that there are in fact four types of limit situation, viz:

   (i) As $x \to \infty$, so does y. In this case, y becomes bigger and bigger as x becomes bigger and bigger.

(ii) As $x \rightarrow$ some finite value—a, say—$y \rightarrow \infty$. Here y increases indefinitely in value as x approaches closer and closer to the value a.

(iii) As $x \rightarrow \infty$, $y \rightarrow$ some finite value.

(iv) As $x \rightarrow$ some finite value, $y \rightarrow$ some finite value. As x approaches closer and closer to its limiting value, y correspondingly moves nearer and nearer to *its* limiting value.

However, we have so far dealt with the concept of a limit in a rather empirical way. *The mathematical* definition of a limit arises directly from the kind of considerations we have been dealing with, but the reasoning is subtle and involves defining precisely what is meant by such statements as 'bigger and bigger', 'smaller and smaller', 'approaches closer and closer to the value a', etc. To show the kind of approach used, we will give the formal definition of one of the four types of limiting situation which can arise, and deal with the others in general terms; for further information on the mathematical definition of a limit the reader is referred to texts on mathematical analysis (e.g. Hardy (1967)).

5.4.1 $y \rightarrow \infty$ *as* $x \rightarrow \infty$

The meaning of this is that we should be able to make y as big as we like by a suitable choice of x, and that this choice of x will get bigger and bigger as we ask that y get bigger and bigger. Note the order of action, which is very important, and lies at the foundations of all limit definitions. It is not that we choose x and then see how big y has become; on the contrary, we decide first of all how big we wish y to be and then see if we find an x which will bring this about. The important thing is to fix the behaviour of the *dependent* variable, which after all is our main concern. Having done this, we then consider how to assign the independent variable so as to ensure this required behaviour.

Now if y is to tend to infinity with x, this means that y has to become greater than any number we care to name, and this has to happen in harness with x also becoming greater than any imaginable number. But if y is to be $> N$, say, then the value which x has to be greater than will depend on N. With the function

$$y = x^2$$

for example, if we require $y > N$, then x must be $> \sqrt{N}$. We therefore need for the general case: '$y > N$ if $x > V_N$', the subscript in V_N showing that V depends on N. Furthermore, it is not enough that y should be $> N$ for just *some* values of $x > V_N$; it must continue to be $> N$ for *all* values of $x > V_N$; otherwise we might have the situation in Fig. 5.1:

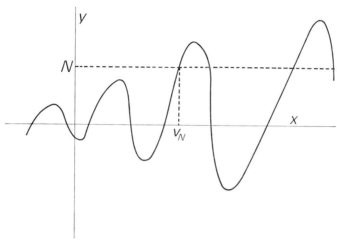

Fig 5.1

In this case, the value of y oscillates more and more wildly, and we certainly cannot say that it tends to ∞, because although it is $>N$ for part of the time, no matter how large we make N, it is very definitely $<N$ at other times.

These and other considerations lead to the following formal definition:

> *The function $y(x)$ is said to tend to $+\infty$ (positive infinity) with x if, given $N>0$, no matter how large N may be, we can determine V_N (i.e. a quantity depending on N) so that $y(x)$ is $>N$ for all $x>V_N$.*

A standard mathematical notation for 'y tends to ∞ with x' is

$$\lim_{x\to\infty} y(x)=\infty$$

Again the reader must not be deceived by the equality sign; it cannot be overemphasized that '$=\infty$' is a shorthand for 'becomes greater than any imaginable number'.

Similar forms of definition to the one just given hold for x and/or $y\to-\infty$.

5.4.2 $y\to\infty$ as $x\to a$

Considerations similar to those of the previous section hold when $y\to\infty$ as $x\to$ a finite value—a, say—rather than becoming infinite. The only difference is that instead of y becoming larger and larger as x becomes larger and larger we require that y should become larger and larger as x comes nearer and nearer to *a*. Clearly, also, this must be true as *x* approaches *a* either from above or below *a*, i.e. we require *y* to →∞ as | *x* − *a* | becomes smaller and smaller. These ideas can be expressed in a precise mathematical form in a somewhat similar manner to the definition in the previous Section (see e.g. Hardy (1967)). The notation used is also similar:

$$\lim_{x \to a} y(x) = \infty$$

with the same caveat about '=∞' as before.

Example:

$$\lim_{x \to 7} \frac{1}{(x-7)^2} = \infty$$

For as *x* approaches 7, either from above or below (i.e. as | *x* − 7 | →0) $1/(x-7)^2$ will become larger and larger, and we can make $1/(x-7)^2$ as large as we like by making | *x* − 7 | sufficiently small.

5.4.3   *y* → *l* as *x* → ∞

In this case, it is the dependent variable which has to approach as close as is desired to a finite value (*l*) as the independent variable becomes indefinitely great; the approach to *l* can be from above or below. More precisely, for *y* to tend to *l* as *x* →∞, it must be possible for | *y* − *l* | to become as small as we please for a suitably large choice of *x*.

We express this as

$$\lim_{x \to \infty} y = l$$

Example:

$$\lim_{x \to \infty} \frac{1}{x} = 0$$

5.4.4   *y* → *l* as *x* → *a*

This implies that *y* can be brought as close as we please to *l* in value (either through a sequence of values >*l* or a sequence of values <*l*) by taking *x* sufficiently near to *a*; more precisely, | *y* − *l* | can be made as small as we like by taking | *x* − *a* | sufficiently small.

The usual notation for this situation is

$$\lim_{x \to a} y = l$$

Examples:

(i) $\lim_{x \to 4} \dfrac{1}{x} = \dfrac{1}{4}$

(ii) $\lim_{x \to 1} \dfrac{\ln x}{2 * (x-1)} = \dfrac{1}{2}$

In all these examples and situations, remember that we may not be able to actually give x or y their limiting values; we may only be able to conceive of approaching them as closely as we please.

5.5   Oscillating functions

It can happen that in the limit, none of the criteria given in Sections 5.4.1–5.4.4. will hold. For example, consider the 'square wave' function:

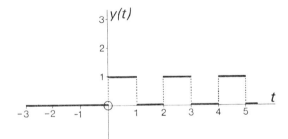

Fig 5.2

It is obvious that this function neither becomes infinite nor tends to a limit as $t \to \infty$. On the other hand, the function $y(t)$ is quite specifically defined:

$y(t) = 0, \quad t < 0$

$y(t) = 1, \quad 0 \leqslant t < 1$

$y(t) = 0, \quad 1 \leqslant t < 2$

$y(t) = 1, \quad 2 \leqslant t < 3$

etc.

This can be expressed in general terms as

$$y(t)=0, \quad t<0$$

$$y(t)=\frac{1-(-1)^n}{2}, \quad (n-1)\leqslant t<n, \quad n=1, 2, 3, 4, \ldots$$

This function cannot be pinned down to a limiting value, but nor does it ever become >1. It is an example of a function *oscillating finitely* in the limit. It is also possible to have functions *oscillating infinitely* in the limit, e.g.

$$y(t)=0, \quad t<0$$

$$y(t)=\frac{1-(-1)^n}{2}*t, \quad (n-1)\leqslant t<n, \quad n=1, 2, 3, 4, \ldots$$

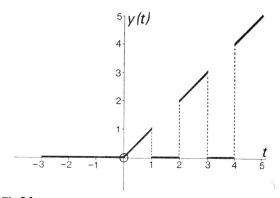

Fig 5.3

These are not completely artificial functions; square-wave functions, for example, occur frequently in electronics and, if one is not careful, so do functions which oscillate more and more wildly with increasing time.

5.6   Theorems on limits

From formal mathematical definitions of a limit, it is possible to prove various useful theorems concerning limits in general, though one must be very careful to distinguish between cases involving only finite limits and those involving infinite ones.

5.6.1   Finite limit theorems

Let $u(x)$ and $v(x)$ be two functions of x, and let

$$\lim_{x \to a} u(x) = l, \quad \lim_{x \to a} v(x) = m$$

(*a* may in fact be infinite, but *l* and *m* must be finite)
Then:

(i) $\lim_{x \to a} [u(x) \pm v(x)] = \lim_{x \to a} u(x) \pm \lim_{x \to a} v(x) = l \pm m$

i.e. **the limit of the sum (or difference) of two functions, each with a finite limit, is equal to the sum (or difference) of the individual limits.**

(ii) $\lim_{x \to a} [u(x) * v(x)] = \lim_{x \to a} u(x) * \lim_{x \to a} v(x) = lm$

i.e. **the limit of the product of two functions, each with a finite limit, equals the product of the limits.**

(iii) $\lim_{x \to a} \left[\dfrac{u(x)}{v(x)} \right] = \dfrac{\lim_{x \to a} u(x)}{\lim_{x \to a} v(x)} = \dfrac{l}{m}$ if $m \neq 0$

i.e. **the limit of the quotient of two functions, each with a finite limit of which that of the divisor is non-zero, equals the quotient of the limits.**

Notice the important difference to all the other results—we have to examine as a special case the situation when $m = 0$.

Examples:

(i) The limit of a constant is itself.
So, e.g. using $u(x)$ and l as before,

$$\lim_{x \to a} u(x) \pm K = l \pm K, \quad K \text{ a constant}$$

$$\lim_{x \to a} K * u(x) = K * \lim_{x \to a} u(x) = Kl$$

$$\lim_{x \to a} \frac{K}{u(x)} = \frac{K}{l}, \quad l \neq 0$$

$$\lim_{x \to a} \frac{u(x)}{K} = \frac{l}{K}$$

(ii) Let us look again at the function $x(t)$ discussed in Section 5.3.1; we state without formal proof that

$$\lim_{t \to \infty} \exp \left(-(f + E) \, t / V \right) = 0$$

We have

$$\lim_{t \to \infty} x(t) = \lim_{t \to \infty} \left(\frac{f + 0 \cdot 21E - 0 \cdot 79 f \exp\left(-(f+E)\, t/V\right)}{f+E} \right)$$

$$= \lim_{t \to \infty} \left(\frac{f + 0 \cdot 21E}{f+E} - \frac{0 \cdot 79 f \exp\left(-(f+E)\, t/V\right)}{f+E} \right)$$

$$= \frac{f + 0 \cdot 21E}{f+E}$$

5.6.2   Infinite limit theorems

With infinite limits, a little more care is needed; theorems which are true for finite limits are not necessarily true for infinite ones. For example, if $u(x) = x + 1/x$ and $v(x) = x - 1/x$, then

$$\lim_{x \to \infty} u(x) = \infty, \quad \lim_{x \to \infty} v(x) = \infty$$

but
$$\lim_{x \to \infty} [u(x) - v(x)] = \lim_{x \to \infty} \left[x + \frac{1}{x} - x + \frac{1}{x} \right] = \lim_{x \to \infty} \frac{2}{x} = 0$$

We cannot rely on being able to subtract 'infinities' to get zero, however tempting it may be in the above example to say that the result is due to '$\infty - \infty$'$=0$. For if $u(x)$ had been $= 2x + 1/x$ and $v(x) = x - 1/x$, then again

$$\lim_{x \to \infty} u(x) = \infty, \quad \lim_{x \to \infty} v(x) = \infty$$

but now

$$\lim_{x \to \infty} [u(x) - v(x)] = \lim_{x \to \infty} \left[2x + \frac{1}{x} - x + \frac{1}{x} \right] = \lim_{x \to \infty} \left[x + \frac{2}{x} \right] = \infty$$

With expressions whose limits may become infinite, or contain terms which tend to ∞, it is always necessary to reduce the expression down as far as possible, gathering like terms together and cancelling out such terms as one can, *before* going to the limit.

There are a number of different possibilities for the sum, difference, product or quotient of two or more functions which tend to infinity in the limit. What they amount to is that as we said above, the theorems for finite limits cannot be assumed to hold with infinite ones; each case has to be handled on its merits. Some general statements can be made, however; e.g.:

If $\lim_{x \to a} u(x) = \infty \quad$ and $\quad \lim_{x \to a} v(x) = \infty$

then $\lim_{x \to a} [u(x) + v(x)] = \infty$

We have already seen that no statement can be made about $\lim_{x \to a} [u(x) - v(x)]$.

Again, if

$$\lim_{x \to a} u(x) = +\infty \quad \text{and} \quad \lim_{x \to a} v(x) = -\infty$$

then $\lim_{x \to a} [u(x) v * (x)] = -\infty$

Analogous results can be formulated for cases where $u(x) \to \infty$ and $v(x) \to l$ (finite).

5.7   Speed of the limiting process

We saw earlier (Section 5.3.2) in the case of the function x/e^x that although both x and e^x were tending to infinity, $x/e^x \to 0$. Examination of the behaviour of both x and e^x shows that the limit zero seems to arise because e^x is clearly increasing at a much faster rate than x (cf. Table 5.4), and that no matter how large x becomes, its value is swamped by that of e^x. This idea of one function or variable tending to ∞ or zero 'faster' than another can be refined into a precise mathematical concept, but we will content ourselves with simply drawing the reader's attention to it; the section following this one gives some examples of this mechanism in action.

5.8   Limits of some common simple functions

For practical use, certain limits are worth listing. We do not intend to give proofs; the reader, if interested, can have a try at supplying these for himself or else consult any standard textbook on mathematical analysis (e.g. Hardy (1967)). In these examples, n is an *integer variable*, i.e. one which can take only integer values. The phrase '$n \to l$' means that n tends to l through a succession of integer values.

$$(i) \quad \lim_{n \to \infty} x^n = \begin{cases} \infty & \text{if } x > 1 \\ 1 & \text{if } x = 1 \\ 0 & \text{if } -1 < x < 1 \end{cases}$$

If $x = -1$, $\lim_{n \to \infty} x^n$ does not exist; x^n oscillates finitely between ± 1 as $n \to \infty$. If $x < -1$, x^n oscillates infinitely as $n \to \infty$.

(ii) $\lim\limits_{n \to \infty} \dfrac{1}{x^n} = \begin{cases} 0 & \text{if } x > 1 \\ 1 & \text{if } x = 1 \\ \infty & \text{if } 0 < x < 1 \end{cases}$

As with x^n, $1/x^n$ oscillates finitely between ± 1 as $n \to \infty$ for $x = -1$. But unlike x^n, $1/x^n \to 0$ as $n \to \infty$ if $x < -1$. For $-1 < x < 0$, $1/x^n$ oscillates infinitely as $n \to \infty$.

(iii) $\lim\limits_{n \to \infty} n^{1/n} = 1$

(iv) $\lim\limits_{n \to \infty} \dfrac{x^n}{n!} = 0$ for any x (i.e. $n! \to \infty$ with n more rapidly than x^n)

(v) $\lim\limits_{n \to \infty} n^r x^n$ (r any positive integer) $= \begin{cases} \infty & \text{if } x \geqslant 1 \\ 0 & \text{if } -1 < x < 1 \end{cases}$

If $x \leqslant -1$, $n^r x^n$ oscillates infinitely as $n \to \infty$.

(vi) $\lim\limits_{n \to \infty} n^{-r} x^n$ (r any positive integer) $= \begin{cases} \infty & \text{if } x > 1 \\ 0 & \text{if } -1 \leqslant x \leqslant 1 \end{cases}$

If $x < -1$, $n^{-r} x^n$ oscillates infinitely as $n \to \infty$.

(vii) $\lim\limits_{t \to \infty} t^r e^{-t} \to 0 \quad (r \geqslant 0)$

(i.e. $e^{-t} \to 0$ more quickly than any positive power of $t \to \infty$).

(viii) $\lim\limits_{t \to \infty} \ln t = \infty, \quad \lim\limits_{t \to 0} \ln t = -\infty$

(ix) $\lim\limits_{t \to 0} t^r \ln t = 0 \quad (r > 0)$

(i.e. $t^r \to 0$ more quickly than $\ln t \to -\infty$)

5.9 Limits of rational functions

Two important limit problems are

$$\lim_{x \to 0} \frac{a_n x^n + a_{n-1} x^{n-1} + a_{n-2} x^{n-2} + \ldots + a_0}{b_m x^m + b_{m-1} x^{m-1} + \ldots + b_0}$$

and $\quad \lim\limits_{x \to \infty} \dfrac{a_n x^n + a_{n-1} x^{n-1} + a_{n-2} x^{n-2} + \ldots + a_0}{b_m x^m + b_{m-1} x^{m-1} + \ldots + b_0}$

i.e. the limits of a rational function of x.

5.9.1 $x \to 0$

As long as $b_0 \neq 0$, this case is covered by result (iii) of Section 5.6.1, on the limit of the quotients of two functions. This gives us

$$\lim_{x \to 0} \frac{a_n x^n + a_{n-1} x^{n-1} + a_{n-2} x^{n-2} + \ldots + a_0}{b_m x^m + b_{m-1} x^{m-1} + b_{m-2} x^{m-2} + \ldots + b_0} = \frac{a_0}{b_0} \quad \text{if} \quad b_0 \neq 0$$

If $b_0 = 0$, and $a_0 \neq 0$, the limit is ∞; if both a_0 and $b_0 = 0$, the limit is a_1/b_1 unless $b_1 = 0$. This arises from the consideration that if $a_0 = b_0 = 0$, then the function is

$$\frac{a_n x^n + a_{n-1} x^{n-1} + a_{n-2} x^{n-2} + \ldots + a_1 x}{b_m x^m + b_{m-1} x^{m-1} + b_{m-2} x^{m-2} + \ldots + b_1 x}$$

$$= \frac{x}{x} * \frac{a_n x^{n-1} + a_{n-1} x^{n-2} + \ldots + a_1}{b_m x^{m-1} + b_{m-1} x^{m-2} + \ldots + b_1}$$

and in this, $\lim_{x \to 0} (x/x) = 1$† while the limit of the rational fraction part $= a_1/b_1$.
Analogous results hold if e.g. $a_0 = a_1 = b_0 = b_1 = 0$.

5.9.2 $x \to \infty$

With $x \to 0$, the behaviour of our rational function depended on the absolute terms a_0 and b_0 or at least on the coefficients of the lowest powers of x in numerator and denominator. With $x \to \infty$, it is the coefficients of the *highest* powers of x which are of importance. We write the function as

$$y(x) = \frac{x^n \left[a_n + \dfrac{a_{n-1}}{x} + \dfrac{a_{n-2}}{x^2} + \ldots + \dfrac{a_0}{x^n} \right]}{x^m \left[b_m + \dfrac{b_{m-1}}{x} + \dfrac{b_{m-2}}{x^2} + \ldots + \dfrac{b_0}{x^m} \right]}$$

The limits of the expressions in the brackets, as $x \to \infty$, are a_n and b_m respectively. (We can assume that neither of these are zero—if they are, it simply means that different powers of x will appear outside the brackets.) The limit is thus determined entirely by the behaviour of x^n/x^m.
There are various cases:

If $n > m$, $\displaystyle \lim_{x \to \infty} y(x) = \lim_{x \to \infty} x^{n-m} \frac{a_n}{b_m} = \begin{cases} \infty & \text{if } \dfrac{a_n}{b_m} > 0 \\[2ex] -\infty & \text{if } \dfrac{a_n}{b_m} < 0 \end{cases}$

---

† Since $x/x = 1$ for any non-zero value of x, no matter how small.

If $n=m$, $\lim\limits_{x\to\infty} y(x)=\dfrac{a_n}{b_m}$

If $n<m$, $\lim\limits_{x\to\infty} y(x)= \lim\limits_{x\to\infty} x^{n-m}\dfrac{a_n}{b_m}=0$

Examples:

(i) $\lim\limits_{x\to\infty}\dfrac{x+a}{x+b}=1$

(ii) $\lim\limits_{x\to 0}\dfrac{x+a}{2x^3-x+b}=\dfrac{a}{b}$

(iii) $\lim\limits_{x\to 0}\dfrac{x^3-7x+3}{x^3+4x+1}=3$

(iv) $\lim\limits_{x\to\infty}\dfrac{12x^4-7}{3x^4-4x^2+2x-1}=4$

(v) $\lim\limits_{x\to\infty}\dfrac{x^3-3x^2+7}{x^4-2x^3+5x-9}=0$

5.10   Continuous functions

Consider the following graphs regarded as graphs of functions:

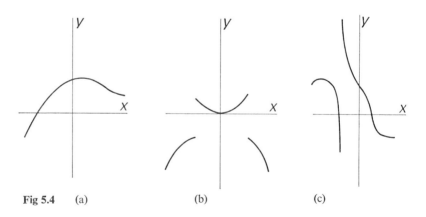

Fig 5.4   (a)   (b)   (c)

The first one (Fig 5.4a) differs from the other two in that there are no breaks in it; as the independent variable undergoes a steady change, so the dependent variable does also. In the other graphs, there are abrupt changes in the dependent variable at certain values of the independent one.

Purely descriptively, the first curve is *continuous*, in the dictionary† sense of the word: 'joined together without interruption', while the others are *discontinuous*.

It is mathematically convenient to distinguish between those functions whose graphs are continuous in the above sense, and those whose are not. This is because functions with continuous graphs, or *continuous functions*, as they are known, have certain very useful properties. For example, if f(x) is a continuous function, and f(a) is positive while f(b) is negative, then at least one solution of

$$f(x) = 0$$

lies between a and b, i.e. f(x) has a *root* (Section 3.14) between a and b. (Strictly speaking, f(x) must have an odd number of roots between a and b.) This kind of result is made great use of in solving equations involving continuous functions.

However, before we can make use of these properties, we must have a more precise definition of continuity, so that we can be sure of being able to recognize a continuous function without being dependent on drawing its graph—which in practice will be an interpolation through a finite number of plotted points, and which could be wrong (cf. Section 3.7).

5.11   Mathematical definition of continuity

5.11.1   *Continuity at a point*

The essential feature of a continuous graph is that any point on it can be reached from any other point on it by moving along the graph. This is not true of a discontinuous graph:

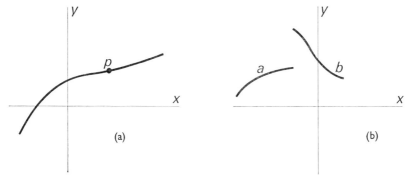

(a)   (b)

Fig 5.5   (a) A continuous graph. Any point *p* can be reached from any other point by moving along the graph. (b) A discontinuous graph. We cannot get to points on *b* by moving along *a*.

† Chambers's 20th Century Dictionary.

In other words, we can get as close as we please to any point on a continuous curve, from either side, and finally arrive there. In terms of the function represented by the graph, if this is $y=y(x)$, then we can get as close as we please to y_0 corresponding to x_0 by allowing x to take values closer and closer to x_0, and furthermore, if x actually $=x_0$, then $y_0=y(x_0)$, i.e. the value of y at x_0 equals the result of substituting x_0 for x in the mathematical definition of $y(x)$. In case this seems obvious from the definition of a function, consider again

$$y(x)=\frac{\ln x}{2*(x-1)}$$

for which the value of y at $x=1$ is *not* obtainable by simply substituting $x=1$ in

$$\frac{\ln x}{2*(x-1)}.$$

We see that in terms of the ideas used in developing the concept of a limit, we are saying that a continuous function $y(x)$ is one for which

$$\lim_{x\to x_0} y(x)=y(x_0)$$

This is actually the mathematical definition of *continuity at a point*—in this case the point $x=x_0$. We really need the idea of continuity over a range of values for practical use of the idea. But first, some examples.

(i) $\dfrac{1}{x+3}$ is continuous at e.g. $x=5$, at $x=0$, and everywhere except at
$x=-3$. This is for two reasons: (a) ∞ is *not* a value, and (b)
$\dfrac{1}{x+3}\to-\infty$ from below $x=-3$ and to $+\infty$ from above $x=-3$
(Fig 5.6).

The first reason, (a), illustrates the point that anywhere that a function becomes infinite is regarded as a *discontinuity*, i.e. a point where the function is not continuous.

(ii) The function in Fig 5.2 has discontinuities at $t=0, 1, 2, 3, 4, \ldots$

(iii) $\dfrac{x^2}{x^2-3}$ is continuous at $x=0$ and discontinuous at $x=\pm\sqrt{3}$.

It is the case that true discontinuities do not occur in Nature—they would imply instantaneous changes, which do not happen. But changes often do happen extremely rapidly, either in distance or in time, and it is often quite an acceptable approximation to regard such changes as discontinuities.

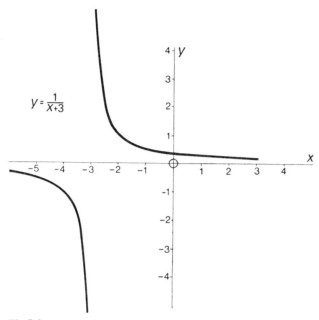

$y = \frac{1}{x+3}$

Fig 5.6

5.11.2   *Continuity over an interval*

To enlarge our idea of continuity, it is convenient to introduce the idea of an *interval*.

An interval is the set of all possible values between given limits or end-points. There are various kinds of interval, depending on whether the end-points are to be included or not:

(1)   The set of values of x such that $a \leqslant x \leqslant b$ is called the *closed* interval a, b and is written $[a, b]$.

(2)   The set of values of x such that $a < x < b$ is called the *open* interval a, b and is written (a, b).

(3)   The set of values of x such that $a < x \leqslant b$ is called the *semi-open* interval a, b and is written $(a, b]$. The set $a \leqslant x < b$, written $[a, b)$, is also a semi-open interval.

The words 'open' and 'closed' simply refer to the exclusion or inclusion of end points in the interval. The distinction is quite often an important one, mathematically.

We can now extend our definition of continuity quite simply by saying that a function continuous at all points of an interval is said to be continuous over the interval. A function continuous for all and any values of the independent variable is said to be *continuous everywhere*.

Examples of continuous functions:

(In these examples x is a variable, a is a constant.)

(1) All polynomials (Chapter 3) are continuous everywhere. So, e.g.
$$\lim_{x \to a} (4x^3 - 7x^2 + 2x - 1) = 4a^3 - 7a^2 + 2a - 1$$

(2) $\sqrt{x}$ is continuous for positive or zero x; it is not defined for $x < 0$.

(3) x^a is continuous where it is defined ($\sqrt{x}$ is a special case of this).

(4) a^x is continuous everywhere for $a > 0$.

(5) $\log_a x$ is continuous except at $x = 0$; it is not defined for $x < 0$.

5.12   'Continuous' functions in which $\lim_{x \to a} y(x) \neq y(a)$

As we have previously seen, it sometimes happens that a function is not defined by its mathematical expression at a particular point, and therefore on our previous definition would be regarded as discontinuous at that point. However, it is sometimes possible to use the limit of the function at the point, if it exists, to define the function there so as to satisfy the conditions of continuity.

This is done as follows. Suppose $f(x)$ is not defined for $x = a$, say, but that $\lim_{x \to a} f(x) = l$. Then we *define* the value of $f(x)$ at $x = a$ as l, i.e. we *define*: $f(a) = l$. This then makes the function continuous at $x = a$.

For example, we have seen that

$$\frac{\ln x}{2 * (x - 1)}$$

is not defined at $x = 1$, but

$$\lim_{x \to 1} \frac{\ln x}{2 * (x - 1)} = \tfrac{1}{2};$$

we therefore *define* the value of

$$\frac{\ln x}{2 * (x - 1)}$$

at $x = 1$ as being $\tfrac{1}{2}$, which makes the function continuous there.

The point may seem a little hair-splitting, but the benefits of continuity make it worth-while trying to get rid of points of non-definition or discontinuity if possible.

5.13   Discontinuities in rational functions

If a rational function takes the form $0/0$ for $x=a$, say, it can be shown that $(x-a)$ divides both the numerator and the denominator without remainder.

To avoid the discontinuity, the procedure is to cancel the common factor and then take the limit. (The situation is actually rather more subtle than this rule indicates, but the result is the same in the end.)

Example:

$$f(x) = \frac{x^2+4x+3}{x^2+3x+2}$$

then at $x = -1$,

$$f(x) \text{ takes the form } \frac{0}{0}$$

This means $(x+1)$ is a factor of numerator and denominator, and indeed it is:

$$f(x) = \frac{(x+3)(x+1)}{(x+2)(x+1)}$$

If we cancel $(x+1)$ above and below, we get:

$$f(x) = \frac{(x+3)}{(x+2)}$$

and $\qquad \lim\limits_{x \to -1} \dfrac{x+3}{x+2} = \dfrac{-1+3}{-1+2} = 2.$

With this value for $f(-1)$, $f(x)$ becomes continuous at $x = -1$.

5.14   The definition of e; the exponential function

The number $e = 2 \cdot 71828 \ldots$, which has occurred several times already, is an important mathematical constant. It arises in many branches of pure and applied mathematics, because of its various properties. In particular, it arises naturally when we try to find the *differential coefficient* (Chapter 9) of $\log_a x$

(*a* being any base), and it is frequently used in the mathematical description of growth and decay processes (see e.g. Chapter 12).

Its definition is at first sight a rather bizarre one:

$$e = \lim_{n \to \infty} \left(1 + \frac{1}{n}\right)^n \qquad (5.4)$$

The fact that this tends to a limit at all is not a straightforward matter, and to the novice, the idea that this limit is not 1 but $2 \cdot 71828 \ldots$ is often incomprehensible. Since

$$\lim_{n \to \infty} \frac{1}{n} = 0$$

he argues, and $1^n = 1$ for any n, surely the limit as $n \to \infty$ of

$$\left(1 + \frac{1}{n}\right)^n$$

must be 1? The reply to this is simply that as with so many limit problems, the answer is not as obvious as it looks. Careful mathematical analysis shows, in fact, that the limit must lie between 2 and 3, and calculation shows it to be the value given.

From the definition, a useful property of e can be deduced. This is that

$$e^x = \lim_{n \to \infty} \left(1 + \frac{x}{n}\right)^n \qquad (5.5)$$

e^x is called the *exponential function*, and written: exp (x). This notation is common in formulae, especially where (x) is in fact a complicated expression. It is also easier for the printer.

5.14.1   Alternative expressions for e and e^x

The functions

$$\left(1 + \frac{1}{n}\right)^n$$

and

$$\left(1 + \frac{x}{n}\right)^n$$

which occur in the definitions of e and e^x can be expanded by the Binomial Theorem (Section 4.2). We have:

$$\left(1+\frac{1}{n}\right)^n = 1+n*\frac{1}{n}+\frac{n(n-1)}{2!}*\left(\frac{1}{n}\right)^2+\frac{n(n-1)(n-2)}{3!}*\left(\frac{1}{n}\right)^3+..+\left(\frac{1}{n}\right)^n$$

$$\left(1+\frac{x}{n}\right)^n = 1+n*\frac{x}{n}+\frac{n(n-1)}{2!}*\left(\frac{x}{n}\right)^2+\frac{n(n-1)(n-2)}{3!}*\left(\frac{x}{n}\right)^3+..+\left(\frac{x}{n}\right)^n$$

$$(5.6)$$

It can be shown by careful analysis of limits that as $n \to \infty$, the expressions (5.6) tend to the *infinite series*

$$e = \lim_{n \to \infty}\left(1+\frac{1}{n}\right)^n = 1+1+\frac{1}{2!}+\frac{1}{3!}+\frac{1}{4!}+\dots \textit{ ad infinitum}$$

$$= 2\cdot71828\dots \tag{5.7a}$$

$$e^x = \lim_{n \to \infty}\left(1+\frac{x}{n}\right)^n = 1+x+\frac{x^2}{2!}+\frac{x^3}{3!}+\frac{x^2}{4!}+\dots \textit{ ad infinitum} \tag{5.7b}$$

As before we ask the reader to accept that infinite series such as these can have finite sums; this topic is considered in Chapter 10.

5.15   Examples from the medical literature

As a further illustration of points arising in limiting processes we consider two examples from recent medical literature. The first is from a paper by Ekins, Newman & O'Riordan (1968) on immuno-assay methods.

It concerns the values of $K*q$ given by

$$\epsilon^2 SVT * \left(q-\frac{1}{K}\right)^2 + 2*\left(q-\frac{1}{K}\right) - \frac{4}{K} = 0, \tag{5.8}$$

in particular, the value of $K*q$ as $\epsilon \to 0$.

Now, it is very tempting to say that since

$$\lim_{\varepsilon \to 0}\left[\epsilon^2 SVT * \left(q-\frac{1}{K}\right)^2 + 2*\left(q-\frac{1}{K}\right) - \frac{4}{K}\right]$$

is

$$2*\left(q-\frac{1}{K}\right)-\frac{4}{K}$$

therefore the value of $K \ast q$ from (5.8) for $\epsilon \to 0$ is given by

$$2 \ast \left(q - \frac{1}{K}\right) - \frac{4}{K} = 0 \qquad (5.9)$$

i.e. $K \ast q - 1 - 2 = 0$ (multiplying the equation (5.9) across by $K/2$)

i.e. $K \ast q = 3$

This is indeed the correct answer *in the physical context of the problem*—but an important point is missed by deriving it in this way.

The point is that (5.8) is in fact a quadratic equation, with two roots. When $\epsilon \to 0$ our procedure above leaves us with a single root. What has happened to the other root?

Let us discuss the matter in terms of the general quadratic

$$ax^2 + bx + c = 0 \qquad (5.10)$$

If the coefficient a becomes zero, we have apparently

$$bx + c = 0$$

i.e. $x = \dfrac{-c}{b}$

—this corresponds to our result $K \ast q = 3$.

But let us use a mathematical trick to isolate the behaviour of a. Write

$$y = \frac{1}{x}$$

Substituting in (5.10) we have

$$\frac{a}{y^2} + \frac{b}{y} + c = 0,$$

i.e. $cy^2 + by + a = 0$

If $a = 0$, the roots of this are given by

$$cy^2 + by = 0$$

i.e. $y \ast (cy + b) - 0$

i.e. $y = 0$ or $y = -b/c$

If $y = -b/c$, $x = 1/y = -c/b$, the root we already have. But if $y = 0$, $x = 1/y$ becomes infinite. Hence the result of $a \to 0$ in (5.10) is that one root $\to -c/b$ *and one root* $\to \infty$ (or to $-\infty$, depending on the sign of b and the direction from which $a \to 0$).

Physically speaking, an infinite root sounds nonsensical and ignorable. In the context of the problem being considered by Ekins, Newman and O'Riordan it is. But it may not always be so; an infinite root (or a root tending to infinity, to be precise) could mean a breakdown of some kind in the conditions of the system being observed, and should in general not be ignored. In terms of the equation

$$ax^2 + bx + c = 0$$

it is the root

$$\frac{-b + \sqrt{(b^2 - 4ac)}}{2a} \quad \text{which} \quad \to -\frac{c}{b} \quad \text{as} \quad a \to 0$$

and the root

$$\frac{-b - \sqrt{(b^2 - 4ac)}}{2a} \quad \text{which} \quad \to \pm \infty \quad \text{as} \quad a \to 0$$

The second example is one of a number which arose in an investigation by Samuel *et al* (1968) into the effect of neomycin on exchangeable pools of cholesterol. They are more complex than those we have dealt with so far in that they are *double limit* problems; there are two variables both simultaneously tending to limiting values.

Double limit problems need to be handled with care; if we have a function of two variables

say, $f(x, y)$

it is *not* always the case by any means that

$$\lim_{x \to a} \left[\lim_{y \to b} f(x, y) \right] = \lim_{y \to b} \left[\lim_{x \to a} f(x, y) \right]$$

Frequently, the order in which the limits are taken is important, and it may well be that the final results are different. As a simple example, consider

$$f(x, y) = \frac{x^2}{x^2 + y^2}$$

$$\lim_{y \to 0} \left[\lim_{x \to 0} f(x, y) \right] = \lim_{y \to 0} \frac{0}{y^2} = 0\dagger$$

but $$\lim_{x \to 0} \left[\lim_{y \to 0} f(x, y) \right] = \lim_{x \to 0} \frac{x^2}{x^2} = 1 \quad \text{(cf. Section 5.9.1)}$$

---

† Because no matter how small y becomes, $0/y^2$ is always zero. Hence $\lim_{y \to 0} 0/y^2 = 0$.

And if y and x tend to zero simultaneously, say in such a way that $y = \alpha * x$, $x \to 0$, the result will be different again:

$$\lim_{\substack{x \to 0 \\ y = \alpha x}} \left[\frac{x^2}{x^2 + y^2} \right] = \lim_{x \to 0} \left[\frac{x^2}{x^2(1 + \alpha)} \right] = \frac{1}{1 + \alpha}$$

The brackets are often dropped, and we write, e.g. $\lim_{x \to 0} \lim_{y \to 0} f(x, y)$ meaning that $\lim_{y \to 0}$ is taken first and $\lim_{x \to 0}$ on the result. Where the order or way in which the limits are taken does not matter, we write, e.g. $\lim_{\substack{x \to 0 \\ y \to 0}} f(x, y)$.

In the particular example we are about to discuss, the variables tend independently to their limits, and as it happens the order of the limits does not matter. But it is as well to be aware of the fact that it *can* matter, and there are techniques for deciding whether a given function is sensitive to limit order or not.

The system considered by Samuel *et al.* was:

$$b = [(\xi - \eta) - \beta * (1 - \xi \eta)]/(1 + \eta) \tag{5.11}$$

$$c = -\beta \xi \tag{5.12}$$

and the root

$$u = \frac{-b + \sqrt{(b^2 - 4c)}}{2} \tag{5.13}$$

of the equation

$$u^2 + bu + c = 0$$

The variables are ξ and η, β being a constant, and the question at issue is the limiting value of u as ξ and $\eta \to 0$ simultaneously.

Now

$$\lim_{\xi \to 0} u = \lim_{\xi \to 0} \left[\frac{-b + \sqrt{(b^2 - 4c)}}{2} \right]$$

$$= \lim_{\xi \to 0} \left(\frac{-b}{2} \right) + \lim_{\xi \to 0} \left[\frac{\sqrt{(b^2 - 4c)}}{2} \right]$$

$$= \lim \left(\frac{-b}{2} \right) + \frac{\sqrt{\left[\lim_{\xi \to 0} (b^2 - 4c) \right]}}{2}$$

i.e.
$$\lim_{\xi \to 0} u = \lim_{\xi \to 0} \frac{-b}{2} + \sqrt{\frac{\left[\lim_{\xi \to 0} b^2 - \lim_{\xi \to 0} 4c\right]}{2}} \qquad (5.14)$$

—provided that the conditions laid down in Sections 5.6.1 and 5.6.2 for evaluating limits of sums, products, etc., are not violated. As it happens, they are not.

Now
$$\lim_{\xi \to 0} b = \lim_{\xi \to 0} [(\xi - \eta) - \beta * (1 - \xi\eta)]/(1 + \eta)$$

$$= \frac{-\eta - \beta}{1 + \eta}$$

$$\lim_{\xi \to 0} c = \lim_{\xi \to 0} (-\beta\xi)$$

$$= 0$$

Whence, from (5.14),
$$\lim_{\xi \to 0} u = -\tfrac{1}{2}\left(\frac{-\eta - \beta}{1 + \eta}\right) + \tfrac{1}{2}\sqrt{\left[\left(\frac{-\eta - \beta}{1 + \eta}\right)^2\right]}$$

$$= -\tfrac{1}{2}\left(\frac{-\eta - \beta}{1 + \eta}\right) + \tfrac{1}{2}\left(\frac{\eta + \beta}{1 + \eta}\right)$$

$$= \frac{\eta + \beta}{1 + \eta} \qquad (5.15)$$

Therefore
$$\lim_{\eta \to 0}\lim_{\xi \to 0} u = \lim_{\eta \to 0}\left(\frac{\eta + \beta}{1 + \eta}\right)$$

$$= \beta \qquad (5.16)$$

It is instructive to see what happens if we reverse the order of taking limits.

From (5.11)
$$\lim_{\eta \to 0} b = \lim_{\eta \to 0} [(\xi - \eta) - \beta * (1 - \xi\eta)]/(1 + \eta)$$

$$= \xi - \beta$$

and since from (5.12) we see that c is unaffected by changes in η, we have from (5.13)

$$\lim_{\eta \to 0} u = \frac{-(\xi - \beta) + \sqrt{[(\xi - \beta)^2 + 4\beta\xi]}}{2} \tag{5.17}$$

Whence

$$\lim_{\xi \to 0} \lim_{\eta \to 0} u = \lim_{\xi \to 0} \frac{-(\xi - \beta) + \sqrt{[(\xi - \beta)^2 + 4\beta\xi]}}{2}$$

$$= \frac{\beta + \sqrt{[(-\beta)^2]}}{2}$$

$$= \beta \tag{5.18}$$

Comparing this with the result (5.16), we see that in this instance, as ξ and $\eta \to 0$, the order of taking limits is immaterial.

Chapter 6
The Functions of Trigonometry

6.1   Introduction

The reader will certainly have been introduced to trigonometry at school. Unfortunately, however, orthodox school teaching of this subject tends to be dominated by its historical background, which is rooted in geodesey and surveying, and the reader might well ask why space should be devoted to trigonometry in a text-book concerned with medical applications of mathematics.

There are two main reasons for doing so. In the first place, trigonometric situations do arise in medical work—for example in radiotherapy, cardiology and physiology. Secondly, the oscillatory nature of the simpler trigonometric functions and their functional interrelationships make them useful tools in the study of oscillatory systems. The *sine* and *cosine* functions (q.v.) are the simplest and most elementary oscillatory solutions which can arise in the solution of *differential equations* (Chapter 12) and because of this they are of great importance in electronics, and arise also in epidemiological work and in genetics.

These two different aspects—the geometrical and the functional—both deal with quantities which in one way or another can be regarded as *angles*, though often in a purely abstract way. We deal first, therefore, with angular measurement.

6.2   Measurement of angles

There are two systems of angular measurement in use. The first is the well-known one in which the unit of angle is the *degree* (°), defined as 1/360th part of a full revolution. There is also *radian measure* (sometimes known as *circular measure*) in which the unit of angle is the *radian*, defined as *the angle subtended at the centre of a circle by an arc equal in length to the radius of the circle* (Fig. 6.1).

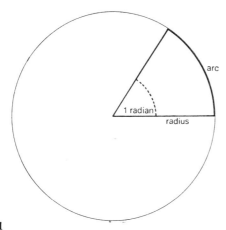

Fig 6.1

It can be shown that the angle so defined is independent of the size of circle used; in other words, if we have two concentric circles, centre O, then (Fig 6.2) if the angle is 1 radian, the arc AB=the radius OA of the smaller circle, and the arc $A'B'$=the radius OA' of the larger circle.

Conversely for any circle centre O, an arc equal to the radius will subtend an angle of 1 radian at the centre. It can also be shown that the radian measure of the angle subtended at the centre of a circle by any arc is

$$\frac{\text{length of the arc}}{\text{radius of the circle}} \quad \text{(See Fig. 6.3)}.$$

As with the radian itself, the radian measure of an angle is independent of the size of the circle used. Hence radian measure is a consistent system of angular measurement, and the number of radians in a given angle depends only on the angle itself.

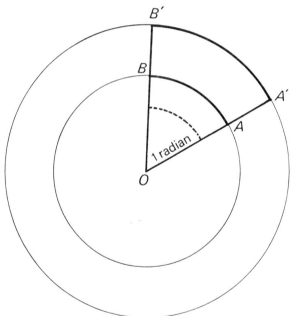

Fig 6.2

Due to the purely geometrical way in which radian measure is defined, and its lack of dependence on arbitrary numerical quantities—such as the constant 360 which lies at the base of the degree system—radian measure has some properties which are extremely useful in mathematical manipulation, though all expressions involving radians can be expressed in equivalent forms with measurements given in degrees.

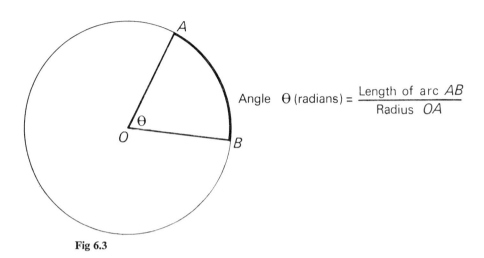

$$\text{Angle} \quad \Theta \text{ (radians)} = \frac{\text{Length of arc } AB}{\text{Radius } OA}$$

Fig 6.3

There is not an exact number of radians in a full revolution; a full revolution $= 2\pi$ radians, where π is the familiar constant $3 \cdot 14159 \ldots$ Since 2π radians and $360°$ represent the same angle, we have:

$$1° = \frac{2\pi}{360} \text{ radians} = 0 \cdot 017 \text{ radians}$$

$$1 \text{ radian} = \left(\frac{360}{2\pi}\right) \text{ degrees} = 57 \cdot 296°$$

$\left.\right\}$ approximately

Radian measure is sometimes indicated by r or superscript c, viz: 1r or 1^c, but it is usual to write the radian measure of an angle without any indication, the convention being that angles so written are being measured in radians. Thus if the three angles of a triangle are indicated by α, β, and γ respectively, then the well-known proposition that the three angles of a triangle add up to two right angles ($= 180°$) would be stated as

$$\alpha + \beta + \gamma = \pi$$

in radian terms. (A right angle is $90°$ or $\pi/2$ radians; a full revolution is 4 right angles.)

Degrees are subdivided into *minutes* and *seconds*. One minute $= 1/60$th of a degree, and is written as $1'$, and one second $= 1/60$th of a minute, and is written

F

as 1″. Radians have no subunits, fractions of a radian being written as decimals or fractions. Equivalents are:

$$1' = 0\cdot0003 \text{ radians}$$
$$1'' = 0\cdot000005 \text{ radians}$$
approximately.

6.3   Signed magnitudes

Before we can define the trigonometric functions we need some definitions and conventions.

6.3.1   Sign of an angle

We regard an angle as being generated by the rotation of a line about its point of intersection with a fixed line. Now any given position of the moving line can be reached by rotations in different directions and of different amounts:

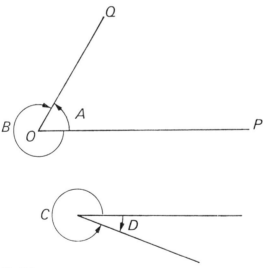

Fig 6.4

These fall into two classes; the *clockwise* rotations (e.g. through angles *B*, *D*, in Fig 6.4) and the *anticlockwise* rotations (e.g. through angles *A*, *C*). It may not be enough therefore, to say that the moving line has a particular position relative to the fixed line; we may need to know what movement brought it to the given position. The convention is that *clockwise rotations are negative, anticlockwise rotations are positive.* For example, if in Fig 6.4 we rotate the moving line from OP to OQ, this can be achieved in two ways: either through the angle A—which is positive, say $+75°$—or through the angle B, which is negative, and which will have the value $-285°$ if A is $+75°$. (The values of the angles A and B are related by the fact that their absolute values (i.e. values without signs) add up to a complete revolution: $75° + 285° = 360°$.) Thus we can regard the angle POQ as either $+75°$ or $-285°$. We see also that angles which differ by a multiple of $\pm 360°$ ($= \pm 2\pi$ radians) are geometrically equivalent, and so normally refer to an angle by those positive or negative values less than $360°$ in magnitude, with a slight preference in practice for positive values. (We would therefore refer to an angle as, e.g. $192°$ rather than as $-168°$.)

It is unfortunate that clockwise motion, which is regarded as positive in so many physical applications, should have a negative sign attached to it in this mathematical one. However, the conventions are now set and one has simply to make the best of the situation.

6.3.2 Projections

Consider two lines, AB and CD, say; and let AA' be the perpendicular from A to CD, BB' the perpendicular from B to CD (i.e. the angle between BB' and CD is a right angle, as is that between AA' and CD).

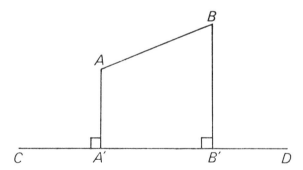

Fig 6.5   (a) (N.B. In this and other diagrams, ⌐ indicates a right angle).

Then $A'B'$ is called the *projection* of AB on CD. Note that one cannot reverse this; AB is not the projection of $A'B'$ on AB, in general, since AA' and BB' will not usually be perpendicular to both AB and CD at the same time—this will only happen if AB and CD are parallel. Note also that we may need to lengthen CD (Fig 6.5b).

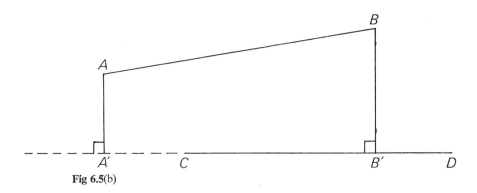

Fig 6.5(b)

From the definition above, we see that if two lines OA and OB intersect at O, the projection of OA on OB is OA', where AA' is perpendicular to OB:

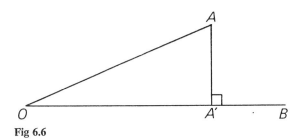

Fig 6.6

Now consider again the rotation of a line about its point of intersection with a fixed reference line, but this time let us take the moving line to be of some fixed length. Such a rotating line is called a *radius vector*.

With each position of the rotating line, there will be associated a projection on the fixed line:

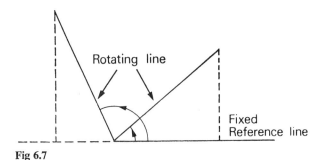

Fig 6.7

However, a projection of any given size will have *four* possible positions of the radius vector associated with it.

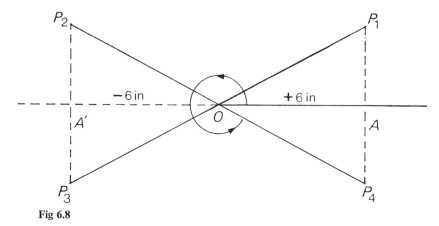

Fig 6.8

These are divided into two pairs by the convention that projections which fall to the right of the centre of rotation are said to be *positive*, and those which fall to the left of the centre of rotation are called *negative*. Thus if OA and OA' (Fig 6.8) are each 6 in. in length, we say that OA is $+6$ in. and OA' is -6 in.

It is also found to be necessary to distinguish between directions *perpendicular* to the fixed reference line. The convention is that perpendiculars lying above the fixed reference line are called *positive* and those below are called *negative*. So in Fig 6.9 OM, PQ are positive while ON, RS are negative.

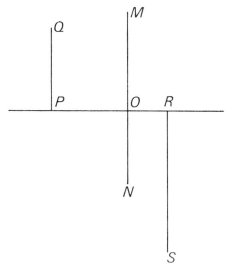

Fig 6.9

The radius vector is regarded as positive at all times, even when it coincides with a direction with negative sign.

A summary of the conventions listed in this and the previous section will be found in the Appendix, page 395. Note that the conventions are exactly the same as those for graphs (Chapter 2) and co-ordinate geometry (Chapter 8).

6.4   Trigonometric functions: geometrical definitions

The reader may well be used to the definitions of the trigonometric functions in terms of right-angled triangles (e.g. 'sine = opposite/hypotenuse'), with extensions to angles greater than 90°. In order to emphasize that these functions are defined basically for all angles, and not just those possible in triangles, we will deliberately avoid this approach in favour of definitions based on signed projections and perpendiculars as defined in Section 6.3. The emphasis is thus placed where it belongs, i.e. on the angle, and not on some triangle in which it happens to find itself.

Consider an angle X:

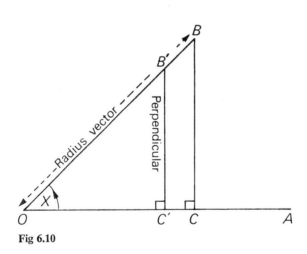

Fig 6.10

Let us regard OA as the fixed line, and OB as the radius vector. If we take any other point B' on OB, and drop perpendiculars BC, $B'C'$ onto OA then the triangles OBC, $OB'C'$ will be *similar*, i.e. they will have the same angles, and corresponding sides will be in proportion.

Now OC is the projection of OB on OA, and OC' that of OB' on OA. The geometrical properties of similar triangles tell us that

$$\frac{BC}{OB}=\frac{B'C'}{OB'}$$ (6.1)

(allowing in this for the signs of projections and perpendiculars). This is true no matter where we take the point B' (and this determines C'). The only circumstance which will alter the value of the ratios in (6.1) is if the angle X should change. In other words, the ratio

$$\frac{\text{(signed) length of the perpendicular to } OA \text{ from any point on } OB}{\text{length of the radius vector from } O \text{ to that point}}$$

(6.2)

is a constant for a given angle. It is known as the *sine* of the angle X. Note that since the position of the radius vector can be reached by rotation from coincidence with OA *negatively* through an angle $-(360°-X)$, it follows that (6.2) can be regarded also as the sine of the angle $-(360°-X$ or of $-(2\pi-X)$ if we measure X in radians.

Keeping Fig 6.10 in mind, the definition of sine is usually abbreviated to

$$\text{Sine}=\frac{\text{perpendicular}}{\text{radius vector}}.$$ (6.3)

Because it depends solely on the angle, the sine is a function of the angle to which it refers, and we denote this by writing—e.g. in the present case—sin (X). In practice an abbreviation of this is used, and the brackets are dropped if ambiguity is not introduced as a result; we write: sin X†. Note that we have no means yet of computing sin X, given X; we are restricted entirely to geometrical constructions for the moment.

The value and definition of sin X is unchanged if we take the perpendicular from a point on OB to OA as the radius vector (Fig 6.11—D is any point on OA, and OE is the projection of OD on OB.)

The geometry of the situation ensures that

$$\frac{B'C'}{OB'}=\frac{DE}{OD}$$

i.e. sin X still depends only on X.

Other ratios dependent only on X—i.e. other functions of X—can be defined for the situation shown in Fig 6.10. We give below (Table 6.1) a list of definitions,

† As with log x, we will make use of both notations in this book. This applies to all the trigonometric functions, not just to the sine function.

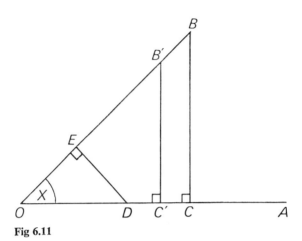

Fig 6.11

equivalents and abbreviations for the six trigonometric functions in common use:

Table 6.1   The functions of trigonometry

Function	Definition	Equivalents		Abbreviations
sine	$\dfrac{\text{perpendicular}}{\text{radius vector}}$	—		sin
cosine	$\dfrac{\text{projection}}{\text{radius vector}}$	—		cos
tangent	$\dfrac{\text{perpendicular}}{\text{projection}}$	$\dfrac{\text{sine}}{\text{cosine}}$		tan
cotangent	$\dfrac{\text{projection}}{\text{perpendicular}}$	$\dfrac{1}{\text{tangent}}$,	$\dfrac{\text{cosine}}{\text{sine}}$	cot
secant	$\dfrac{\text{radius vector}}{\text{projection}}$	$\dfrac{1}{\text{cosine}}$		sec
cosecant	$\dfrac{\text{radius vector}}{\text{perpendicular}}$	$\dfrac{1}{\text{sine}}$		cosec, csc

Note that the last four functions can be defined in terms of sine and cosine, which are the really fundamental entities.

The theorem of Pythagoras, i.e.

$$(\text{projection})^2 + (\text{perpendicular})^2 = (\text{radius vector})^2$$

is often of use in computing the ratios and in deriving inter-relationships.

Equivalent forms of this, e.g.

perpendicular $= \sqrt{\{(\text{radius vector})^2 - (\text{projection})^2\}}$
projection $= \sqrt{\{(\text{radius vector})^2 - (\text{perpendicular})^2\}}$

are also helpful.

Examples:

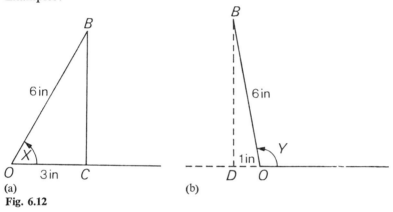

(a)   (b)

Fig. 6.12

Suppose that:

OB is of length 6 in.	(all figures)
OC ,, ,, ,, 3 in.	(Fig 6.12a)
OD ,, ,, ,, 1 in.	(Fig 6.12b)
OE ,, ,, ,, 2 in.	(Fig 6.12c)
OF ,, ,, ,, 5 in.	(Fig 6.12d)

Then allowing for the sign convention of Section 6.3, we have:

Fig 6.12a:

$$\sin X = \frac{BC}{OB} = \frac{\sqrt{(OB^2 - OC^2)}}{OB} \quad \text{(Pythagoras' theorem)}$$

$$= \frac{\sqrt{(36 - 9)}}{6} = \frac{\sqrt{3}}{2} = 0 \cdot 866 \ldots$$

Fig 6.12b:

$$\cos Y = \frac{OD}{OB} = \frac{-1}{6} = -0 \cdot 166 \ldots$$

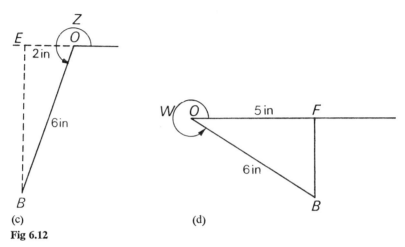

(c)   (d)

Fig 6.12

Fig 6.12c:

$$\tan Z = \frac{EB}{OE} = \frac{-\sqrt{(36-4)}}{-2} = \frac{\sqrt{32}}{2} = 2\cdot828\ldots$$

Fig 6.12d:

$$\cot W = \frac{OF}{FB} = \frac{5}{-\sqrt{(36-25)}} = -\frac{5}{\sqrt{11}} = -1\cdot508\ldots$$

We see that none of these are terminating decimals, and this is characteristic of the sines, cosines, etc., generally met with. We see also that some of the values

Second Quadrant		First Quadrant	
SIN	+	SIN	+
COS	−	COS	+
TAN	−	TAN	+
Third Quadrant		Fourth Quadrant	
SIN	−	SIN	−
COS	−	COS	+
TAN	+.	TAN	−

Fig 6.13

are positive and some, negative. The sign of the value of a trigonometric function depends on the quadrant (Chapter 2) in which lies the radius vector defining its angle. Figure 6.13 gives the signs of the sine, cosine and tangent functions for each quadrant (for convenience, this diagram is reproduced in the Appendix, page 396). Thus, for example, we would expect sin 141° to be positive, since the radius vector for 141° lies in the second quadrant:

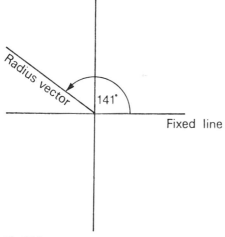

Fig 6.14

Similarly cos (−215°) is negative, since the radius vector for −215° also lies in the second quadrant:

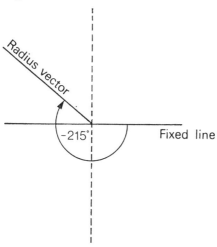

Fig 6.15

Because of their geometrical basis, the trigonometric functions are sometimes called the *trigonometric ratios*, but this is not common. They are also known as the *circular functions* because of their close connection with rotations and the geometry of the circle. We will see later (Section 6.7) that it is possible to compute the values of the trigonometric functions of any angle without recourse to drawing, and tables of these values have been in existence for a long time.

6.5

Our definitions, and trigonometric formulae in general, are independent of the system of measurement being used, and for instance in the sections which follow, the reader can assume that the angular units are immaterial unless there is a specific warning to the contrary. However, this independence cannot always be assumed—see for example Section 6.7 and also the differentiation formulae of Chapter 9—and one must always check that the formula or functional relationship being used is valid if specific units of measurement are involved.

There are one or two conventions in use with regard to units. Generally, radian measure is used when indicating fractions of a complete revolution or *period* (see Section 6.9) and also for mathematical theory, while the degree system is used for practical geometrical work and for calculations from tables. Note that computer sub-programs for calculating sines, cosines, etc., tend to require the angles to be given in radians, so that in situations where it is natural to the problem in hand to use the degree system, it is usually necessary to include a conversion from degrees to radians in the main program.

6.6   Projection and the trigonometric functions

In the previous section we have regarded radius vector, projection and perpendicular as the primary elements in determining the trigonometric functions. However, it very often happens that we know the angle—or a function of it— and one of the basic lengths, and from these, wish to deduce the value of one of the other lengths. The following formulae are useful in this connection—the angle is that formed by the projection and the radius vector.

$$\text{perpendicular} = \begin{cases} \text{radius vector} * \text{sine} \\ \text{projection} * \text{tangent} \\ \text{projection/cotangent} \\ \text{radius vector/cosecant} \end{cases}$$

$$\text{projection} = \begin{cases} \text{radius vector} * \text{cosine} \\ \text{perpendicular/tangent} \\ \text{perpendicular} * \text{cotangent} \\ \text{radius vector/secant} \end{cases}$$

$$\text{radius vector} = \begin{cases} \text{perpendicular/sine} \\ \text{projection/cosine} \\ \text{projection} * \text{secant} \\ \text{perpendicular} * \text{cosecant} \end{cases}$$

Example:

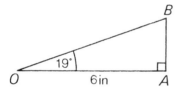

Fig 6.16

If $OA = 6$ in.,

we have:

OB (the radius vector) $= OA$ (the projection)$/\cos 19°$

$= 6$ in.$/0\cdot9455 = 6\cdot35$ in.

The connection between the trigonometric functions and the projections of a radius vector generalizes a little to a relation between any line segment and its projection on any other line, whether they intersect or not (Fig. 6.17).

It can be shown that in each of the diagrams in Fig 6.17,

$$CD = AB \cos \theta \quad \text{(i.e. } AB * \cos \theta) \tag{6.4}$$

In the case of the non-intersecting lines, the angle between them is taken to be that which would occur if the lines were produced until they did intersect.

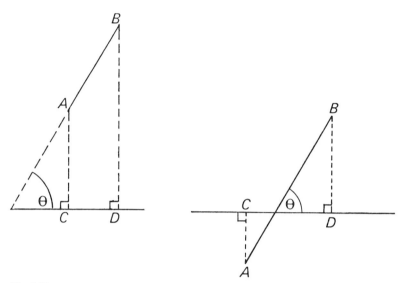

Fig 6.17

6.7   Functional definitions

So far, we have discussed the functions purely as geometrical ratios. On this basis, to find, e.g., cos X means drawing the angle X and measuring various lines. This is obviously a clumsy, inaccurate and impractical method for computing these functions.

However, mathematical investigation shows that when we try to define them purely in terms of a sequence of operations on their arguments, so that given X, we can compute sin X, etc., the result is that none of these functions can be defined by a finite sequence of such operations. So, for example, we cannot find constants a, b, c, d such that

$$\sin X = \frac{aX+b}{cX+d}$$

or $$\cos X = a + bX + cX^2 + dX^3$$

are true.

Sines, cosines, etc. can be *approximated* by expressions of this kind, but an unlimited number of terms is needed for an exact equivalent.

The formulae concerned are usually quoted for angles in *radians*. The two most important are:

$$\sin X = X - \frac{X^3}{3!} + \frac{X^5}{5!} - \frac{X^7}{7!} + \ldots \text{ad infinitum}$$

$$\cos X = 1 - \frac{X^2}{2!} + \frac{X^4}{4!} - \frac{X^6}{6!} + \ldots \text{ad infinitum}$$

Remember, *in these formulae X is assumed to be measured in radians.*

As we have said in earlier chapters, series of this kind are called *infinite series*, and they pose special problems of their own—indeed, the idea that an unlimited number of terms added and subtracted together can sometimes have a finite total is perhaps a surprising one. This topic is discussed in Chapter 10.

It is also possible to define the sine and cosine functions (and therefore all the other trigonometric functions) as the solutions of *differential equations* (Chapter 12), from which their properties and values can be obtained.

Mathematical formulations have been developed for all the trigonometric functions, and we ask the reader to accept that given any angle, the values of its sine, cosine, etc. can be computed to any desired degree of accuracy as mathematical functions, and without the need to resort to drawing diagrams. It is on these methods that the familiar tables of sines, cosines, etc. are based.

6.8   Trigonometric functions of related angles

Although the functions of any given angle have definite and unique values (except in certain special cases—see Section 6.9) it is not necessary to construct tables of them for all possible angles, but only for angles in the range 0°–90°, since it is possible to deduce relationships between the trigonometric functions of angles in this range and those outside it. For example, it can be shown that

$$\sin (180° + A°) = -\sin A°; \tag{6.5}$$

hence sin 217°, for instance, which $= \sin (180° + 37°)$,
must $= -\sin 37° = -0 \cdot 6018$.

Again

$$\cos (\pi - \alpha) = -\cos \alpha$$

so that e.g.

$$\cos (\pi - 0 \cdot 3) = -\cos (0 \cdot 3) = -0 \cdot 9553$$

In fact, since there are also connections between the functions of any angle A and the angle $90° - A$, a table of trigonometric functions really needs to cover only the range 0°–45°, and this is sometimes all that is given. However, for convenience, tables are normally constructed over the range 0°−90°.

A full table of equivalences similar to (6.5) is given in the Appendix (page 397).

6.9   Oscillation and periodicity

If we plot sin X and cos X against X, we obtain the well-known oscillatory curves: ·

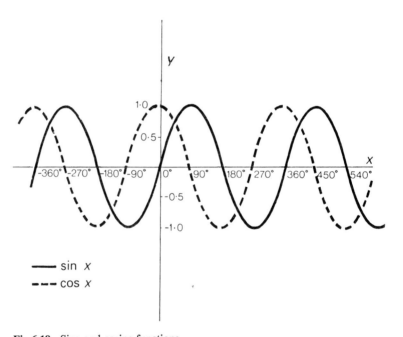

Fig 6.18   Sine and cosine functions.

The values of each curve repeat over an interval of 2π (or 360° if using degrees); e.g.

$$\sin X = \sin (X+2\pi) = \sin (X+4\pi) = \sin (X+6\pi) = \ldots = \sin (X+2n\pi)$$

where n is any positive integer. Similar results hold for sec X and cosec X. Tan X and cot X, however, repeat over an interval of π (180°). Note that sin X and cos X both lie in the range $[-1, 1]$.

A function $f(x)$ such that $f(x)=f(x+\omega)$ for any x, where ω is the smallest number giving $f(x)$ this property, is said to be *periodic* with period ω. Substituting the value of $x+\omega$ for x, we have

$$f(x+\omega)=f((x+\omega)+\omega)=f(x+2\omega)$$

and hence

$$f(x)=f(x+\omega)=f(x+2\omega)=f(x+3\omega)=\ldots=f(x\pm n\omega),$$

n a positive integer. It is usual to quote the period as *radians*.

The functions sin, cos, sec, and cosec are periodic with period 2π (360°), while tan and cot are periodic with period π (180°). But while sin and cos are *continuous* oscillatory functions, the other four trigonometric functions are neither continuous nor oscillatory—for example, tan x:

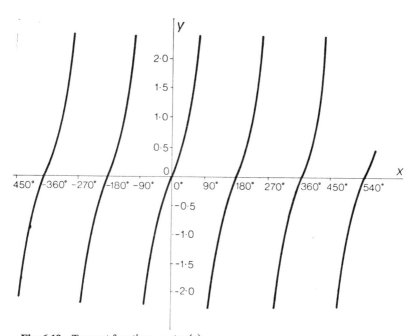

Fig. 6.19   Tangent function: $y=\tan(x)$.

Tan X and sec X are discontinuous at $X=\pm\pi/2,\ \pm3\pi/2,\ \pm5\pi/2\ldots$ etc. ($\pm90°$, $\pm270°$, $\pm450°$, $\ldots$ etc.) while cot X and cosec X are discontinuous at $X=0,\ \pm\pi,\ \pm2\pi,\ \pm3\pi,\ldots$ etc. ($0°$, $\pm180°$, $\pm360°$, $\pm540°$, $\ldots$ etc.).

Some further points concerning periodic functions are given in Section 6.17.

6.10   Special angles

From considerations of elementary geometry, it is possible to calculate the values of the trigonometric functions of certain angles without using infinite series or other functional methods. For example it can be shown that

$$\tan 45° = 1, \quad \sin \frac{\pi}{3} = \frac{\sqrt{3}}{2}, \quad \text{etc.}$$

A table of function values for the more important angles is given on page 398.

6.11   Functional relationships

From the definitions given in Table 6.1, and using Pythagoras' theorem (Section 6.4), it can be shown that for any angle, A, say:

$$\sin^2 A + \cos^2 A = 1 \tag{6.6}$$

$$\sec^2 A = 1 + \tan^2 A \tag{6.7}$$

$$\operatorname{cosec}^2 A = 1 + \cot^2 A \tag{6.8}$$

where $\sin^2 A$ *is the notation used for* $(\sin A) * (\sin A)$, *i.e.* $(\sin A)^2$, *and similarly for* $\sec^2 A$, $\tan^2 A$ *etc.*

Note that $\sin A^2$ will normally be taken to mean $\sin (A^2)$, so do not write this when really meaning $\sin^2 A$. A similar caveat applies to the other functions.

6.12   Limits of trigonometric functions

If we have a small angle, x say (measured in radians for this application), then we see that the projection approximates in length to the radius vector:

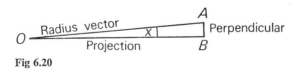

Fig 6.20

As x becomes smaller and smaller, so does the perpendicular AB, while the length of the projection OB comes closer and closer to that of the radius OA.

If x is small enough, we can regard OA and OB as being essentially the same length, and AB can then be considered as a very small arc of a circle of radius $OA=OB$. Now since the radian measure of an angle = arc/radius (Section 6.2), we will have

$$x=AB/OA$$

approximately. But $AB/OA=\sin x$ by definition. Thus *for small x, $\sin x$ and x are approximately equal.*

Similarly, *$\tan x$ is approximately equal to x for small x*:

Table 6.2 x, $\sin x$ and $\tan x$ for small x

x	$\sin x$	$\tan x$
·1000	0·09983	0·10033
·0500	0·04998	0·50004
·0100	0·01000	0·01000
·0050	0·00500	0·00500

The unsophisticated geometrical arguments given above can be refined into two statements involving limits as $x\to0$. These are:

$$\lim_{x\to0}\left(\frac{\sin x}{x}\right)=1 \qquad\qquad (6.9)$$

$$\lim_{x\to0}\left(\frac{\tan x}{x}\right)=1 \qquad\qquad (6.10)$$

Further examples of such limits are given in the Appendix (page 395). Remember that *in these formulae x is in radians.*

6.13   Compound and multiple angle formulae

It often happens that we have to deal with trigonometrical functions of angles which are themselves sums or differences of other angles. There are formulae for these which are also used to reduce or manipulate complex expressions. We give the formulae without proof; the proofs are tedious and not very relevant to our purpose—for details consult e.g. Hall & Knight (1946).

6.13.1   Compound angles

Given two angles, A and B, we have:

$$\sin(A+B)=(\sin A)*(\cos B)+(\cos A)*(\sin B)$$

usually written without brackets or multiplication signs on the right hand side as

$$\sin (A+B) = \sin A \cos B + \cos A \sin B \qquad (6.11)$$

Using similar notation:

$$\sin (A-B) = \sin A \cos B - \cos A \sin B \qquad (6.12)$$

$$\cos (A+B) = \cos A \cos B - \sin A \sin B \qquad (6.13)$$

$$\cos (A-B) = \cos A \cos B + \sin A \sin B \qquad (6.14)$$

Notice that the signs on both sides of a sine formulae correspond whereas those in cosine formulae are opposites. It is very easy to make a mistake in these!

There are corresponding formulae for tangent, cotangent etc. The only ones of any real importance are those for $\tan (A \pm B)$, which are used in co-ordinate geometry (Chapter 8). They are:

$$\tan (A+B) = \frac{\tan A + \tan B}{1 - \tan A \tan B} \qquad (6.15)$$

$$\tan (A-B) = \frac{\tan A - \tan B}{1 + \tan A \tan B} \qquad (6.16)$$

Examples:

(i) $\sin 15° = \sin (45° - 30°)$

$$= \sin 45° \cos 30° - \cos 45° \sin 30°$$

$$= \frac{1}{\sqrt{2}} * \frac{\sqrt{3}}{2} - \frac{1}{\sqrt{2}} * \frac{1}{2} \quad \text{(see Appendix, page 398)}$$

$$= \frac{0·7321}{2·8284}$$

$$= 0·2588$$

(ii) This is an example illustrating techniques used in obtaining the *differential coefficients* (Chapter 9) of the trigonometric functions. We have:

$$\tan (A+B) - \tan A = \frac{\tan A + \tan B}{1 - \tan A \tan B} - \tan A$$

$$= \frac{\tan A + \tan B - \tan A + \tan^2 A \tan B}{1 - \tan A \tan B}$$

$$= \frac{(\tan B) * (1 + \tan^2 A)}{1 - \tan A \tan B}$$

$$= \frac{\tan B \sec^2 A}{1 - \tan A \tan B} \quad \text{(see Section 6.11)}$$

from which it follows that

$$\frac{\tan (A+B)-\tan A}{B}=\frac{\tan B}{B} \ast \frac{\sec^2 A}{1-\tan A \tan B}$$

If we assume A and B are in radians, we can use the limiting result

$$\lim_{B \to 0} \left(\frac{\tan B}{B}\right)=1 \quad (\text{Section } 6.12)$$

to obtain

$$\lim_{B \to 0} \frac{\tan (A+B)-\tan A}{B}=\sec^2 A,$$

a result of use in the differential calculus.

6.13.2   *Multiple and sub-multiple angles*

By putting $A=B$, or replacing A and B by $A/2$ in the formulae of Section 6.13.1, a number of formulae connecting the trigonometric functions of angles with those of angles twice, or alternatively half, their size, can be deduced. For example, putting $A=B$ in formula (6.11) gives

$$\sin (2A)=\sin (A+A)$$

$$=\sin A \cos A+\cos A \sin A$$

$$=2 \sin A \cos A$$

Similarly, putting $A=B=C/2$ in (6.15) gives

$$\tan C=\frac{2 \tan C/2}{1-\tan^2 C/2}$$

A list of such formulae is given in the Appendix (page 399).

6.13.3

Although there are many formulae connecting trigonometric functions of sums and differences of angles, there are, curiously enough, none for such functions of products or quotients (other than multiplication or division by integer constants). For example, there is no straightforward expression for $\sin (xy)$ or $\cos (x/y)$ in terms of $\sin x$, $\sin y$ or any other trigonometric functions of x or y.

A large collection of formulae and series, etc., for the trigonometric functions is given in Abramovitz and Stegun (1965).

6.14   General values and principal values

6.14.1   General values

We have seen that, given X, we can obtain specific and unique values for sin X, cos X etc. However, sometimes the position is reversed: we have, e.g. cos X, and wish to find X. The question arises, is there a unique value for X? For example, what value of X is such that cos $X=0\cdot21$, and is there only one such value?

Let us for the moment confine ourselves to sin X and cos X. If we examine the graphs of these two functions (Fig 6.18), we see that they do not take values outside the range $[-1, 1]$. Thus there are no solutions to the equations

$$\sin X = 16$$

or $$\cos X = -7\cdot5$$

since there are no values of X which would make them true.

On the other hand, if we draw a line parallel to the X-axis at a height h, where $h \leqslant 1$, we see that this line cuts the graph of, e.g., sin X in an unlimited number of points:

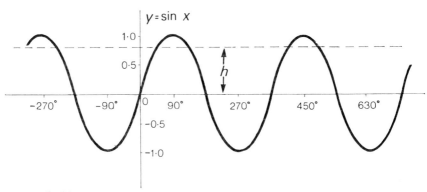

Fig 6.21

Each of these points corresponds to a value of X for which sin $X=h$. So for example, if $h=\frac{1}{2}$, we have Fig 6.22.

i.e. $X=30°, 150°, 390°, 510° \dots$

all satisfy sin $X=\frac{1}{2}$.   Similarly

$$X=60°, 300°, 420°, 660° \dots$$

all satisfy cos $X=\frac{1}{2}$.

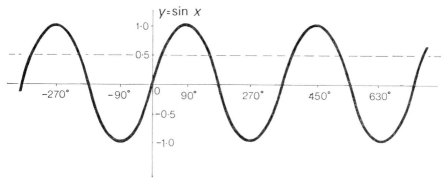

Fig 6.22

The clue to these values lies in page 397 of the Appendix. From this we see that

$$\sin A = \sin (180° - A) = \sin (360° + A) = \sin (360° + 180° - A)$$
$$= \sin (-180° - A) = \sin (-360° + A) = \ldots$$

etc.

Thus if $X = A°$ is a solution of $\sin X = \frac{1}{2}$, then the angles $180° - A°$, $360° + A°$, $540° - A°$, $-180° - A°$, $-360° + A°$, ... etc. will also satisfy $\sin X = \frac{1}{2}$. But (page 398) $\sin 30° = \frac{1}{2}$, and therefore the angles $30°$, $150°$, $390°$, $510°$, ..., $-210°$, $-330°$, ... etc., all satisfy $\sin X = \frac{1}{2}$.

6.14.2 Principal values

Of all the angles satisfying $t(X) = y$, where $t(X)$ denotes a trigonometric function of X, one angle will be the smallest in absolute value. This particular angle is called the *principal* value of the solution. So for example the principal value of the solution of $\sin X = \frac{1}{2}$ is $X = 30°$.

These results are expressed in the following general formulae:

(i) If $\sin X = y$, where X is the principal value then

$\sin (180° * n + (-1)^n * X°)$ also $= y$

where n is either zero or a positive or negative integer. More concisely, we can say:

The angle $180° * n + (-1)^n * X°$

has the same sine as $X°$. In radian terms, the angle

$n\pi + (-1)^n * X$

has the same sine as X.

By similar processes, we have:

   (ii) The angle

$$n * 360° \pm X°$$

      has the same cosine as $X°$. In radian terms,

$$2n\pi \pm X$$

      has the same cosine as X.

   (iii) The angle

$$n * 180° + X°$$

      has the same tangent as $X°$. In radian terms,

$$\tan(n\pi + X) = \tan X$$

      Results for the other three trigonometric functions can be deduced from these.

    The values to use in any particular situation will depend on the conditions defining the problem. Usually, however, it is the principal value which is used.

6.15   The inverse circular functions

We will use radian measure in this section as it is the more common representation in the topic we are about to discuss; the corresponding results in terms of degrees are not difficult to deduce.

    If $\sin X = y$, we have already seen that X can be any of an unlimited number of angles whose sine equals y. This fact is written as

$$\arcsin y = X$$

meaning in words: 'X is the angle whose sine is y'. If x is the principal value of X, then the general value of $\arcsin y$ is $n\pi + (-1)^n x$ in radians (or $n * 180° + (-1)^n x°$ in degrees).

    Similarly

$$\theta = \arctan(1)$$

and

$$\theta = n\pi + \frac{\pi}{4} \quad (n=0, \pm 1, \pm 2, \pm 3, \ldots)$$

express the same fact in two different ways.

The expressions arcsin, arccos, arctan, arccot, arcsec, arccosec are called the *inverse circular functions*. It is important to remember that they are all *angles*.

From Section 6.14, we see that the inverse circular functions have an unlimited number of values. The principal value (Section 6.14.2) is usually the one of interest. If y is positive, the principal values of arcsin y, arccos y and arctan y lie between 0 and $\pi/2$; if y is negative, the principal values of arcsin y and arctan y lie between 0 and $-\pi/2$ and the principal value of arccos y lies between $\pi/2$ and π. The convention for arccos y when $y<0$ gets over the fact that cos $X=y$ has two smallest solutions for X—equal in absolute magnitude but opposite in sign—by taking the positive solution:

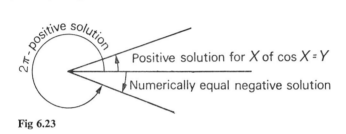

Fig 6.23

When using computer programs to evaluate inverse circular functions, make sure to find out which of the possible values is being produced by the program. Normally it will be the principal value, but occasionally this is not so.

N.B. The reader may occasionally meet an alternative notation for the inverse circular functions, viz:

$\sin^{-1} y$ for arcsin y

$\cos^{-1} y$ for arccos y

$\tan^{-1} y$ for arctan y etc.

There is obviously a great risk of confusing this notation with the algebraic index -1, meaning reciprocation. For this reason the notation is falling into disuse, but it is as well to remember that $\sin^{-1} y$, $\cos^{-1} y$, etc. have the meanings given above and do not mean $1/\sin y$, $1/\cos y$, etc. (which would be written either as cosec y, sec y, ... or as $(\sin y)^{-1}$, $(\cos y)^{-1}$, ... etc.).

The circular functions have an obvious role to play in the mathematical handling of geometrical problems and in computations relevant to position in space. However, their functional properties make them extremely useful in mathematical work generally; because of these properties, they are of widespread occurrence in mathematics, and the student should become familiar with them as part of his basic mathematical knowledge.

6.16   Hyperbolic functions

Related to the circular functions of angle are the *hyperbolic functions*. These bear something of the same relationship to the *rectangular hyperbola* (see Section 8.2) as the circular functions of angle do to the circle. As with the sine, cosine, tangent, ... etc., functions we have been discussing in this chapter, there are the *hyperbolic sine*, *hyperbolic cosine*, etc. There are written sinh, cosh, tanh, etc., and sometimes pronounced 'shine', 'cosh', 'tanch', and also as 'sin-h', 'cos-h', 'tan-h', ...

They are normally used only as functions, however; their definitions and some of their properties are given in the Appendix, page 400, but apart from this they are not considered further in this book.

6.17   A further note on periodic functions

Since with a periodic function $f(x)$, we have

$$f(x)=f(x+\omega)=f(x+2\omega)=\ldots$$

where ω is the period, it can be seen that the graph of $f(x)$ can be regarded as a series of repetitions of any section of total length ω (Figs. 6.24(a) and (b)).

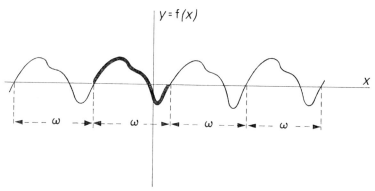

Fig 6.24(a)

When we are dealing with periodic functions of time (see *e.g.* Section 10.5) the quantity $1/\omega$ is called the *frequency* (ω in radians). It is the number of repetitions per second (or per unit time) of the basic section from which the function is regarded as constructed.

Note that it is the independent variable itself which increases by the period, not the overall argument. For example, while the period of $\sin(t)$ is 2π, and its

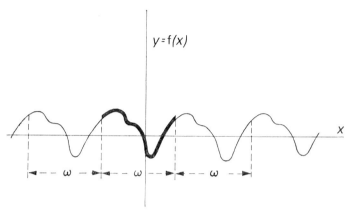

$y = f(x)$

Fig 6.24(b)

frequency is $1/2\pi$, the period of $\sin(pt)$ is $2\pi/p$, since

$$\sin\{p(t+2\pi/p)\} = \sin(pt+2\pi) = \sin(pt)$$

and $2\pi/p$ is the smallest quantity with this property vis-a-vis $\sin(pt)$. Thus the frequency of $\sin(pt)$ is $p/(2\pi)$. For example,

$$\sin(4\pi t) \quad (t \text{ in seconds})$$

has a period of $2\pi/(4\pi) = 0\cdot5$ sec., and a frequency of $1/0\cdot5 = 2$ repetitions (or beats) per second:

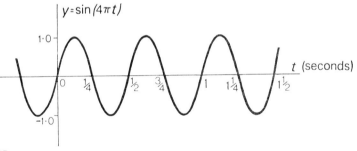

$y = \sin(4\pi t)$

Fig 6.25

Chapter 7
Ordered Sets of Data
Vector and Matrix Algebra

7.1 Introduction

The medical reader is most likely to meet *vectors* and *matrices* in the statistical study of large amounts of data, particularly analysis involving several different types of measurement on the same individual (*multivariate analysis.*) Many of the publications of statistical methods assume a knowledge of *matrix algebra*, as the manipulation of matrices is called. Matrices are also used when we need to handle systems of linear functions of several variables. Such systems occur in statistics, in the dynamics of vibrating systems (both mechanical and electrical), in the solution of differential equations (Chapter 12) in co-ordinate geometric transformations (Chapter 8), and in the study of physiological problems such as the release of insulin and the performance of the kidney. Because of this multiple role, matrices provide one of the many means whereby the concepts of one mathematical topic can be used to analyse results in another; for example, they enable us to make geometrical analogies in statistics and differential equations.

It is simplest to consider this topic as a convenient notation for handling large amounts of data. The subject seems to have acquired a considerable jargon in which ordinary English words (e.g. space, dimension, identity, complex) are given a special technical meaning. In this Chapter we can do little more than introduce the ideas of matrix algebra and define some of its special words and operations. Knowledge of these definitions can be important when reading texts which use vector and matrix notation or when attempting to use computer programs for carrying out matrix operations.

7.2 Vector notation

In many instances it is convenient to gather data together in ordered sets. For example, a set of biochemical tests (calcium, phosphate, total protein, albumin) may be performed on a large number of blood samples. For each sample the concentrations of Calcium (mg/100 ml), Phosphate (mg/100 ml), Total Protein (g/100 ml) and Albumin (g/100 ml) would be recorded, giving for one sample say, $(9 \cdot 5, 3 \cdot 5, 7, 4)$ *respectively*, while for another sample the results might be $(10 \cdot 2, 4 \cdot 1, 7 \cdot 2, 4 \cdot 8)$ respectively. For convenience we write the results down in a fixed order separated by commas and enclosed in brackets. Such an ordered set of values is called a *vector*. If we wish to refer to the vector $(9 \cdot 5, 3 \cdot 5, 7, 4)$ it is tedious to have to continually write $(9 \cdot 5, 3 \cdot 5, 7, 4)$, so by an extension of algebraic notation we write $\mathbf{x} = (9 \cdot 5, 3 \cdot 5, 7, 4)$; now whenever we refer to $\mathbf{x}$ we refer to the *vector* of results given in the order (Calcium, Phosphate, Total Protein, Albumin).

The results above refer to particular blood samples, but by analogy with the single variable, we may use the vector **x** to represent a set of readings whose values are unknown. The use of **x** here results in a considerable condensation in the discussion of the set of biochemical tests (Calcium, Phosphate, Total Protein, Albumin).

The vector **x** is often written in heavy type, or underlined, to help distinguish it from a variable x representing a single value. A variable representing a single value is called a *scalar*. There is no special convention about the choice of letter to represent different vectors, though the vectors **i**, **j**, and **k** sometimes have a special meaning (Section 7.8.1). Numbers in **x** are called the *elements* of **x** and are denoted by means of a suffix (also called a subscript) on the corresponding small letter x. In our example

>the Calcium value would be referred to as x_1
>
>the Phosphate value as x_2
>
>the Total Protein value as x_3
>
>the Albumin value as x_4

and in the first sample given above

$$x_1 = 9 \cdot 5$$
$$x_2 = 3 \cdot 5$$
$$x_3 = 7$$
$$x_4 = 4$$

Notice the obvious extension of this notation to any number of tests. The number of elements in a vector is called the *dimension* of the vector. Our four biochemical tests Calcium, Phosphate, Total Protein and Albumin have been represented by a *four-dimensional* vector **x**. Each element of the vector takes on a conventional numerical value, and so x_1, or x_2 etc. can be used in algebraic formulae.

For example:

>Globulin = Total Protein − Albumin

may be written

>Globulin = $x_3 - x_4$

When a four-dimensional vector is used in a computer program the program has to allocate four separate storage locations to hold its value.

7.2.1   Distance and dimensions

In discussing positions of points on a page (two dimensions) we may determine any point A by its distance across the page—denoted by a_1, and up the page—

denoted by a_2, so the point can be represented by the vector $\mathbf{a} = (a_1, a_2)$, a two-dimensional vector (cf. Chapter 2).

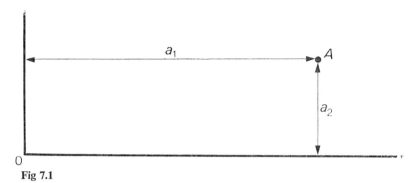

Fig 7.1

Similarly we may represent any point in a room (three-dimensional space) as determined by the distances a_1 and a_2 from the two walls and a_3 from the floor, so the point can be represented by the vector $\mathbf{a} = (a_1, a_2, a_3)$, a three-dimensional vector.

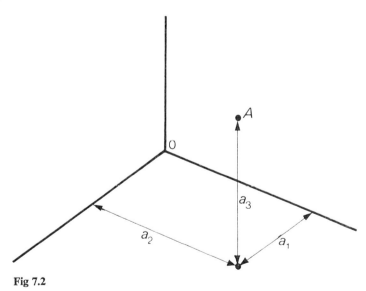

Fig 7.2

Our four biochemical tests are said to represent a *point* in *four dimensional space*. We cannot draw or see four-dimensional space but we imagine it to have a similar relationship to three-dimensional space as the familiar three-dimensional space has to that of two dimensions. We will illustrate this idea by considering a generalization of the concept of distance between two points A and B. In one dimension A is (a_1) and B is (b_1)

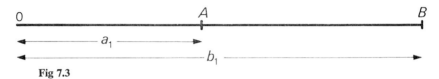

Fig 7.3

The distance between A and B is $b_1 - a_1$.
This may also be written as

$$\sqrt{\{(b_1 - a_1)^2\}};\tag{7.1}$$

the reason for writing it this way will become clear in what follows.
In two dimensions

A is $\mathbf{a} = (a_1, a_2)$, B is $\mathbf{b} = (b_1, b_2)$

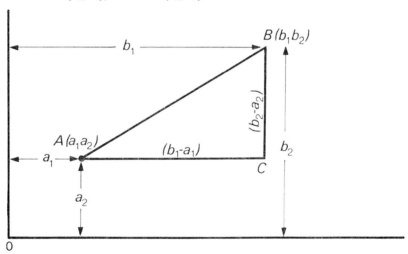

Fig 7.4

and the distances

$$AC = b_1 - a_1, \quad BC = b_2 - a_2.$$

By Pythagoras' theorem:

(distance AB)^2 = (distance AC)^2 + (distance BC)^2

so   (distance AB)^2 = $(b_1 - a_1)^2 + (b_2 - a_2)^2$

Hence

distance $AB=\sqrt{\{(b_1-a_1)^2+(b_2-a_2)^2\}}$ (7.2)

In three dimensions

A is $\mathbf{a}=(a_1, a_2, a_3)$ B is $\mathbf{b}=(b_1, b_2, b_3)$.

The distance between A and B can be obtained by repeated application of Pythagoras' theorem, giving

distance $AB=\sqrt{\{(b_1-a_1)^2+(b_2-a_2)^2+(b_3-a_3)^2\}}$ (7.3)

Notice the progression from one to two, to three dimensions:

distance $AB=\sqrt{\{b_1-a_1)^2\}}$ in one dimension

or $=\sqrt{\{(b_1-a_1)^2+(b_2-a_2)^2\}}$ in two dimensions

or $=\sqrt{\{(b_1-a_1)^2+(b_2-a_2)^2+(b_3-a_3)^2\}}$

in three dimensions

It is natural to *define* for four-dimensional vectors that the 'distance' between A and B is

distance $AB=\sqrt{\{(b_1-a_1)^2+(b_2-a_2)^2+(b_3-a_3)^2+(b_4-a_4)^2\}}$ (7.4)

This 'distance' can be calculated but it cannot be measured with a ruler; it is a *mathematical analogy*.

The distance defined in this way has many of the properties of ordinary physical distance. When $AB=0$ then A and B must be the same point, and as AB gets bigger so the points in some sense get farther apart.

For example, consider three blood samples A, B and C, the elements being defined as at the beginning of this section:

A is $\mathbf{a}=(9\cdot5, 3\cdot5, 7, 4)$

B is $\mathbf{b}=(10\cdot2, 4\cdot1, 7\cdot2, 4\cdot8)$ (7.5)

C is $\mathbf{c}=(8\cdot5, 3\cdot5, 5, 2\cdot6)$

then the 'distance'

$$AC=\sqrt{\{(9\cdot5-8\cdot5)^2+(3\cdot5-3\cdot5)^2+(7-5)^2+(4-2\cdot6)^2\}}$$
$$=\sqrt{\{1^2+0^2+2^2+1\cdot4^2\}}=2\cdot638;$$

the other 'distances' are

$AB=1\cdot237$

$BC=3\cdot596,$

suggesting that sample A is 'closer' to sample B than to sample C.

G

It is interesting to see what happens when we change the scale of measurement. Suppose we measure total protein and albumin in mg/100 ml instead of grams/100 ml, then the last two elements in each vector would be multiplied by 1000,

i.e. $A = (9 \cdot 5, 3 \cdot 5, 7000, 4000)$ distance $AC = 2441$

$B = (10 \cdot 2, 4 \cdot 1, 7200, 4800)$ distance $AB = 825$

$C = (8 \cdot 5, 3 \cdot 5, 5000, 2600)$ distance $BC = 3111$

and the relative distances change. So distance as defined by (7.4) is scale dependent. In the practical use of distance to distinguish between multi-dimensional measurements, we normally choose the scale of measurement to give comparable sizes to the ranges of our observations. Techniques similar to these were used by Day & Wood (1968) to distinguish small bones of Hominid 8 talus found in the Olduvai Gorge, Tanzania, from those of modern man and apes.

The biochemical example above considered four dimensions; in general we refer to an n-dimensional vector $\mathbf{x}$ with elements x_i. The actual numerical values of n and i are substituted when they are known (e.g. 'a four-dimensional vector with elements x_1, x_2, x_3, x_4').

7.3 Matrix notation

The vector is a particular case of an array of data. If we consider the same biochemical tests and results as given in Section (7.2.1) on three different blood samples, we may write the results as follows:

	1st sample	2nd sample	3rd sample	
Calcium	9·5	10·2	8·5	
Phosphate	3·5	4·1	3·5	
Protein	7	7·2	5	(7.6)
Albumin	4	4·8	2·6	

This rectangular array of numbers is referred to as a *matrix*; if it has *m rows* and *n columns* it is called an $m \times n$ *matrix*†. We can notationally identify this matrix by a letter, say A, and the elements of A by $a_{i,j}$ where this represents the element in the ith row and the jth column. In the example above $a_{4,2}$ is $4 \cdot 8$. The notation a_{ij}—i.e. dropping the comma between the subscripts—is also used. Matrices are often distinguished by the use of capital letters in bold type $\mathbf{A}$ or underlining $\underline{A}$ and a preference for the letters A–C, L, M, P–W. Some texts use the notation (a_{ij}) to represent the whole matrix $\mathbf{A}$. The matrix $\mathbf{I}$ has a special meaning (Section 7.4). Note that $\mathbf{X}$, $\mathbf{Y}$, $\mathbf{Z}$ usually represent vectors.

---

† Normally spoken of as an 'm by n matrix'.

A vector can be regarded as a *one column* matrix or a *one row* matrix. It is often easier to write a vector as a one row matrix (*a row vector*) but when working with vectors it is conventional to regard them as one column matrices (*a column vector*). An element of a column vector can be written as $x_{i,1}$ and of a row vector as $x_{1,j}$.

The progression from a vector with element x_i to a matrix with element $a_{i,j}$ could be continued to produce an *array* of data ordered on three features, with elements $w_{i,j,k}$, i.e. with three suffices; and so on for four, five, or more suffices. (In computer programming, all ordered arrays of data are called *arrays* and sometimes one refers to a *three-dimensional* array meaning an array with three suffices, but the number of values each suffix can have is still regarded as the suffix's dimension.)

The formal mathematical rules for handling arrays are mostly confined to vectors and matrices. It was convenient to create a new form of arithmetic to handle the more common calculations which arose in the use of vectors and matrices. The rules of this arithmetic and some of their consequences are given in the following sections. Throughout these sections we shall give the elements of the matrices very simple numerical values but the reader should remember that in practice, the numbers will not be so easy and we will normally require mechanical or electronic computers to perform the operations. After all, it is one of the aims of matrix algebra to represent complicated arithmetical operations in a simple way. Most digital computer systems have special programs for dealing with matrix operations. A matrix with only one element, i.e. a single number, is called a *scalar*.

7.3.1   Equality

We say that two matrices are equal if they are the same matrix of values, e.g. if $\mathbf{A} = \mathbf{B}$ then $a_{i,j} = b_{i,j}$ for all i and j.

7.4   Types of matrix

In this Section we introduce further names given to different types of matrix. The names are mostly descriptive, e.g. a *square matrix* is a matrix with an equal number of rows and columns; a *rectangular matrix* has a different number of rows from the number of columns. In all the examples below the matrices will be illustrated with three or four dimensions; in practice the dimension of each matrix will be appropriate to the problem.

Some definitions applicable to square matrices are:

(i) Diagonal

e.g. $\begin{pmatrix} 6 & 0 & 0 \\ 0 & 5 & 0 \\ 0 & 0 & 2 \end{pmatrix}$, $\begin{pmatrix} 2 & 0 & 0 & 0 \\ 0 & 9 & 0 & 0 \\ 0 & 0 & 4 & 0 \\ 0 & 0 & 0 & 1 \end{pmatrix}$

General elements: $a_{i,j}=0$ for $i \neq j$. The elements $a_{i,i}$ of a matrix are called the *diagonal*.

(ii) Symmetric

e.g. $\begin{pmatrix} 1 & 3 & 9 \\ 3 & 5 & 2 \\ 9 & 2 & 6 \end{pmatrix}$, $\begin{pmatrix} 0 \cdot 9 & 0 \cdot 1 & 0 \cdot 3 & 0 \cdot 2 \\ 0 \cdot 1 & 0 \cdot 8 & 0 \cdot 4 & 0 \cdot 6 \\ 0 \cdot 3 & 0 \cdot 4 & 0 \cdot 5 & 0 \cdot 7 \\ 0 \cdot 2 & 0 \cdot 6 & 0 \cdot 7 & 0 \cdot 1 \end{pmatrix}$

General elements: $a_{i,j}=a_{j,i}$, i.e. elements are 'reflected' in the diagonal.

(iii) Zero **0**

e.g. $\begin{pmatrix} 0 & 0 & 0 \\ 0 & 0 & 0 \\ 0 & 0 & 0 \end{pmatrix}$, $\begin{pmatrix} 0 & 0 & 0 & 0 \\ 0 & 0 & 0 & 0 \\ 0 & 0 & 0 & 0 \\ 0 & 0 & 0 & 0 \end{pmatrix}$

All elements are zero; this definition also applies to rectangular matrices and vectors.

(iv) Identity **I**

e.g. $\begin{pmatrix} 1 & 0 & 0 \\ 0 & 1 & 0 \\ 0 & 0 & 1 \end{pmatrix}$, $\begin{pmatrix} 1 & 0 & 0 & 0 \\ 0 & 1 & 0 & 0 \\ 0 & 0 & 1 & 0 \\ 0 & 0 & 0 & 1 \end{pmatrix}$

General element: $i_{j,k}=0$ if $j \neq k$
$$=1 \text{ if } j=k$$

This matrix fulfils the role of unity in matrix algebra. Its general element is often referred to as $\delta_{j,k}$ using $\delta_{j,k}$ to indicate a quantity that is zero when $j \neq k$, and 1 when $j=k$.

There are other types of matrix referred to when some feature may present a computational advantage or difficulty, e.g. *sparse matrices*, which have mostly zero elements; *band matrices* which have their non-zero elements confined to a narrow band either side of the diagonal; *upper triangular matrices* which have all their elements below the diagonal equal to zero, and *lower triangular matrices,* which have all their elements above the diagonal equal to zero.

7.4.1 Partitioned matrices

We can form a large matrix by putting together a suitably matched set of smaller matrices, for example

$$A=\begin{pmatrix}1 & 2\\3 & 4\end{pmatrix} \quad B=\begin{pmatrix}5 & 6 & 7\\8 & 9 & 10\end{pmatrix} \quad C=\begin{pmatrix}11 & 12\\13 & 14\end{pmatrix} \quad D=\begin{pmatrix}15 & 16 & 17\\18 & 19 & 20\end{pmatrix}.$$

Then we can create a new matrix **F** as

$$F=\begin{pmatrix}A & B\\ \hline C & D\end{pmatrix}=\begin{pmatrix}1 & 2 & 5 & 6 & 7\\3 & 4 & 8 & 9 & 10\\11 & 12 & 15 & 16 & 17\\13 & 14 & 18 & 19 & 20\end{pmatrix}$$

Such matrices are called *partitioned matrices* and are particularly useful when manipulating very large matrices on computers. Rules for handling partitioned matrices have been worked out and some are given in the Appendix. A particular case of the partitioned matrix is one in which the new matrix **F** is formed by adding a further row and column to a matrix **A**; this is called a *bordered matrix*. It is used in statistical work when we introduce additional variables into a problem. The advantage of having a bordered matrix is that it is sometimes possible to make use of earlier calculations on the matrix **A**, when computing with the new matrix **F**.

7.5 Operations on matrices

7.5.1 The transpose

An operation which will prove useful in conjunction with matrix multiplication (to be discussed later) is the *transpose*. The effect of this is to interchange the role of rows and columns. In the transpose of matrix **A** the element in the ith row, jth column of the transpose is the element in the jth row and ith column of the matrix **A**. The transpose of **A** is usually written A^T or A', and the elements of the transpose as $a_{i,j}^T$ or $a'_{i,j}$, and so

$$a_{i,j}^T=a_{j,i}. \tag{7.7}$$

For example:

$$\mathbf{A} = \begin{pmatrix} 9 \cdot 5 & 10 \cdot 2 & 8 \cdot 5 \\ 3 \cdot 5 & 4 \cdot 1 & 3 \cdot 5 \\ 7 & 7 \cdot 1 & 5 \\ 4 & 4 \cdot 8 & 2 \cdot 6 \end{pmatrix}, \mathbf{A}^{\mathrm{T}} = \begin{pmatrix} 9 \cdot 5 & 3 \cdot 5 & 7 & 4 \\ 10 \cdot 2 & 4 \cdot 1 & 7 \cdot 1 & 4 \cdot 8 \\ 8 \cdot 5 & 3 \cdot 5 & 5 & 2 \cdot 6 \end{pmatrix}$$

A symmetric matrix is unaltered by transposition:

$$\mathbf{S} = \begin{pmatrix} 1 & 3 & 9 \\ 3 & 5 & 2 \\ 9 & 2 & 6 \end{pmatrix}, \mathbf{S}^{\mathrm{T}} = \begin{pmatrix} 1 & 3 & 9 \\ 3 & 5 & 2 \\ 9 & 2 & 6 \end{pmatrix}$$

A column vector with element $x_{i, 1}$ transposes to a row vector with element $x_{1, i}$ and a row vector transposes to a column vector:

$$\mathbf{x} = \begin{pmatrix} 9 \cdot 5 \\ 3 \cdot 5 \\ 7 \\ 4 \end{pmatrix}, \mathbf{x}^{\mathrm{T}} = (9 \cdot 5, \ 3 \cdot 5, \ 7, \ 4)$$

7.5.2 Addition and subtraction

In addition and subtraction we simply add or subtract the matching elements of the two matrices:

$$\text{If} \quad \mathbf{C} = \mathbf{A} + \mathbf{B} \quad \text{then} \quad c_{i, j} = a_{i, j} + b_{i, j}; \tag{7.8}$$

$$\text{if} \quad \mathbf{C} = \mathbf{A} - \mathbf{B} \quad \text{then} \quad c_{i, j} = a_{i, j} - b_{i, j}$$

For example consider the three samples of biochemical tests given in Section 7.3.

$$\mathbf{A} = \begin{pmatrix} 9 \cdot 5 & 10 \cdot 2 & 8 \cdot 5 \\ 3 \cdot 5 & 4 \cdot 1 & 3 \cdot 5 \\ 7 & 7 \cdot 2 & 5 \\ 4 & 4 \cdot 8 & 2 \cdot 6 \end{pmatrix} \qquad \text{see (7.6)}$$

Let $\mathbf{B}$ be the matrix in which each column has elements equal to the average values of the Calcium, Phosphate, etc.

$$\mathbf{B} = \begin{pmatrix} 9 \cdot 4 & 9 \cdot 4 & 9 \cdot 4 \\ 3 \cdot 7 & 3 \cdot 7 & 3 \cdot 7 \\ 6 \cdot 4 & 6 \cdot 4 & 6 \cdot 4 \\ 3 \cdot 8 & 3 \cdot 8 & 3 \cdot 8 \end{pmatrix} \tag{7.9}$$

The matrix $C = A - B$ is the difference of the concentrations from their averages, a common statistical calculation.

$$C = A - B = \begin{pmatrix} 0 \cdot 1 & 0 \cdot 8 & -0 \cdot 9 \\ -0 \cdot 2 & 0 \cdot 4 & -0 \cdot 2 \\ 0 \cdot 6 & 0 \cdot 8 & -1 \cdot 4 \\ 0 \cdot 2 & 1 \cdot 0 & -1 \cdot 2 \end{pmatrix} \tag{7.10}$$

This is just a simple extension of ordinary arithmetic. To have any meaning, all the matrices must be the same size, for if say A is a 4×3 matrix but B was a 4×4 matrix it would be impossible to compute $c_{1,\,4}$ or $c_{2,\,4}$ or $c_{3,\,4}$ or $c_{4,\,4}$.

The notation $A - B$ proves a convenient way of handling the representation of a large number of differences. In handling matrix algebra we use a system for matrix expressions exactly the same as ordinary algebra; in particular we can use brackets and indices. If A and B are defined as the matrices (7.6) and (7.9) then $(A - B)$ is the matrix C in (7.10) and $(A - B)^T$ denotes the transpose of the matrix C in (7.10).

7.6   Matrix multiplication

The process called *matrix multiplication* is not so obviously analogous to conventional multiplication of scalar quantities. We shall begin by defining the process, and then give examples of its use. Matrix multiplication may appear to the reader to represent a rather complicated and bizarre collection of multiplications and additions among the elements of the matrices involved. However, this rule was not thought up to confuse the non-mathematician; it has proved the most convenient notation to represent a particular computational process which occurs repeatedly in geometry, statistics, and the other fields of study mentioned in the introduction to this Chapter.

Multiplication of a matrix by a constant or variable, that is, by a scalar quantity, is perfectly straightforward; we just multiply *every* element in the matrix by the scalar. For example:

$$3 * \begin{pmatrix} 1 & 2 \\ 3 & 4 \end{pmatrix} = \begin{pmatrix} 3 & 6 \\ 9 & 12 \end{pmatrix}$$

We still use the symbol $*$ for multiplication; however in most mathematical texts it is either omitted or the symbol $\cdot$ is used. Multiplication of one matrix by another has a much more complicated definition. Basically we form an *element* of the new matrix by taking a *row* of the *first* matrix with a *column* of the *second* matrix, and adding up the products of matching elements.

For example:

$$\mathbf{A} = \begin{pmatrix} 1 & 2 \\ 3 & 4 \end{pmatrix} \quad \text{and} \quad \mathbf{B} = \begin{pmatrix} 10 & 20 \\ 30 & 40 \end{pmatrix}$$

Then $\mathbf{A} * \mathbf{B} = \begin{pmatrix} 1 & 2 \\ 3 & 4 \end{pmatrix} * \begin{pmatrix} 10 & 20 \\ 30 & 40 \end{pmatrix}$

1st row of $\mathbf{A}$ ＊ 1st column of $\mathbf{B}$ 1st row of $\mathbf{A}$ ＊ 2nd column of $\mathbf{B}$

i.e. $\mathbf{A} * \mathbf{B} = \begin{pmatrix} (1 * 10 + 2 * 30) & (1 * 20 + 2 * 40) \\ (3 * 10 + 4 * 30) & (3 * 20 + 4 * 40) \end{pmatrix};$

2nd row of $\mathbf{A}$ ＊ 1st column of $\mathbf{B}$ 2nd row of $\mathbf{A}$ ＊ 2nd column of $\mathbf{B}$

after carrying out the multiplications and additions this becomes:

$$\mathbf{A} * \mathbf{B} = \begin{pmatrix} 70 & 100 \\ 150 & 220 \end{pmatrix}$$

We may formally define a new matrix $\mathbf{C}$ to be the product of $\mathbf{A}$ and $\mathbf{B}$ as follows:

If $\mathbf{C} = \mathbf{A} * \mathbf{B}$ where $\mathbf{A}$ has q columns

and $\mathbf{B}$ has q rows

then $c_{i,j} = \sum\limits_{k=1}^{q} a_{i,k} * b_{k,j}$ (7.11)

For example, the element in the 2nd row and 3rd column of $\mathbf{C}$ is:

$$c_{2,3} = a_{2,1} * b_{1,3} + a_{2,2} * b_{2,3} + a_{2,3} * b_{3,3} + a_{2,4} * b_{4,3} + \text{ etc.}$$

Note how in formula (7.11) we repeat the neighbouring suffix k and add up the products $a_{i,k} * b_{k,j}$ for all the values of k. Formulae which appear in this form can often be handled by matrix multiplication.

A formula of the form

$$\sum\limits_{k=1}^{q} a_{i,k} * b_{j,k}$$

can be represented as $\mathbf{A} * \mathbf{B}^{\mathrm{T}}$.

The matrices do not have to be square; for example:

$$\mathbf{E} = \begin{pmatrix} 0 \cdot 6 & 0 \cdot 8 \\ -8 & 6 \end{pmatrix} \quad \mathbf{F} = \begin{pmatrix} 1 & 3 & 4 \\ 0 & 2 & 5 \end{pmatrix} \tag{7.12}$$

$\mathbf{G} = \mathbf{E} * \mathbf{F}$

$g_{1,1} = 0 \cdot 6 * 1 + 0 \cdot 8 * 0 = 0 \cdot 6,$ $g_{1,2} = 0 \cdot 6 * 3 + 0 \cdot 8 * 2 = 3 \cdot 4,$

$g_{1,3} = 0 \cdot 6 * 4 + 0 \cdot 8 * 5 = 6 \cdot 4,$ $g_{2,1} = -8 * 1 + 6 * 0 = -8,$

$g_{2,2} = -8 * 3 + 6 * 2 = -12,$ $g_{2,3} = -8 * 4 + 6 * 5 = -2$

$$\mathbf{G} = \begin{pmatrix} 0 \cdot 6 & 3 \cdot 4 & 6 \cdot 4 \\ -8 & -12 & -2 \end{pmatrix} \tag{7.13}$$

The resulting matrix **G** has the same number of *rows as the first* matrix and the same number of *columns as the second* matrix, and the number of columns in the first matrix must be the same as the number of rows in the second matrix. In summary:

G=**E** * **F**

number of rows of **G**=number of rows of **E**

number of columns of **G**=number of columns of **F**

number of rows of **F**=number of columns of **E**.

Thus a 4×5 matrix times a 5×4 matrix gives a 4×4 matrix, while a 3×4 matrix cannot be multiplied by a 6×5 matrix. Note also that *the order of multiplication is important*; **E** * **F** is not the same as **F** * **E** (see example in Section 7.7.1).

7.6.1   The product of column and row vectors

There are two different products between row and column vectors.
    If we take the *column* vector

$$\mathbf{x} = \begin{pmatrix} 1 \\ 2 \\ 3 \\ 4 \end{pmatrix}$$

and the *row* vector

$$\mathbf{x}^T = (1, \ 2, \ 3, \ 4)$$

then

$$\mathbf{H} = \mathbf{x}^T * \mathbf{x} = (1, \ 2, \ 3, \ 4) * \begin{pmatrix} 1 \\ 2 \\ 3 \\ 4 \end{pmatrix}$$

The first matrix has one row and four columns, the second matrix has four rows and one column, so the result is a matrix with just one row and one column, i.e. a single value or scalar, and is given by the sum of squares of the numbers:

$$h_{1, \ 1} = 1^2 + 2^2 + 3^2 + 4^2 = 30$$

This notation is a convenient way of handling the sums of squares or cross products which frequently occur in statistical work:

$$\mathbf{x}^T * \mathbf{x} = \sum x_i^2 \qquad \mathbf{x}^T * \mathbf{y} = \sum x_i * y_i \tag{7.14}$$

If we write the product with the row vector after the column vector our definition of multiplication gives a quite different answer:

$$J = x * x^T = \begin{pmatrix} 1 \\ 2 \\ 3 \\ 4 \end{pmatrix} (1, \ 2, \ 3, \ 4)$$

The first matrix has four rows and one column, the second matrix has one row and four columns, so the result is a matrix with four rows and four columns representing the products of all possible pairs of numbers in the two vectors:

$$J = \begin{pmatrix} 1 & 2 & 3 & 4 \\ 2 & 4 & 6 & 8 \\ 3 & 6 & 9 & 12 \\ 4 & 8 & 12 & 16 \end{pmatrix}$$

So the notation $x * y^T$ can be a simple way of generating a matrix whose elements are all possible products of an element of x with an element of y.

7.6.2   Applications of matrix multiplication

When considering addition and subtraction of matrices we showed matrix A in (7.5.2) whose rows represented the results of different biochemical tests on three samples and the matrix B whose rows were the average values of these test results. The matrix $C = A - B$ was then the matrix of the test values measured from their mean. A related matrix frequently used in statistical work is called the 'variance/covariance matrix'. If V is this matrix then

$V_{i, i}$ estimates the variance of the ith test results

$S_i = \sqrt{(V_{i, i})}$ estimates the standard deviation of the ith test results

$V_{i, j}$ estimates the covariance of the ith and jth test results

$r_{i, j} = \dfrac{V_{i, j}}{\sqrt{(V_{i, i} * V_{j, j})}}$ estimates the correlation coefficient of the ith and jth test results

Assuming that there are n samples, i.e. A, B and C have n columns, the formula for V is expressed in matrix notation as:

$$V = \left(\frac{1}{n-1}\right) * C * C^T \quad \text{i.e.} \quad V = \left(\frac{1}{n-1}\right) * (A - B) * (A - B)^T \qquad (7.15)$$

In the example given in Section 7.5.2

$$V_{1,\,1}=\tfrac{1}{2} * (0\cdot1^2+0\cdot8^2+(-0\cdot9)^2)=0\cdot73$$

$$V_{1,\,2}=V_{2,\,1}=\tfrac{1}{2} * (0\cdot1 * (-0\cdot2)+0\cdot8 * 0\cdot4+(-0\cdot9) * (-0\cdot2))$$

$$=0\cdot24$$

and so on, giving

$$\mathbf{V}=\begin{pmatrix} 0\cdot73 & 0\cdot24 & 0\cdot98 & 0\cdot95 \\ 0\cdot24 & 0\cdot12 & 0\cdot24 & 0\cdot30 \\ 0\cdot98 & 0\cdot24 & 1\cdot48 & 1\cdot30 \\ 0\cdot95 & 0\cdot30 & 1\cdot30 & 1\cdot24 \end{pmatrix}$$

Note that $\mathbf{V}$ is a symmetric matrix.

The important thing about this notation is that the formula (7.15) remains simple, however large the vectors and matrices. We avoid having to record hundreds of suffixed variables representing the elements in our *mathematical* manipulations. It is a notational convenience, however, and ultimately all the elements have to be used in the computations. If we had twelve biochemical tests on 200 samples—a reasonable size for the daily load of a routine biochemical screening laboratory—then the simple formula given in (7.15) above represents over 30,000 arithmetic operations!

Another important application of matrix multiplication occurs when the columns of a matrix are considered to represent points on a graph or an object in three-dimensional space. Matrix multiplication corresponds to the arithmetic processes necessary to find the position of the points when the axes of reference are rotated or scales are changed. This aspect is considered in more detail in Chapter 8 but it is the properties of matrices in this tangible application that are usually used as the basis of analogy, when similar arithmetic processes are found in other topics.

The columns of matrix $\mathbf{F}$ in (7.12) can be considered to represent three points on a graph, the points having co-ordinates (1, 0) (3, 2) and (4, 5). Let us say that we wish to rotate the axes of reference through $53°$ (cos $(53°)=0\cdot6$, sin $(53°)=0\cdot8$) and then change the scale of the second element of each vector by a factor of 10. It is possible to compute new values for the co-ordinates of the three points (1, 0), (3, 2), (4, 5) with reference to the new axes; they become $(0\cdot6, -8)$, $(3\cdot4, -12)$ and $(6\cdot4, -2)$. The computations correspond exactly to matrix multiplication of matrix $\mathbf{F}$ by matrix $\mathbf{E}$ in (7.12) so the matrix $\mathbf{E}$ could be regarded as representing this rotation and change of scale. The precise derivation of matrices for known angles of rotation of the axes is given in Section 8.6.3.

7.7   Matrix algebra

In this Section we give some of the rules for handling matrix operations. Most of them can be demonstrated by tediously setting out the matrices element by element and applying the rules of addition, subtraction and multiplication. We do not go through this process and the reader should remember that the simple formulae given below can represent, or conceal, a tremendous number of arithmetic operations in any practical application.

7.7.1   Matrix expressions

It is possible to handle matrix expressions exactly as algebraic expressions provided the operations are feasible in terms of rows and columns matching, e.g.

$$\mathbf{A} * (\mathbf{B}+\mathbf{C}) - (\mathbf{A}+\mathbf{C}) * \mathbf{B} = \mathbf{A} * \mathbf{B} + \mathbf{A} * \mathbf{C} - \mathbf{A} * \mathbf{B} - \mathbf{C} * \mathbf{B}$$

$$= \mathbf{A} * \mathbf{C} - \mathbf{C} * \mathbf{B}$$

The important exception is that *the order of multiplication is important—* $\mathbf{A} * \mathbf{B}$ does not have to be equal to $\mathbf{B} * \mathbf{A}$.

For example

$$\mathbf{A} = \begin{pmatrix} 1 & 2 \\ 3 & 4 \end{pmatrix}, \qquad \mathbf{B} = \begin{pmatrix} 5 & 7 \\ 6 & 8 \end{pmatrix}$$

$$\mathbf{A} * \mathbf{B} = \begin{pmatrix} 17 & 23 \\ 39 & 53 \end{pmatrix}, \qquad \mathbf{B} * \mathbf{A} = \begin{pmatrix} 26 & 38 \\ 30 & 44 \end{pmatrix}$$

We talk of *pre-multiplication* of $\mathbf{B}$ by $\mathbf{A}$ for $\mathbf{A} * \mathbf{B}$ and *post-multiplication* of $\mathbf{B}$ by $\mathbf{A}$ for $\mathbf{B} * \mathbf{A}$.

7.7.2   The identity matrix and the inverse

The matrix $\mathbf{I}$, i.e. all $\mathbf{I}$'s down the diagonal, performs the role of unity:

$$\mathbf{I} * \mathbf{A} = \mathbf{A} \quad \text{and} \quad \mathbf{A} * \mathbf{I} = \mathbf{A} \qquad (7.16)$$

i.e. multiplication of a matrix by $\mathbf{I}$ leaves the matrix unchanged.

A form which frequently occurs is $(\mathbf{A} - \lambda * \mathbf{I})$ where λ is a scalar; this represents matrix $\mathbf{A}$ with λ subtracted from each diagonal element of $\mathbf{A}$.

Example:

$$A=\begin{pmatrix}1&2\\3&4\end{pmatrix}, \qquad A-\lambda I=\begin{pmatrix}1-\lambda&2\\3&4-\lambda\end{pmatrix}$$

Sometimes it is possible to find two matrices which when multiplied together produce **I**. For example

(i) $A=\begin{pmatrix}3&1\\4&2\end{pmatrix}, \qquad B=\begin{pmatrix}1&-0\cdot5\\-2&1\cdot5\end{pmatrix}$

then $\qquad A*B=\begin{pmatrix}1&0\\0&1\end{pmatrix} \qquad$ i.e. $\quad$ **I**

(ii) $A=\begin{pmatrix}\cos\theta&\sin\theta\\-\sin\theta&\cos\theta\end{pmatrix} \qquad B=\begin{pmatrix}\cos\theta&-\sin\theta\\\sin\theta&\cos\theta\end{pmatrix}$

then $\qquad A*B=I \qquad$ (because $\cos^2(\theta)+\sin^2(\theta)=1$)

Similarly $\quad B*A=I$

When for a given matrix **A** there is only one matrix **B** with this property it is convenient to regard **B** as the *inverse* of **A** or 1/A, and write it as A^{-1},

i.e. $\qquad A*A^{-1}=I \qquad\qquad A^{-1}*A=I$

Consider the matrix set of simultaneous linear equations which defines **x** by:

$$a_{1,1}*x_1+a_{1,2}*x_2+a_{1,3}*x_3+\ldots+a_{1,n}*x_n=y_1$$
$$a_{2,1}*x_1+a_{2,2}*x_2+a_{2,3}*x_3+\ldots+a_{2,n}*x_n=y_2$$
$$\cdot\quad\cdot\quad\cdot\quad\cdot\quad\cdot\quad\cdot\quad\cdot\quad\cdot\quad\cdot\quad\cdot$$
$$a_{n,1}*x_1+a_{n,2}*x_2+a_{n,3}*x_3+\ldots+a_{n,n}*x_n=y_n$$

The actual values of n, the a's and y's are assumed to be known.
In matrix notation this may be written

$$A*x=y \tag{7.17}$$

where **A** and **y** are known.
Pre-multiply each side of the equation by A^{-1}

then $\qquad A^{-1}*A*x=A^{-1}*y$

i.e. $\qquad\qquad I*x=A^{-1}*y \tag{7.18}$

i.e. $\qquad\qquad x=A^{-1}*y$

which gives an explicit expression for **x**.
The unique inverse exists only for some square matrices. Those square

matrices which do not have an inverse are called *singular* matrices, and in the example just given a singular matrix **A** would mean that there is not a unique solution to **x** from equation (7.17) unless the elements of **y** are all zero.

The rules for finding the inverse are very complicated; they are given for 2×2 and 3×3 matrices in the Appendix. Computer programs usually exist to do the operation and reference may be made to Ralston & Wilf (1960).

7.7.3   Rules for inverse and transpose of products

(i) $(A * B)^{-1} = B^{-1} * A^{-1}$ (7.19)

Note the reversed order of the multiplication.

(ii) $(A * B)^T = B^T * A^T$ (7.20)

Note again the reversal of order.

7.7.4   Orthogonal matrices

A square matrix **C** such that

$$C^T * C = I,$$ (7.21)

i.e. $C^{-1} = C^T$, is called *orthogonal*.

In Section 7.2.1 we defined the (distance)^2 between two vectors **A** and **B** to be $(a_1 - b_1)^2 + (a_2 - b_2)^2 + (a_3 - b_3)^2 + \ldots$ etc. so that by formula (7.14)

$$(\text{distance})^2 = (A - B)^T * (A - B)$$

Also we noted that a rotation of axes of reference can be represented by a matrix multiplication, say by the matrix **E**, so that

A becomes $E * A$

and   **B** becomes $E * B$

Referred to the new axes of reference

$$(\text{distance on new axes})^2 = (E * A - E * B)^T * (E * A - E * B)$$

which by application of the rules just given becomes

$$(E * (A - B))^T * (E * (A - B))$$

i.e. $$= (A - B)^T * E^T * E * (A - B)$$

If $\mathbf{E}$ is orthogonal $\mathbf{E}^T * \mathbf{E} = \mathbf{I}$ and the distance referred to the new axes of reference is $(\mathbf{A} - \mathbf{B})^T * (\mathbf{A} - \mathbf{B})$, the same as with the old axes of reference. An orthogonal matrix thus represents a transformation which 'preserves distance'. The matrix $\mathbf{E}$ in (7.12) is not orthogonal, and the corresponding geometrical interpretation does not preserve distance due to the change of scale by a factor of 10 in the second element. The matrix

$$\begin{pmatrix} 0\cdot6 & 0\cdot8 \\ -0\cdot8 & 0\cdot6 \end{pmatrix}$$

corresponds to a rotation by $53°$ with no change of scale and it can easily be checked by formula (7.21) to be orthogonal, as is to be expected, for a simple rotation of the axes of reference has no effect on the distances between points.

7.8   Directional vectors and complex numbers

7.8.1   Vector methods

The term *vector methods* is sometimes used to refer to a particular use of two- or three-dimensional vectors. This occurs in problems involving directed forces in mechanics or electricity where a force, tension, magnetic field, etc. is said to have a strength and direction. These forces can be represented by a line drawn in the direction of the force and with length proportional to the strength of the

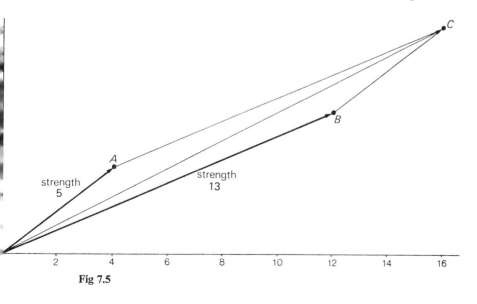

Fig 7.5

force. In this notation it is usual to reserve the three symbols **i**, **j** and **k** for the three forces of strength unity acting along the directions of the axes of reference. They are called *unit vectors* in this case. If we regard all the forces as acting through the origin of the reference axes we could represent the lines of force by the co-ordinates of the end of the lines.

In Fig 7.5 we have represented two forces, one acting from the origin O to the point A with co-ordinates (4, 3) and the other to the point B with co-ordinates (12, 5). The physical laws which govern the behaviour of forces say that the resultant force will be equivalent to a line from O to the point C with co-ordinates (16, 8). Note that in the previous notation of this Chapter, $\mathbf{c}=\mathbf{a}+\mathbf{b}$, where $\mathbf{a}=(4, 3)$, $\mathbf{b}=(12, 5)$ and $\mathbf{c}=(16, 8)$. This may be more familiar to readers as the 'parallelogram of forces'.

In vector methods it is often useful and convenient to express vectors in terms of **i**, **j** and **k**. For example, the vector (4, 3) above could be represented as $4\mathbf{i}+3\mathbf{j}$.

7.8.2   Scalar product

Let us replace the points $A=(4, 3)$, $B=(12, 5)$ of the previous section by general points $\mathbf{a}=(a_1, a_2)$ and $\mathbf{b}=(b_1, b_2)$. In this notation, the product

$$\mathbf{a}^{\mathrm{T}} * \mathbf{a} = a_1^2 + a_2^2 \tag{7.22}$$

i.e. (the length of $OA)^2$ is called the *dot* or *scalar* product and written $\mathbf{a}.\mathbf{a}$ Similarly the product

$$\mathbf{a}^{\mathrm{T}} * \mathbf{b}(=a_1 * b_1 + a_2 * b_2) \quad \text{is written} \quad \mathbf{a}.\mathbf{b}.$$

The dot product is related to the angle between the lines OA and OB for it can be shown that

$$\cos (\text{angle } AOB) = \frac{\mathbf{a}.\mathbf{b}}{\sqrt{\{(\mathbf{a}.\mathbf{a})\,(\mathbf{b}.\mathbf{b})\}}}$$

or in the previous notation of this Chapter

$$\frac{\mathbf{a}^{\mathrm{T}} * \mathbf{b}}{\sqrt{\{(\mathbf{a}^{\mathrm{T}} * \mathbf{a}) * (\mathbf{b}^{\mathrm{T}} * \mathbf{b})\}}} \tag{7.23}$$

Further development of this notation which is extremely convenient for many physical applications involving movement and forces may be found in Weatherburn (1950).

7.8.3   Complex numbers

Another representation for two-dimensional vectors is called a *complex number*. This is a two-dimensional vector in which the rule for multiplication is different from that given earlier in this Chapter; it has many applications, particularly in electronics. The complex number uses an alternative notation to separate the two elements of the vector. They are usually written

$$x_1 + ix_2 \quad \text{or} \quad x_1 + jx_2$$

instead of

$$\begin{pmatrix} x_1 \\ x_2 \end{pmatrix}$$

The complex number notation does not usually employ the conventions of bold type or underlining; instead it treats the vector as an ordinary algebraic expression, relying on the i or j to keep the elements apart. For example

$$(6+j3)+(4+j2)=10+j5$$

instead of

$$\begin{pmatrix} 6 \\ 3 \end{pmatrix} + \begin{pmatrix} 4 \\ 2 \end{pmatrix} = \begin{pmatrix} 10 \\ 5 \end{pmatrix}$$

The mathematician normally uses the symbol i; however in electronics i is already bespoken as the conventional symbol for current and we will follow this convention in using the symbol j to separate the elements. The letter z is often used to represent a complex number.

The multiplication rule is rather different from that given for ordinary two-dimensional vectors, for vector times a vector now gives a vector and the order of multiplication does not matter. The reason for this rule will be given later but complex number notation will only be appropriate in applications such as electronics where the multiplication rule corresponds to computations which have a particular physical interpretation.

The rule for multiplication is

$$(x_1+jx_2) * (y_1+jy_2)=(x_1 * y_1 - x_2 * y_2)+j(x_2 * y_1+x_1 * y_2) \quad (7.24)$$

Example:

$$(6+j3) * (4+j2)=18+j24$$

There are two points to note about the rules for multiplication, addition and subtraction. First, *when the second elements of the vectors are zero* $(x_2=y_2=0)$ the results of these operations with the first elements only are identical to the answer one obtains with real numbers. For example:

$$(6+j0) * (4+j0) = 24+j0$$
$$(6+j0) + (4+j0) = 10+j0$$

Secondly, the rules given above can be easily reproduced by treating j as an ordinary scalar variable and performing normal algebraic multiplication, addition, etc. but whenever we have

j^2, j^6, j^{10}, j^{14} etc. we replace it by -1

j^3, j^7, j^{11}, j^{15} etc. we replace it by $-j$

j^4, j^8, j^{12}, j^{16} etc. we replace it by $+1$

j^5, j^9, j^{13}, j^{17} etc we replace it by $+j$

That is we make j behave as if $j^2 = -1$. (j is called the *square root of -1* though obviously no such quantity could be computed as a real number.) Because of this technique for handling these vectors they are usually regarded as an extension to the ordinary number system and any zero element is omitted when writing the numbers. For example $6+j0$ is written and treated as the real number 6; $0+j4$ is written and treated like $j * 4$ or $4 * j$. The element not qualified by j is called the *real part* and the element qualified by j is called the *imaginary part*.

The complex number notation is a powerful technique for handling both elements of a vector simultaneously by ordinary algebraic manipulation, and some computer languages, e.g. Fortran IV, accept complex numbers and adjust the rules of multiplication, addition, etc. accordingly.

For mathematicians the definition of the multiplication rule followed from the idea of making a variable j behave as if j^2 could equal -1, and they found it added considerable generality to their ideas and eased the task of manipulating certain algebraic relationships. They found some particularly useful consequences from this idea, notably when the vector was expressed in the form

$$\cos(\theta) + j \sin(\theta).$$

Three of these were:

(i) $(\cos(\theta) + j\sin(\theta)) * (\cos(\phi) + j\sin(\phi)) = \cos(\theta+\phi)$
$$+ j\sin(\theta+\phi) \quad (7.25)$$

(ii) $(\cos(\theta) + j\sin(\theta))^n = \cos(n\theta) + j\sin(n\theta)$

e.g. $(\cos(\pi/4) + j\sin(\pi/4))^4 = \cos(\pi) + j\sin(\pi) = -1+j0 \quad (7.26)$

That is, multiplication of complex numbers expressed in terms of angles corresponds to addition of the angles.

(iii) If we handle the expression $e^{j\theta}$ as if j and θ were variables multiplied together then it behaves in exactly the same way as $\cos(\theta) + j\sin(\theta)$ (θ being measured in radians). This is a very simple notation and one which is easy to handle. One will often find $e^{j\theta}$ or $e^{i\theta}$ used to indicate the complex number $\cos(\theta) + j\sin(\theta)$.

For further examples of the use of complex numbers the reader is referred to Shaw (1962) who uses them for studying electronic circuits.

7.9   Determinants

We come now to a further calculation which continually occurs in different applications of square matrices. It is sufficiently common to be given a name. It is a single value associated with the matrix and the rule for computing it is quite complicated. The value is called the *determinant* and the determinant of $\mathbf{A}$ is written $\det(\mathbf{A})$ or $|\mathbf{A}|$. For the most part the value associated with different matrices will be different but this is not always the case; for example, matrices which only differ from each other by the interchange of whole rows or whole columns will have the same absolute value for their determinant, though possibly the sign will be different.

With a simple 2×2 matrix, for example:

$$\mathbf{L} = \begin{pmatrix} 1 \cdot 0 & 0 \cdot 3 \\ 0 \cdot 5 & 7 \cdot 0 \end{pmatrix}$$

we will have

$$|\mathbf{L}| = 1 \cdot 0 * 7 \cdot 0 - 0 \cdot 3 * 0 \cdot 5 = 6 \cdot 85$$

In general, if

$$\mathbf{L} = \begin{pmatrix} l_1 & l_2 \\ l_3 & l_4 \end{pmatrix} \quad \text{then} \quad |\mathbf{L}| = l_1 * l_4 - l_2 * l_3 \tag{7.27}$$

With a 3×3 matrix, for example

$$\mathbf{M} = \begin{pmatrix} 4 & 8 & 2 \\ 0 \cdot 6 & 1 & 0 \cdot 3 \\ 9 & 0 \cdot 5 & 7 \end{pmatrix}$$

we will have:

$$|\mathbf{M}| = 4 * (1 * 7 - 0 \cdot 3 * 0 \cdot 5) - 8 * (0 \cdot 6 * 7 - 0 \cdot 3 * 9)$$
$$+ 2 * (0 \cdot 6 * 0 \cdot 5 - 1 * 9)$$
$$= \qquad 4 * 6 \cdot 85 \qquad - \quad 8 * 1 \cdot 5 \quad + \qquad 2 * (-8 \cdot 7)$$
$$= -2 \cdot 0$$

In general, if

$$\mathbf{M} = \begin{pmatrix} m_{1,1} & m_{1,2} & m_{1,3} \\ m_{2,1} & m_{2,2} & m_{2,3} \\ m_{3,1} & m_{3,2} & m_{3,3} \end{pmatrix}$$

then the rule for obtaining the determinant is:

$$|\mathbf{M}| = m_{1,1} * \begin{vmatrix} m_{2,2} & m_{2,3} \\ m_{3,2} & m_{3,3} \end{vmatrix} - m_{1,2} * \begin{vmatrix} m_{2,1} & m_{2,3} \\ m_{3,1} & m_{3,3} \end{vmatrix}$$
$$+ m_{1,3} * \begin{vmatrix} m_{2,1} & m_{2,2} \\ m_{3,1} & m_{3,2} \end{vmatrix}$$

The determinant may be generalized to an $n \times n$ matrix in a similar fashion, by taking each element of the first row, excluding the column it is in, and multiplying it by the determinant of the $(n-1) \times (n-1)$ matrix formed by the remaining rows and columns. The terms are then alternately added and subtracted to form the value known as the determinant.

7.9.1   Meaning and application of determinants

Determinants have many practical applications. For example, the determinant of the covariance matrix mentioned in Section 7.6.2 represents the generalization of the statistical concept of variance to n variables or n dimensions, and frequently occurs in statistical calculations.

Again, when the columns or rows of a 2×2 matrix represent the two directional vectors OA and OB through the origin of co-ordinates O as in Fig 7.5,

e.g. $\mathbf{L} = \begin{pmatrix} 4 & 12 \\ 3 & 5 \end{pmatrix}$

then the modulus of the determinant of $\mathbf{L}$ is the area enclosed by the parallelogram $OACB$. So the area of $OACB$ in Fig 7.5 is the modulus of $| 4 * 5 - 12 * 3 |$, that is 16. Similarly it can be shown that if a 3×3 matrix represents three directional vectors through the origin in three-dimensional space, then the determinant of the matrix is equal to the volume of the parallelepiped—the three-dimensional analogue of a parallelogram—with these vectors as edges (Birkhoff & MacLane, 1953). Extending this process, the determinant represents the generalization from area to volume to *hypervolume*, as the n dimensional analogue of this concept is called.

7.10   Singular and ill-conditioned matrices

Particularly important are situations in which the determinant is zero or very near zero. This situation invariably leads to trouble in computations.

If the determinant of a 2×2 matrix is zero and if the columns of the matrix represent points on a graph, then the points can be shown to lie on a straight line, i.e. they lie in one dimension; similarly, if the columns of a 3×3 matrix represent points in three-dimensional space, and the determinant is zero, then the points lie in a plane, i.e. we have again points which could be represented with fewer dimensions than have been used. The analogue of this concept generalizes to a $n \times n$ matrix: if its determinant is zero the points are said to lie in a *hyperplane*. A matrix whose determinant is zero is *singular* and A^{-1} does not exist. If the elements of A^{-1} are very large in relation to those of A the matrix is called *ill-conditioned* and these matrices will be very susceptible to error when involved in calculations such as solving simultaneous linear equations or inverting the matrix. Some further remarks on ill-conditioning may be found in Marcus (1960).

7.11   Eigenvectors and eigenvalues

There is another set of values associated with a square matrix which like the determinant represent calculations of frequent practical application. These are a set of values called the *eigenvalues* and a matrix whose *columns* are called the *eigenvectors*. Like so many named mathematical features they occur in a variety of applications and a variety of mathematical forms. We will start with some purely mathematical definitions. Our discussion will be based on two-dimensional matrices but as we use matrix notation the ideas and definitions can easily be generalized to three or more dimensions.

Let **L** be a matrix $\begin{pmatrix} l_{1,1} & l_{2,1} \\ l_{2,1} & l_{2,2} \end{pmatrix}$

and **V** a matrix $\begin{pmatrix} v_{1,1} & v_{1,2} \\ v_{2,1} & v_{2,2} \end{pmatrix}$

then for known values of the $v_{i,j}$ it may be possible to find values of **L** and quantities λ_1, λ_2 such that the following conditions hold (at this point just consider them to be computing rules):

$$\mathbf{L}^{-1} * \mathbf{V} * \mathbf{L} = \begin{pmatrix} \lambda_1 & 0 \\ 0 & \lambda_2 \end{pmatrix} \qquad (7.29)$$

$$\det (\mathbf{V} - \lambda_1 \mathbf{I} *) = 0$$

$$\det (\mathbf{V} - \lambda_2 * \mathbf{I}) = 0$$

(7.30)

$$\left. \begin{array}{l} \begin{pmatrix} v_{1,1} & v_{2,1} \\ v_{2,1} & v_{2,2} \end{pmatrix} * \begin{pmatrix} l_{1,1} \\ l_{2,1} \end{pmatrix} = \begin{pmatrix} \lambda_1 * l_{1,1} \\ \lambda_1 * l_{2,1} \end{pmatrix} \\[2em] \begin{pmatrix} v_{1,1} & v_{2,1} \\ v_{2,1} & v_{2,2} \end{pmatrix} * \begin{pmatrix} l_{1,2} \\ l_{2,2} \end{pmatrix} = \begin{pmatrix} \lambda_2 * l_{1,2} \\ \lambda_2 * l_{2,2} \end{pmatrix} \end{array} \right\}$$

(7.31)

All these conditions are equivalent and when they are satisfied the columns of **L** are vectors called the *eigenvectors* of **V** and the numbers represented by λ_1 and λ_2 are called the *eigenvalues*. It is usual to use the Greek symbol λ for eigenvalues. Each column of **L** is associated with a value of λ by the conditions (7.31). The larger value of λ_1 or λ_2 is called the *principal value* and its associated eigenvector is called the *principal component*. Eigenvalues and eigenvectors are also called *characteristic values* and *characteristic vectors*. They are applicable whenever the mathematical computations lead to one of the conditions (7.29)–(7.31).

If **V** is a symmetric matrix, it is always possible to find eigenvalues and eigenvectors, and furthermore, in this case **L** will be orthogonal, i.e. $\mathbf{L}^{-1} = \mathbf{L}^{\mathrm{T}}$.

The equation

$$(v_{1,\,1} - \lambda) * (v_{2,\,2} - \lambda) - v_{1,\,2} * v_{2,\,1} = 0$$

(7.32)

with roots λ_1, λ_2 is equivalent to the expressions in (7.30), for when we expand the determinants we get the equation given in (7.32); it is known as the *characteristic equation* of the matrix. Such forms sometimes occur in the solution of differential equations (Chapter 12).

If the matrix **V** represented a change of co-ordinates then condition (7.31) gives a vector

$$\begin{pmatrix} l_{1,\,1} \\ l_{2,\,1} \end{pmatrix}$$

whose co-ordinates in the new system are

$$\begin{pmatrix} \lambda_1 l_{1,\,1} \\ \lambda_1 l_{2,\,1} \end{pmatrix}$$

i.e. a simple multiple of the co-ordinates in the old system, and similarly for the vector $\begin{pmatrix} l_{1,\,2} \\ l_{2,\,2} \end{pmatrix}$.

The main interest in eigenvectors in recent medical work has been centred in the properties arising from an application in statistical work called *principal component analysis* (Kendall, 1961). Figure 7.6 shows the heights and weights of a set of medical students. It looks rather random and the phrase 'buckshotogram' has been used to describe such a picture. However there is a quite evident tendency for taller people to be heavier and vice-versa. One can reasonably postulate the idea of 'size' and refer to big students or small students. If we want to quantify 'size' in this context, the mathematician will probably try to use some form of straight line graph going through the middle of the points and use the measurement of points along this line to describe 'size'. There are several criteria he can choose for selecting the best line. The one we will consider here is that sums of squared perpendicular distances of the points from the line is a minimum. The choice of this criterion for best fit is influenced by the fact that this is one of the few situations for which the mathematician knows the answer,

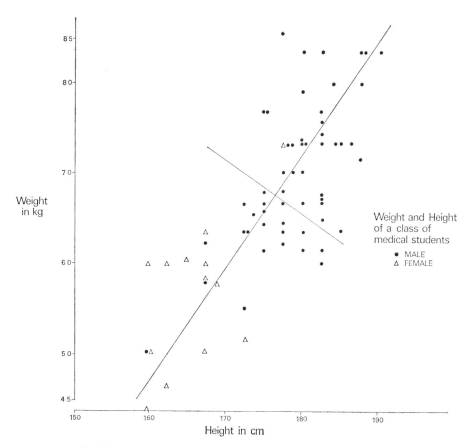

Fig 7.6

and he takes the view that he can give some help, despite the somewhat artificial nature of these conditions. There is however a mechanical analogy, for if we imagine that each spot in Fig 7.6 is really a small piece of lead shot, then this best-fit line will correspond to the axis of rotation about which the system will spin with the minimum inertia and no tendency to wobble. Height and weight measurements may then be referred to a new set of axes, one of which is the desired line (size) and another at right angles to it, which we can call 'shape' because it represents the departure from the main height/weight relationship.

The mathematical solution of this problem is too complex for this book. The answer is to put the origin of the new axes at the centre of gravity, i.e. the point (mean height, mean weight) and to rotate the original axes by an amount which can be represented by the matrix of eigenvectors of the symmetric variance/covariance matrix of the heights and weights. Calling this matrix $\mathbf{V}$, then if a point is

$$\mathbf{x} = \begin{pmatrix} \text{height} \\ \text{weight} \end{pmatrix}$$

we convert to the new axes by the rule

$$\text{size} = l_{1,\,1} * \text{height} + l_{2,\,1} * \text{weight}$$

$$\text{shape} = l_{1,\,2} * \text{height} + l_{2,\,2} * \text{weight}$$

where

$$\begin{pmatrix} l_{1,\,1} \\ l_{2,\,1} \end{pmatrix}$$

is the 'principal component' of $\mathbf{V}$.

The variance/covariance matrix of size and shape can be shown to be

$$\mathbf{L}^{\mathrm{T}} * \mathbf{V} * \mathbf{L} = \begin{pmatrix} \lambda_1 & 0 \\ 0 & \lambda_2 \end{pmatrix} \tag{7.33}$$

Those familiar with multivariate analysis will see from (7.33) that size and shape as defined are uncorrelated and the variances of these new measures correspond to the eigenvalues. If the relationship between height and weight was a perfect straight line then there would be no shape component, that is, the variance in the shape direction would be zero, i.e. $\lambda_2 = 0$; in which case the points could be represented in one dimension only, the 'size' dimension.

We can generalize these results because with matrix notation we have analogous computing rules in three or more dimensions. When dealing with problems represented by many dimensions, e.g. the answers to a large number of psychiatric tests, we hope that all but one or two eigenvalues will be zero so that we can represent the test results in one or two dimensions. We can then do our mathematics to display our points on a flat piece of paper. Note that the new components are derived by a computational trick. Giving a meaning to them, e.g. 'intelligence' is a much more difficult task!

A very similar solution occurs in problems of discriminating between several groups of multi-dimensional measures where the mathematics leads to an equation of the form:

$$\det (\mathbf{B} - \lambda\mathbf{W}) = 0$$

which is clearly similar to the equations (7.30).

The results and formulae of this section yield different answers for different scales of measurement, so careful consideration of the scales of measurement for each of the variables and their effect on the analysis is important.

For further details of the rules of matrix algebra a variety of texts may be consulted—for example Stephenson (1967), Aitken (1948) or Ferrar (1957).

Chapter 8
Co-ordinate Geometry

8.1   Introduction

In previous chapters, we have seen that functions may be visualized by means of graphs. It is possible to reverse the process, and to discuss the shape and characteristics of drawings and figures in terms of mathematical functions, and in the last analysis, therefore, in terms of numbers. Such a process is essential, for instance, when we try to use digital computers to solve problems which are most naturally thought of in visual terms—e.g. in radiotherapy, in molecular biology or in stereotactic surgery.

The ideas used are a fusion of the techniques of the graph on the one hand and the theory of mathematical functions on the other. The result is the subject known variously as *co-ordinate geometry*, *algebraic geometry*, or *analytic geometry*.

8.2   Plane curves: the equation of a curve

Suppose we have a plane curve—that is, a curve lying entirely in a plane. If we choose Cartesian axes of reference (Section 2.2.1) in the plane, then any point on the curve will have co-ordinates relative to these axes (Fig 8.1).

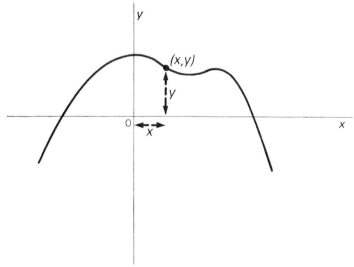

Fig 8.1

Now it is a reasonable supposition that there must be some underlying law governing the curve which determines whether a given point in the plane is on

207

the curve or not—the points on the curve obviously share a special relationship which holds for each of them but does not hold for the other points in the plane. But the position of any point in the plane is defined by its co-ordinates, and so whatever this special relationship may be, it must be expressible in terms of the co-ordinates of the points on the curve, and must be valid for every point on it.

The nature of this relationship can be seen from the following considerations: suppose we choose a value for an x co-ordinate. It is immediately clear that if a point with this x co-ordinate is to lie on the curve then the shape and position of the curve imposes limitations on the possible values of the y co-ordinate of the point (Fig 8.2).

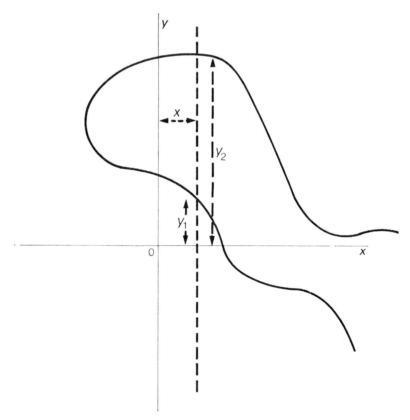

Fig. 8.2 y_1 and y_2 are two possible values of the y co-ordinate for the given value of x

In other words, there is an interrelation between the values of x and y for any point (x, y) on the curve; given x, y is determined, and—by similar reasoning—

given y, x is determined (though there may be more than one value of y possible for a given x and conversely—see Fig 8.2). Thus y and x for any point must be functionally related.

We are thus led to the idea that the shape and properties of a curve can be described by a functional relationship between the x and y co-ordinates of any point on it.

Such relationship is called the *equation of the curve*. More often than not, it is of an implicit rather than an explicit form (Section 3.9).

Examples:

(some of these will be dealt with in detail later):

(i)   The *circle:*

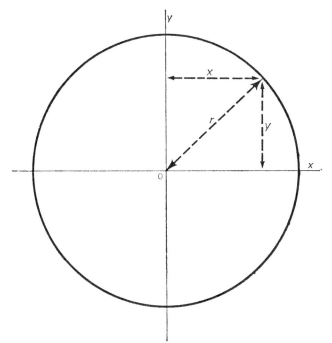

Fig 8.3

Every point has the relation

$$x^2+y^2=r^2$$

between its x and y co-ordinates, where r is the radius and the origin of co-ordinates is the centre of the circle.

(ii) The *cardioid*:

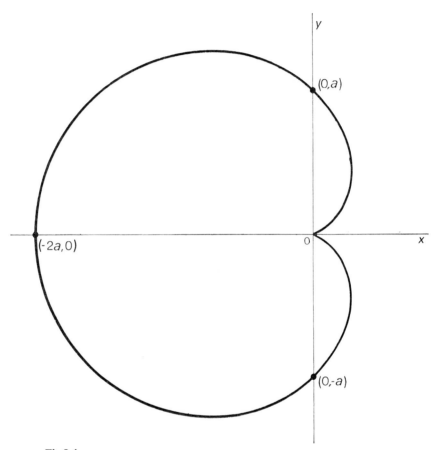

Fig 8.4

The equation

$$x^2 + y^2 + ax = a\sqrt{(x^2 + y^2)}$$

relates the x and y co-ordinates of every point. This example illustrates that quite complicated mathematical expressions may sometimes be needed to describe an apparently simple shape. Conversely, simple mathematical functions can present quite complex curves.

(iii) The *rectangular hyperbola*:

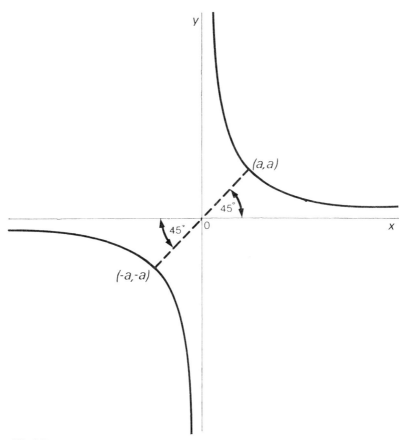

Fig 8.5

The equation of the curve is

$$xy = a^2 \quad \left(\text{or } y = \frac{a^2}{x}\right)$$

— — — — — — — — —

The power of such a representation is that all the techniques of algebra and mathematical analysis can be brought to bear on problems connected with curves and shapes, and the answers expressed as *numbers*. For example, we may be interested in knowing where two curves intersect. Suppose that their equations are $f(x, y)=0$ and $g(x, y)=0$. Now any point of intersection lies by definition on both curves, and therefore its co-ordinates satisfy *both* equations simultaneously. So if the point of intersection is denoted by (x_i, y_i) then we have

$$f(x_i, y_i)=0$$

$$g(x_i, y_i)=0$$

simultaneously. Solution of this pair of simultaneous equations gives the co-ordinates of the intersection point (or points—there may be more than one pair of values possible for (x_i, y_i)).

As an example:

Where does the circle $x^2+y^2=5$ intersect the rectangular hyperbola $xy=1$? If the point of intersection is (x_i, y_i) then we have:

$$x_i^2+y_i^2=5 \quad \text{(since } (x_i, y_i) \text{ lies on the circle)} \tag{8.1}$$

and at the same time:

$$x_i y_i=1 \quad \text{(since } (x_i, y_i) \text{ lies on the rectangular hyperbola)} \tag{8.2}$$

From (8.2),

$$y_i=1/x_i$$

Substituting for y_i in (8.1), we have

$$x_i^2+\frac{1}{x_i^2}=5$$

i.e. $x_i^4-5x_i^2+1=0$

(cross multiplying by x_i^2).

This is a quadratic in x_i^2, with solution:

$$x_i^2=\frac{5\pm\sqrt{(25-4)}}{2}=\frac{5+\sqrt{21}}{2} \quad \text{or} \quad \frac{5-\sqrt{21}}{2}$$

(cf. Section 1.10.2)

i.e. $x_i^2=4\cdot89$ or $0\cdot21$.

There are thus *four* possible values for x_i, namely: $\pm\sqrt{4\cdot89}$ and $\pm\sqrt{0\cdot21}$

i.e. $2\cdot21,\ -2\cdot21,\ 0\cdot47,\ -0\cdot47$

with corresponding values of y_i (from either (8.1) or (8.2)—but (8.2) is easier):

$$0\cdot45,\ -0\cdot45,\ 2\cdot13,\ -2\cdot13.$$

So our analysis tells us immediately that the two curves meet in four points, and also locates them for us exactly:

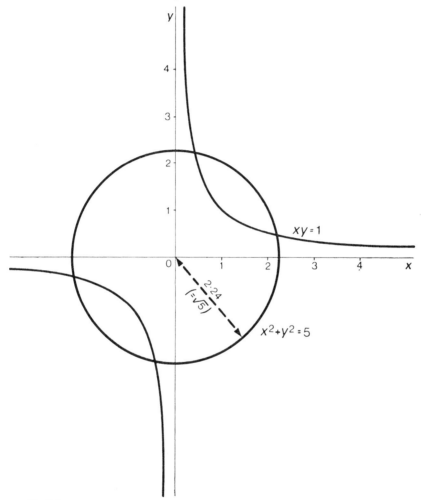

Fig 8.6

It is not always as straightforward as this, but the idea remains the same.

8.3   Points on a curve

An important corollary to our previous development is that if the equation of a curve is satisfied by the co-ordinates of some particular point, then the point

H

lies on the curve. For example, the point

$$(3, 2)$$

lies on the curve defined by

$$x^3 + 3x - 9y^2 = 0$$

because if we substitute $x = 3$, $y = 2$ in the equation of the curve, we get

$$3^3 + 3 * 3 - 9 * 2^2$$

which equals 0. In other words, (3, 2) is a point whose co-ordinates are related in the way demanded by the equation of the curve.

8.4   Three useful results

8.4.1   Division of a line in a given ratio

Situations often occur in which we have to find the point which will divide a given line segment into two parts whose lengths are in a given ratio. Suppose the line is PQ, where P has co-ordinates (x_1, y_1) and Q, (x_2, y_2). The problem then is to find R on PQ such that $PR : RQ$ has a given value—say $k_1 : k_2$ (Fig 8.7a).

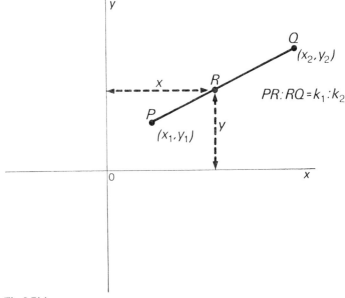

Fig 8.7(a)

If we denote the co-ordinates of the point R by (x, y), then it can be shown that

$$x = \frac{k_2 x_1 + k_1 x_2}{k_1 + k_2}$$

$$y = \frac{k_2 y_1 + k_1 y_2}{k_1 + k_2}$$

(8.3)

These are known as *Joachimsthal's Ratio-Formulae.*

Example:

Find the co-ordinates of the point which divides in the ratio $5:4$ the line joining $(-1, 2)$ and $(3, 5)$

In terms of (8.3), we have

$$k_1 = 5 \qquad k_2 = 4 \qquad x_1 = -1 \qquad y_1 = 2 \qquad x_2 = 3 \qquad y_2 = 5$$

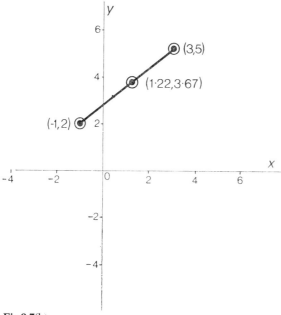

Fig 8.7(b)

and therefore

$$x = \frac{4 * (-1) + 5 * 3}{4 + 5} = \frac{11}{9} = 1 \cdot 22$$

$$y = \frac{4 * 2 + 5 * 5}{4 + 5} = \frac{11}{3} = 3 \cdot 67$$

(cf. Fig 8.7b).

8.4.2   Distance between two points

If (x_1, y_1) and (x_2, y_2) are any two points, then the distance between them is

$$d = \sqrt{\{(x_1 - x_2)^2 + (y_1 - y_2)^2\}} \qquad \text{(Section 7.2.1)}$$

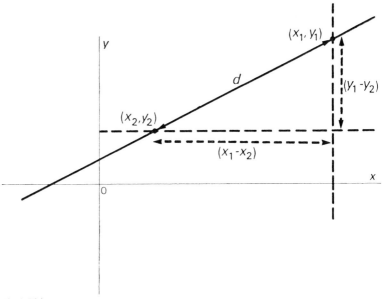

Fig 8.8(a)

Example:

The distance between the points (1, 3) and (6, 4) is

$$\sqrt{\{(1 - 6)^2 + (3 - 4)^2\}} = \sqrt{26} \div 5 \cdot 1$$

(cf. Fig 8.8(b)).

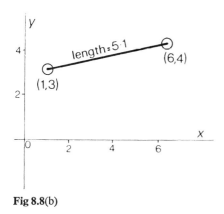

Fig 8.8(b)

8.4.3   Area of a triangle

The area of the triangle with vertices (x_1, y_1), (x_2, y_2) and (x_3, y_3) is given by:

$$\text{Area} = \tfrac{1}{2} * \text{the modulus of the determinant} \begin{vmatrix} x_1 & y_1 & 1 \\ x_2 & y_2 & 1 \\ x_3 & y_3 & 1 \end{vmatrix}$$

$$= \tfrac{1}{2} * | x_1(y_2 - y_3) - y_1(x_2 - x_3) + x_2 y_3 - x_3 y_2 |$$

(This is a generalization of the comment in Section 7.9, in which one of the points is the origin $(0, 0)$.)

Examples:

(i) The area of the triangle with vertices $(1, 4)$, $(2, 1)$ and $(3, 0)$ is the modulus of

$$\tfrac{1}{2} * \begin{vmatrix} 1 & 4 & 1 \\ 2 & 1 & 1 \\ 3 & 0 & 1 \end{vmatrix} = 1$$

(ii) The area of the triangle with vertices $(0, 5)$, $(7, -1)$ and $(-7, 11)$ is the modulus of

$$\tfrac{1}{2} * \begin{vmatrix} 0 & 5 & 1 \\ 7 & -1 & 1 \\ -7 & 11 & 1 \end{vmatrix} = 0$$

Now the only way in which the area of a triangle can be zero is if the three vertices lie on the same straight line. Our three points do, in fact, as can be shown by plotting them (see Fig 8.10b).

Thus a test for the collinearity of three points is that if they have co-ordinates (x_1, y_1), (x_2, y_2), (x_3, y_3) then

$$\begin{vmatrix} x_1 & y_1 & 1 \\ x_2 & y_2 & 1 \\ x_3 & y_3 & 1 \end{vmatrix} = 0$$

Care must be taken, however, in applying this or other techniques in practice, especially if a digital computer is being used, as round-off errors can lead to a wrong result. The value must either be computed exactly or else a tolerance worked out such that if the area as computed is less than this tolerance, the area will be taken as zero.

8.5   The straight line

We have already met various forms of the equation of a straight line when discussing functions (Section 3.10). The general form of the equation of a straight line is

$$lx + my + n = 0 \tag{8.4}$$

or its equivalent.

However, there are special cases and different forms of this equation, each with a different geometrical meaning. These we now discuss without proofs; for these the reader is referred to standard texts (e.g. Sommerville (1949), Kindle (1950), Protter & Morrey (1966)).

8.5.1   Special cases

(i) If $l=0$, the equation (8.4) becomes

$$my + n = 0$$

i.e. $y = -\dfrac{n}{m}$

This represents *a straight line parallel to the x-axis.*

Example:

$2y + 5 = 0$ (Fig 8.9).

(ii) If $m=0$, equation (8.4) becomes

$$lx + n = 0$$

i.e. $x = -n/l$

This represents a line parallel to the y-axis.

Example:

$3x - 4 = 0$ (Fig 8.9)

(iii) If $n = 0$, the equation becomes
$$lx + my = 0$$

The point $(0, 0)$ satisfies this equation, for any values of m and n, and therefore any equation of this form represents *a line through the origin.*

Example:

$2x - 5y = 0$ (Fig 8.9)

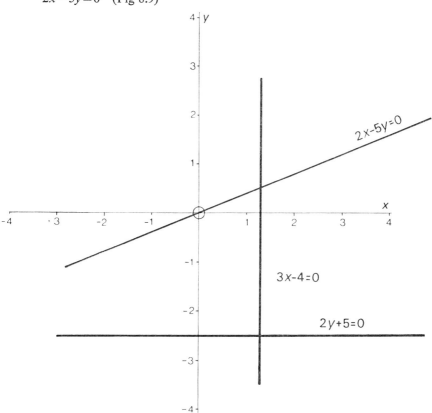

Fig 8.9

8.5.2   *Special forms*

(i) Equation of a straight line through two given points

If the points are (x_1, y_1) and (x_2, y_2) then the equation is

$$\frac{y-y_1}{y_2-y_1}=\frac{x-x_1}{x_2-x_1}\qquad (y_2\neq y_1, x_2\neq x_1)$$

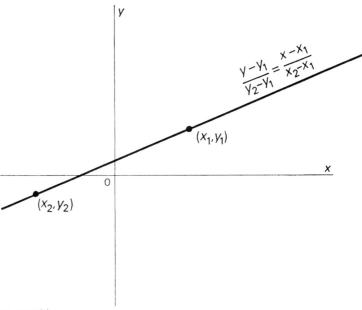

Fig 8.10(a)

N.B. If either $y_2 \doteq y_1$ or $x_2 \doteq x_1$ (Section 1.7.1), this form can lead to computational difficulties.

Example:

The straight line through the points

$$(0, 5) \quad \text{and} \quad (7, -1) \quad \text{is}$$

$$\frac{y-5}{-1-5}=\frac{x-0}{7-0}$$

i.e. $7y+6x-35=0$

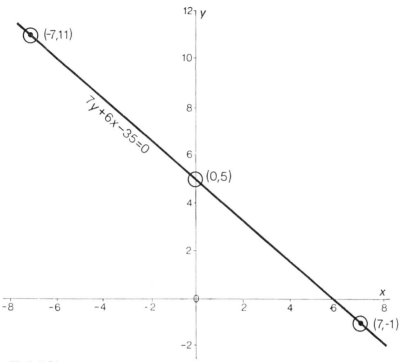

Fig 8.10(b)

The point $(-7, 11)$ also lies on this line (cf. Example (ii), Section 8.4.3) since $7 * 11 + 6 * (-7) - 35 = 0$.

If $y_1 = y_2$, the equation of the line is $y = y_1$, while if $x_1 = x_2$, the equation is $x = x_1$. (Can you see why this should be so? If you cannot, try drawing the lines.)

(ii) Equation of a straight line through a given point in a given direction

Let the direction be specified by the angle θ which the line makes with the x-axis (Figs 8.11a and 8.11b).

The equation is

$$(y - y_1) \cos \theta = (x - x_1) \sin \theta$$

or alternatively (if $\theta \neq 90°$)

$$y - y_1 = (x - x_1) \tan \theta$$

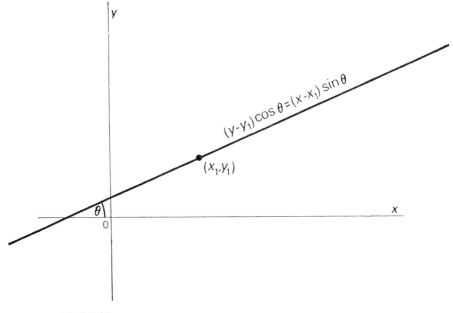

$(y-y_1)\cos\theta = (x-x_1)\sin\theta$

(x_1, y_1)

θ

Fig 8.11(a)

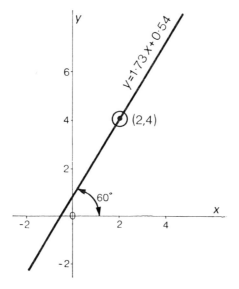

$y = 1.73x + 0.54$

$(2,4)$

60°

Fig 8.11(b)

Example:

The line through (2, 4) making an angle of 60° with the x-axis is

$$(y-4)=(x-2)\sqrt{3} \qquad (\tan 60° = \sqrt{3}\text{—see Appendix, page 398})$$

i.e. $\qquad y=1\cdot73x+0\cdot54$

(Fig 8.11b).

   Notice that although this is not exactly in the form (8.4), it can be thrown into that form by bringing all the terms over to the left-hand side of the = sign. The important thing is that the equation should be linear in x and y, i.e. contain no powers or cross-products of the variables.

(iii) The form $y=mx+c$

This is a frequently-occurring form of straight-line equation. It represents a line which makes an angle arctan (m) with the x-axis and cuts the y-axis at the point $(0, c)$. A useful property of this form is that as we move along the line the change in $y=m$ times the change in x.

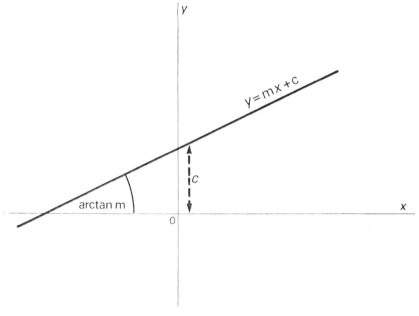

Fig 8.12(a)

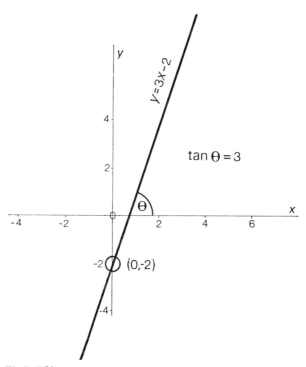

Fig 8.12(b)

The parameter m, in this form of the straight-line equation, is called the *slope* of the line. It is the tangent of the angle which the line makes with the positive x-axis.

Example:

$$y = 3x - 2$$

is a line with slope 3 passing through the point $(0, -2)$ (Fig 8.12b). Note that as a line becomes parallel or nearly parallel to the y-axis, $m \to \infty$. This will cause trouble when using a computer.

(iv) The 'intercept' form

The intercept of a line with a co-ordinate axis is defined as the *signed* distance between the origin of co-ordinates and the point of intersection of the line with the axis. (It follows that the parameter c in (iii) above is the intercept of the line $y = mx + c$ on the y-axis.)

Consider the line which makes an intercept a with the x-axis, and b with the y-axis:

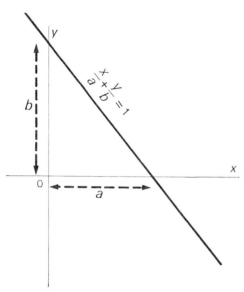

Fig 8.13(a)

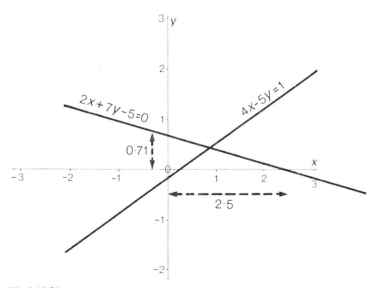

Fig 8.13(b)

Its equation is

$$\frac{x}{a}+\frac{y}{b}=1$$

(This can be deduced from (i) above, since the line passes through the points $(a, 0)$ and $(0, b)$.) It follows that the general straight line $lx+my+n=0$ has intercepts $-n/l$ on the x-axis and $-n/m$ on the y-axis. This is usually the quickest way to draw the line provided that the points of interception are far enough apart (cf. Section 3.10.3).

Examples: (see Fig 8.13b)

(i) The line

$$4x-5y=1$$

has intercepts $\frac{1}{4}$, $-\frac{1}{5}$ on the x- and y-axes respectively.

(ii) The line

$$2x+7y-5=0$$

has intercepts $2\cdot5$, $0\cdot71$ on the x- and y-axes respectively.

(v) The 'perpendicular' form

This is a rather neat form. Suppose we have a line such that the length of the perpendicular from the origin $=p$, say, and this perpendicular makes an angle α, say, with the x-axis (Fig 8.14). Then the equation of the line is

$$x*\cos\alpha+y*\sin\alpha=p$$

8.5.2.1

All the various forms (8.4) and (i)–(v) above can be turned into one another. For instance, if we have a line in the form

$$Ax+By+C=0$$

then dividing across by $\sqrt{(A^2+B^2)}$ gives

$$\frac{A}{\sqrt{(A^2+B^2)}}x+\frac{B}{\sqrt{(A^2+B^2)}}y+\frac{C}{\sqrt{(A^2+B^2)}}=0$$

Now $\frac{A}{\sqrt{(A^2+B^2)}}$

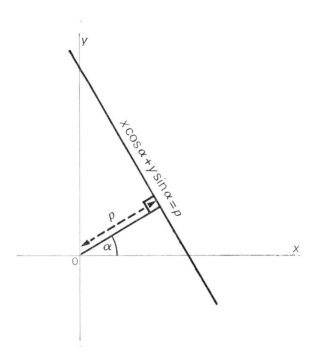

Fig 8.14

and $\dfrac{B}{\sqrt{(A^2+B^2)}}$

can be regarded as the cosine and sine respectively of some angle, since the sum of their squares $=1$, and they are each ≤ 1.

If we call this angle α, we have

$$x \cos \alpha + y \sin \alpha - p = 0$$

writing $-p$ for

$$\dfrac{C}{\sqrt{(A^2+B^2)}}.$$

(N.B. It may be that

$$\dfrac{C}{\sqrt{(A^2+B^2)}}$$

is positive, apparently giving p negative. In this case $-\sqrt{(A^2+B^2)}$ must be used).

Example:

A straight probe is being inserted into the centre of a tumour. This centre is taken to be the origin of a co-ordinate system, and it is planned to pass the probe through a guide point whose co-ordinates are $(7\cdot5\ \text{cm},\ 12\cdot0\ \text{cm})$. At what angle to the x-axis should the probe be inserted?

Since it is to pass through the points $(0, 0)$ and $(7\cdot5, 12)$, the equation of the line of the probe will be

$$\frac{y}{12}=\frac{x}{7\cdot5} \qquad \text{(form (i))}$$

i.e. $\quad y=\dfrac{12}{7\cdot5}x$

$\qquad\ \ =1\cdot6x$

This is of the form $y=mx+c$ with $c=0$.

The angle θ is such that $\tan\theta=1\cdot6$, i.e. $\theta=\arctan 1\cdot6$. From tables (Appendix 441), we find that $\theta=58°$.

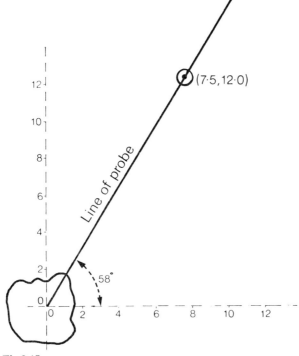

Fig 8.15

8.5.3   Intersection of straight lines

The ideas previously illustrated with respect to intersection of curves apply to straight lines also, of course. Consider the two lines

$$lx + my + n = 0$$
$$Lx + My + N = 0$$

(8.5)

(We will tend to use this form of the straight line, because it is the most general form; the results for the special forms can easily be deduced.)

The point of intersection of these lines—there can only be one, of course—is the solution of the pair of simultaneous equations (8.5).

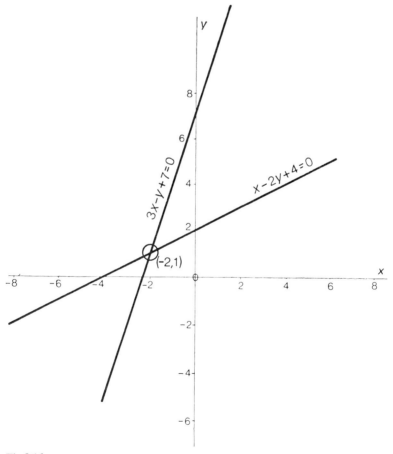

Fig 8.16

This is

$$x = \frac{mN - Mn}{lM - Lm}$$

$$y = -\frac{lN - Ln}{lM - Lm} \qquad \text{(don't forget the negative sign!)}$$

Example:

The two lines

$$3x - y + 7 = 0$$

$$x - 2y + 4 = 0$$

intersect in the point

$$x = \frac{-1 * 4 + 2 * 7}{3 * (-2) - 1 * (-1)} = -2$$

$$y = -\frac{3 * 4 - 1 * 7}{3 * (-2) - 1 * (-1)} = 1$$

(Fig 8.16).

8.5.4   Angles between lines

An important calculation associated with any pair of straight lines is to find the angle at which they intersect. Consider two lines (Figs 8.17a and 8.17b).

Now it is known from considerations of Euclidean geometry that if the angles θ, θ_1, and θ_2 are as shown in Fig 8.17a, then

$$\theta = \theta_2 - \theta_1 \tag{8.6}$$

None of our forms of straight-line equation deal directly with the angles of intersection, θ_1 and θ_2, of the lines with the x-axis, but they do deal with the *tangents* of these angles, i.e. the slopes. From (8.6) we have

$$\tan \theta = \tan (\theta_2 - \theta_1)$$

$$= \frac{\tan \theta_2 - \tan \theta_1}{1 + \tan \theta_2 \tan \theta_1} \qquad \text{(Section 6.13.1)} \tag{8.7}$$

So if our lines are, e.g.

$$y = m_1 x + c_1 \quad \text{where} \quad m_1 = \tan \theta_1$$

$$y = m_2 x + c_2 \quad \text{where} \quad m_2 = \tan \theta_2$$

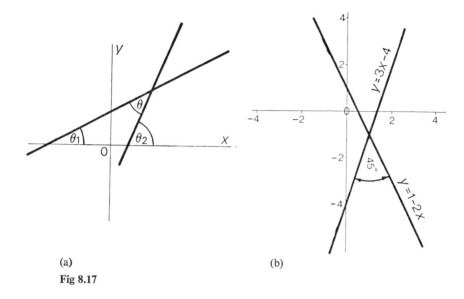

(a)   (b)

Fig 8.17

then from (8.7)

$$\tan \theta = \frac{m_2 - m_1}{1 + m_2 m_1}$$

and therefore

$$\theta = \arctan \left(\frac{m_2 - m_1}{1 + m_2 m_1} \right)$$

Example:

The lines

$$y = 3x - 4$$
$$y = 1 - 2x$$

intersect at an angle of 45°, since

$$\tan \theta = \frac{-2 - 3}{1 + (-2) * 3} = 1$$

(cf. Fig 8.17b)

8.5.5   *Parallel lines*

If two lines are parallel, they have the same slope, i.e. $m_1 = m_2$.

Examples:

(i) The lines
$$y=2x-5$$
$$y=2x+3$$
are parallel (Fig 8.18).

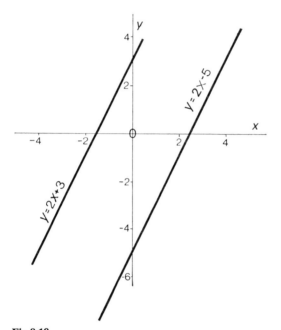

Fig 8.18

(ii) The lines
$$4x-3y+1=0$$
$$4x-3y+17=0$$
are parallel.

(iii) The lines
$$10x-14y+1=0$$
$$5x-7y+16=0$$
are parallel.

8.5.6 Perpendicular lines

By definition, the angle of intersection of perpendicular lines is 90°. From (8.7) this means that $\tan \theta \to \infty$. Now

$$\tan \theta = \frac{\tan \theta_2 - \tan \theta_1}{1 + \tan \theta_2 \tan \theta_1}$$

becomes infinite when

$$1 + \tan \theta_2 \tan \theta_1 = 0$$

or in terms of slopes, when

$$1 + m_1 m_2 = 0 \quad \text{i.e.} \qquad m_1 m_2 = -1$$

In words: *the product of the slopes of perpendicular lines* $= -1$.

There is a corollary to this: if we have a line

$$y = mx + c$$

then any line perpendicular to it must be of the form

$$y = -\frac{1}{m} x + c'$$

$$\text{(because} \quad m * \left(-\frac{1}{m}\right) = -1)$$

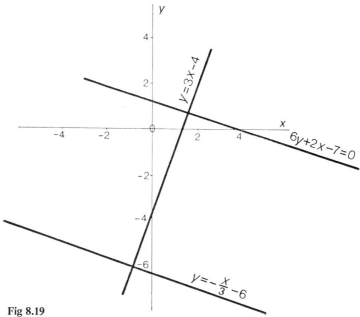

Fig 8.19

Examples:

(i) $y=3x-4$ is perpendicular to $y=-\dfrac{x}{3}-6$

and to $6y+2x-7=0$ (Fig. 8.19).

(ii) To find the line through the point $(-5, 2)$ which is perpendicular to

$y=4x-5$.

The required line must be of the form

$$y=-\frac{x}{4}+c$$

Since it passes through $(-5, 2)$, this point must satisfy the equation
i.e.

$$2=-\left(\frac{-5}{4}\right)+c$$

Hence

$$c=2-\frac{5}{4}=\frac{3}{4}$$

and the required line is

$$y=-\frac{x}{4}+\frac{3}{4}$$

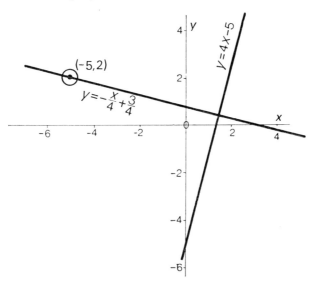

Fig 8.20

8.5.7   *Perpendicular distance of a point from a line*

We state the following result without proof; it follows from consideration of the geometry of the situation when we use the form

$$x \cos \alpha + y \sin \alpha - p = 0 \qquad \text{(Section 8.5.2)}:$$

The perpendicular distance of the point (x_A, y_A) from the line

$$lx + my + n = 0$$

is
$$\frac{lx_A + my_A + n}{\sqrt{(l^2 + m^2)}} \qquad (8.8)$$

The result (8.8) can be used to distinguish between regions of space on opposite sides of a line, for it can be shown that $lx_A + my_A + n$ divides the space in which the line lies into two regions: (1) the region for which all points (x_A, y_A) are such as to make (8.8) positive, which since $\sqrt{(l^2 + m^2)}$ is positive, means the region containing all points (x_A, y_A) such that $lx_A + my_A + n$ is >0; (2) the region for which all points (x_A, y_A) makes (8.8) <0, i.e. $lx_A + my_A + n < 0$. They can be regarded as separated by the region of points (x_A, y_A) such that $lx_A + my_A + n = 0$, i.e. the straight line we started with.

Thus when the co-ordinates of points on the same side of the line

$$lx + my + n = 0$$

are substituted for x and y they will give values with the same sign, while points on opposite sides will give values of opposite signs.

Example (Fig 8.21):

The points $(4, 1)$ and $(-3, 6)$ are on the same side of the line

$$x + 4y + 3 = 0$$

and on the opposite side to the point $(-6, -4)$

For $4 + 4 * 1 + 3 = 11 > 0$

$-3 + 4 * 6 + 3 = 24 > 0$

$-6 + 4 * (-4) + 3 = -19 < 0$

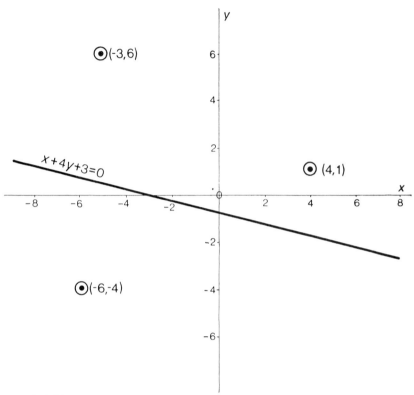

Fig 8.21

8.6   Change of axes and transformation of co-ordinates

In situations where measurements are considered relative to more than one frame of reference (e.g. in radiotherapy dose calculations) the co-ordinates of a point may be known with reference to one set of axes but be required relative to some other set. There are two special cases, which can be combined into the general case.

8.6.1   Change of origin, axes parallel to the original axes

This is also called *translation of axes*.

The problem is, if the co-ordinates of a point P relative to axes OX, OY are (x, y), to determine them relative to $O'X'$, $O'Y'$, where $O'X'$ is parallel to OX,

$O'Y'$ parallel to OY (in which situation OX', OY' are called *parallel axes* to OX, OY):

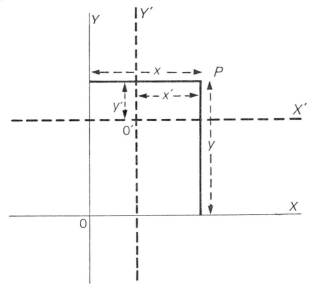

Fig 8.22

That the co-ordinates will be different relative to the new axes will be clear from Fig 8.22. To find them, suppose that the co-ordinates of the point O' are (h, k) relative to the 'old' axes OX, OY (Fig 8.23a). Then it can be shown that relative to $O'X', O'Y'$ the co-ordinates of P are $(x-h, y-k)$.

In other words, if we refer to the co-ordinates of P in the frame $O'X', O'Y'$ as (x', y'), then

$$x' = x - h$$
$$y' = y - k$$
(8.9)

Example   (cf. Fig 8.23b)

The co-ordinates of the point $(3, -4)$ relative to parallel axes through the point $(7, 1)$ are $(3-7, -4-1)$, i.e. $(-4, -5)$.

Equations (8.9) express the new co-ordinates in terms of the old ones; however, expressing the old co-ordinates in terms of the new is often just as useful (v.i. Section 8.9):

$$x = x' + h$$
$$y = y' + k$$
(8.10)

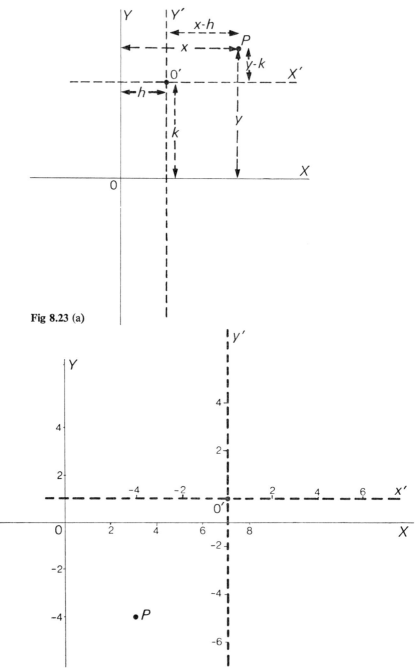

Fig 8.23 (a)

Fig 8.23(b) The co-ordinates of P are $(3, -4)$ relative to OX, OY and $(-4, -5)$ relative to OX', OY'.

8.6.2 *Rotation of axes without change of origin (rotation about a fixed point)*

In this case, the 'new' axes have the same origin as the 'old' ones, but are inclined at an angle to them. The effect is as though the axes had been rotated around the origin.

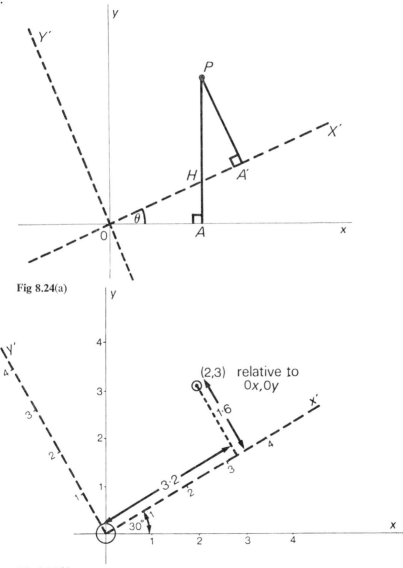

Fig 8.24(a)

Fig 8.24(b)

In Fig 8.24a, OX and OY are the 'old' axes, OX' and OY' the 'new' ones. The angle θ is the amount by which the system OX, OY would have to be rotated to bring it into coincidence with OX', OY'. If P is any point, and PA is perpendicular to OX, PA' perpendicular to OX' (Fig 8.24a), then the lengths OA, AP are the co-ordinates of P relative to OX, OY, and the lengths OA', AP' are the co-ordinates of P relative to OX', OY'. If we refer to (OA, AP) as (x, y) and to $(OA', A'P)$ as (x', y'), then the relationship between them is as follows:

$$x' = x \cos \theta + y \sin \theta \tag{8.11}$$
$$y' = -x \sin \theta + y \cos \theta \tag{8.12}$$

The reverse of this relationship is:

$$x = x' \cos \theta - y' \sin \theta \tag{8.13}$$
$$y = x' \sin \theta + y' \cos \theta \tag{8.14}$$

Example:

The co-ordinates of the point $(2, 3)$ relative to axes rotated through $30°$ are

$$(2 * \cos 30° + 3 * \sin 30°, \; -2 * \sin 30° + 3 * \cos 30°)$$

i.e. $(3·2, 1·6)$.

(See Fig 8.24b).

8.6.3   Matrix representation

The results (8.11)–(8.14) can be expressed in matrix form, a technique which is very useful for digital computer work. We have:

$$\begin{pmatrix} x' \\ y' \end{pmatrix} = \begin{pmatrix} \cos \theta & \sin \theta \\ -\sin \theta & \cos \theta \end{pmatrix} * \begin{pmatrix} x \\ y \end{pmatrix}$$

or alternatively

$$\begin{pmatrix} x \\ y \end{pmatrix} = \begin{pmatrix} \cos \theta & -\sin \theta \\ \sin \theta & \cos \theta \end{pmatrix} * \begin{pmatrix} x' \\ y' \end{pmatrix}$$

Successive rotations are then represented by successive matrix multiplications; e.g. referring again to Fig 8.24a, if x'', y'' represent the co-ordinates of P in a frame of reference further rotated through ϕ relative to OX', OY', then

$$\begin{pmatrix} x'' \\ y'' \end{pmatrix} = \begin{pmatrix} \cos \phi & \sin \phi \\ -\sin \phi & \cos \phi \end{pmatrix} * \begin{pmatrix} x' \\ y' \end{pmatrix}$$

$$= \begin{pmatrix} \cos \phi & \sin \phi \\ -\sin \phi & \cos \phi \end{pmatrix} * \begin{pmatrix} \cos \theta & \sin \theta \\ -\sin \theta & \cos \theta \end{pmatrix} * \begin{pmatrix} x \\ y \end{pmatrix} \tag{8.15}$$

giving the final co-ordinates in terms of the initial ones.

N.B. If we multiply the two trigonometric matrices together in 8.15, we obtain

$$\begin{pmatrix} x'' \\ y'' \end{pmatrix} = \begin{pmatrix} \cos(\phi+\theta) & \sin(\phi+\theta) \\ -\sin(\phi+\theta) & \cos(\phi+\theta) \end{pmatrix} * \begin{pmatrix} x \\ y \end{pmatrix}$$

which is to be expected, since the final axis system is at an angle $(\phi+\theta)$ to the system OX, OY.

8.6.4   General transformation of co-ordinates

The results obtained in the previous sections can be combined. Suppose our 'new' axes are $O'X', O'Y'$, where O' is the new origin and the axes $O'X', O'Y'$ are inclined at an angle θ to the axes OX, OY respectively (Fig 8.25a):

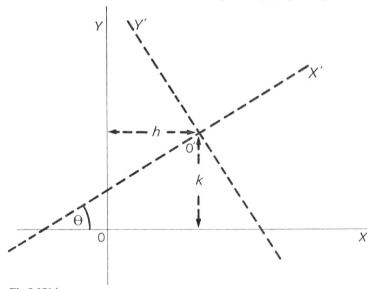

Fig 8.25(a)

If the co-ordinates of O' are (h, k) relative to OX, OY then with the same notation as before, we have:

$$\begin{pmatrix} x' \\ y' \end{pmatrix} = \begin{pmatrix} \cos\theta & \sin\theta \\ -\sin\theta & \cos\theta \end{pmatrix} * \begin{pmatrix} x-h \\ y-k \end{pmatrix} \tag{8.16}$$

If we write

$$\mathbf{X'} = \begin{pmatrix} x' \\ y' \end{pmatrix} \qquad\qquad \mathbf{X} = \begin{pmatrix} x-h \\ y-k \end{pmatrix}$$

and $T = \begin{pmatrix} \cos\theta & \sin\theta \\ -\sin\theta & \cos\theta \end{pmatrix}$

then (8.16) can be written

$$X' = T * X \tag{8.17}$$

Cross pre-multiplying (8.17) by T^{-1}, the inverse of T, we have, formally,

$$T^{-1} * X' = X,$$

i.e. (example ii, Section 7.7.2)

$$\begin{pmatrix} \cos\theta & -\sin\theta \\ \sin\theta & \cos\theta \end{pmatrix} * \begin{pmatrix} x' \\ y' \end{pmatrix} = \begin{pmatrix} x-h \\ y-k \end{pmatrix}, \tag{8.18}$$

another form of the relationship between old and new co-ordinates.

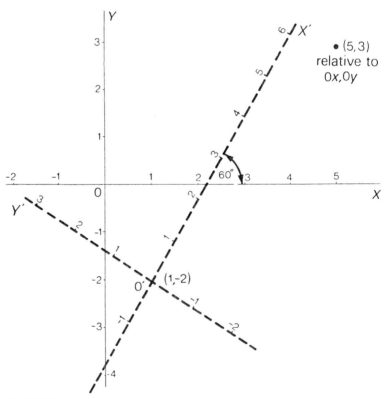

Fig 8.25(b)

Example: (cf. Fig 8.25b)

The co-ordinates of the point (5, 3) relative to axes with origin (1, -2) and inclined at an angle of $60°$ to the old axes are:

$$\begin{pmatrix} x' \\ y' \end{pmatrix} = \begin{pmatrix} \cos 60° & \sin 60° \\ -\sin 60° & \cos 60° \end{pmatrix} * \begin{pmatrix} 5-1 \\ 3-(-2) \end{pmatrix}$$

$$= \begin{pmatrix} 0\cdot500 & 0\cdot866 \\ -0\cdot866 & 0\cdot500 \end{pmatrix} * \begin{pmatrix} 4 \\ 5 \end{pmatrix}$$

$$= \begin{pmatrix} 6\cdot33 \\ -0\cdot96 \end{pmatrix}$$

8.6.5 *Linear transformations*

The relations (8.9)–(8.18) are said to be *linear* in (x, y) and (x', y'), meaning that they contain only the first powers of the variables and not any higher or lower powers or products such as $x'y'$, x^3y, etc. They are examples of *linear transformations*, whose general form is

$$x' = ax + by$$

$$y' = cx + dy$$

where a, b, c, d are constants. Such forms can cover changes of scale as well as rotation and translation (cf. Section 7.7.4, for example).

8.7   Polar co-ordinates

Other co-ordinate systems besides the Cartesian are in use for special purposes; in particular, situations in which there is *rotation round a fixed point* or geometrical situations in which numbers of lines emanate from a fixed point are often best described by *polar* co-ordinates.

Consider a point P, and a fixed line OX through a fixed point O:

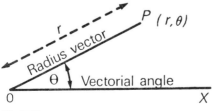

Fig 8.26

If we draw the line OP, then the position of P is determined if we know the angle XOP and the distance OP. The length OP is called the *radius vector*, and is generally denoted by r; the angle XOP is called the *vectorial angle*, and indicated by θ. We then refer to P as the point (r, θ). Note that as with Cartesian co-ordinates, we still need *two* co-ordinates to fix a point. The Greek letter ρ is sometimes used instead of r to denote the radius vector.

θ is considered positive if measured from OX in an anticlockwise direction; r is always considered positive.

Polar co-ordinates can be a very clumsy system to use except when there is a fixed point situation; for example the polar equation of the straight line through the points (r_1, θ_1) and (r_2, θ_2) is

$$r_1 r_2 \sin(\theta_2 - \theta_1) + r_2 r \sin(\theta - \theta_2) + r_1 r \sin(\theta_1 - \theta) = 0$$

But they have their uses; the equations of closed curves (e.g. a circle) are mostly easier to deal with in polar co-ordinates than in Cartesian, and for instance in arc therapy, as used in radiation treatment planning, where a radioactive source is rotated in an arc of a circle with a tumour in the patient as centre, a polar co-ordinate system with the tumour as centre is sometimes used for describing the patient and the beam positions.

Example:

The polar co-ordinates of the beam axis entry point in the cross-sectional outline of a patient undergoing irradiation are $(6, 60°)$ relative to the tumour centre as origin (Fig 8.27); the axis passes through the centre. What are the co-ordinates of the point $(4, 45°)$ when referred to the Cartesian system of an isodose chart, with origin the entry point, positive y-axis along the beam axis into the patient, and x-axis forming a left-handed system with it? (Left-handed co-ordinate systems are often used in radiotherapy calculations.)

Although this problem can be dealt with by axis transformation, it is easier to solve it by using the geometry of the situation. Consider Fig 8.27 in which EX, EY are the left-handed set of axes through the beam axis entry point E, and P is the point with co-ordinates $(4, 45°)$ relative to the fixed line (OZ). If we draw perpendiculars PK, PH to EX, EY respectively, then their lengths will be the co-ordinates of P relative to EX, EY.

Now it can be seen that

(a) $PH = OP \sin(\angle POH)$ (cf. Section 6.6)

(b) $PK = HE$ (because $PHEK$ is a rectangle)

$= OE - OH$

$= OE - OP \cos(\angle POH)$ (Section 6.6)

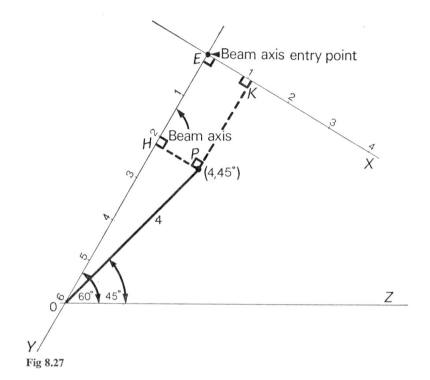

Fig 8.27

But: $OP=4$

$OE=6$

$\angle POH = 60° - 45° = 15°.$

Whence $PH = 4 * \sin 15° = 1\cdot04$

$PK = 6 - 4 * \cos 15° = 2\cdot14$

and these are the required co-ordinates.

8.8   Relation between Cartesian and polar co-ordinates of a point relative to a common origin and axis

Consider a Cartesian frame OX, OY. If we take OX as the reference line for a polar system, then the (x, y) and (r, θ) co-ordinates of any point P are related as follows:

$x = r * \cos \theta$

$y = r * \sin \theta$ (see Fig. 8.28a) or conversely

$$r = \sqrt{(x^2 + y^2)}$$

$$\theta = \text{arc tan } (y/x)$$

(where the value to be taken for θ depends on the quadrant in which the point (x, y) lies—see Appendix page 408).

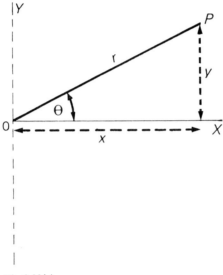

Fig 8.28(a)

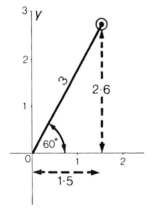

Fig 8.28 (b)

Example:

The Cartesian co-ordinates of the point $(3, 60°)$ are

$$x = 3 * 0·5, \quad y = 3 * 0·866$$

i.e. $(1·5, 2·6)$ (see Fig. 8.28b)

8.9   Change of form under change of axes

Although the shape of any geometrical figure remains the same no matter what set of axes are used in describing its equation, the form of the equation itself will usually change if the axes change. Consider for example, the curve

$$f(x, y) = 0.$$

This is a relation between the x and y co-ordinates of every point on the curve. If we refer to new axes in which the co-ordinates of any point become (x', y') then if our transformation is

$$x = g(x', y')$$
$$y = h(x', y')$$

the equation of the curve relative to the new axes will be obtained by substituting for x and y in $f(x, y) = 0$, i.e.

$$f(g(x', y'), h(x', y')) = 0$$

Although this looks very complicated, the technique can in fact be used to *simplify* expressions. Consider, e.g. the curve

$$x^2 + 4x + y^2 - 8y + 16 = 0 \tag{8.19}$$

Not immediately recognizable perhaps; however, suppose we describe the curve relative to parallel axes through the point $(-2, 4)$—the reason for this particular choice will become apparent in a moment.

We have from Section 8.6.1:

$$x = x' - 2$$
$$y = y' + 4 \tag{8.20}$$

and therefore

$$x^2 + 4x + y^2 - 8y + 16 = 0$$

becomes

$$(x' - 2)^2 + 4(x' - 2) + (y' + 4)^2 - 8(y' + 4) + 16 = 0 \tag{8.21}$$

on substituting for x and y in terms of x' and y' from (8.20).

On multiplying out the terms, (8.21) becomes

$$x'^2 - 4x' + 4 + 4x' - 8 + y'^2 + 8y' + 16 - 8y' - 32 + 16 = 0$$

i.e. $x'^2 + y'^2 = 4$ (8.22)

This is the form of the equation of a circle (see Section 8.2) centre the origin in the x', y' system, and of radius $= 2$. Looking at it another way, we could say that

$$x^2 + 4x + y^2 - 8y + 16 = 0$$

is the equation of a circle of radius 2, centre the point $(-2, 4)$. The figure itself does not change—it cannot, since all that we are doing is using a different descriptive system to describe an unchanging object. Only our mathematical description of it alters. Note that both (8.19) and (8.22) are second-degree expressions; our transformations have not altered the degree of the equation. This is because the transformations (8.20) are linear.

In particular, under translation and rotation of axes, a first degree equation representing a straight line transforms into another first degree equation in the new co-ordinates.

These considerations will be of some importance in the sections which follow.

8.10   Curves of degree greater than one

The equation of a straight line is a first degree equation; it will always contain only terms in x and/or y (or whatever variables are being used), but no powers or products of these variables.

When we come to deal with curves, however, we find that the equations describing them are 'non-linear', i.e. they contain powers and products of the variables. Their mathematical treatment then becomes more complex. We will confine our discussion almost entirely to the case of curves whose equations are of the *second* degree, that is, they may contain terms in x^2, y^2 and xy as well as in x and y. There are two points of general interest to note, however.

First, although in general an equation of degree > 1 represents a curve, in special cases such an equation may 'degenerate' into a set of straight lines (e.g. see Section 8.10.1) Secondly, it is possible to write down equations which do not correspond to a curve at all (or to a set of lines)—in other words, an equation can be such that there is no point in the plane whose co-ordinates will satisfy it. In practice, this latter difficulty is unlikely to arise, but the theoretical possibility of its happening is the reason behind the restrictions on coefficients which we will see are imposed on some of the equations to be discussed.

8.10.1   Equations of the second degree

These are the simplest of the curves whose equations are of integer degree >1. The general equation of the second degree will contain terms in x^2, y^2, xy, x, y and a so-called *absolute term*—that is, a constant term involving neither variable; it is usually written as

$$ax^2 + 2hxy + by^2 + 2gx + 2fy + c = 0 \tag{8.23}$$

where a, h, b, f, g and c are constants, c being the absolute term. The traditional use of the factor 2 in (8.23) is due to the fact that it simplifies various algebraic procedures involving this equation.

Since the constants can have any values, in all possible combinations, it would seem at first sight that (8.23) could represent almost anything. However, just as the general equation of the first degree always represents a straight line, it can be shown that—when a curve can be drawn for it—(8.23) must represent one or other of a very limited variety of curves. This comes about from examination of the ways in which the form of the equation alters when referred to different origin and axes of co-ordinates. We have already seen (Section 8.9) how such transformations can reduce to a simpler form an equation representing a circle. Theoretical considerations along similar lines show that (8.23), when it can be drawn, must be reducible to one of the following *five* forms:

(1) $Ax^2 + 2Hxy + By^2 = 0$ $(AB - H^2 \leq 0)$

This represents a *pair of straight lines through the origin*. The two lines are

$$y - m_1 x = 0, \quad y - m_2 x = 0$$

where m_1 and m_2 are the roots of the quadratic in m

$$Bm^2 + 2Hm + A = 0$$

(hence the restriction $AB - H^2 \leq 0$, since otherwise the equation has no real roots).

Example (Fig 8.29):

$$x^2 - 3xy - 4y^2 = 0$$

corresponds to the two lines

$$y + x = 0$$

$$4y - x = 0$$

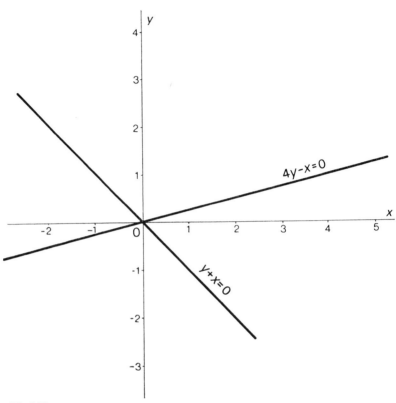

Fig 8.29

The conditions for the general equation of the second degree to represent two straight lines are given in the Appendix (page 409).

(2) $x^2 + y^2 = R^2$

This is a circle of radius R, centre the origin. We have already seen how suitable translations of axes can produce this form. The most general form of second-degree equation representing a circle is

$$ax^2 + ay^2 + 2gx + 2fy + c = 0 \quad (f^2 + g^2 - ac > 0) \tag{8.24}$$

e.g. $3x^2 + 3y^2 + 16x - 5y - 8 = 0$

In practice the coefficients of x^2 and y^2 are made $= 1$ by dividing all terms in the equation by the coefficient of x^2 and y^2, and the general equation of the circle is usually written in the form

$$x^2 + y^2 + 2gx + 2fy + c = 0 \quad (f^2 + g^2 - c > 0) \tag{8.25}$$

The characteristics of (8.24) or (8.25) are: (a) the coefficients of x^2 and y^2 are equal, (b) there is no term in xy.

In the form (8.25), the equation represents a circle centre the point $(-g, -f)$, radius $\sqrt{(f^2+g^2-c)}$ (hence the restriction that $f^2+g^2-c>0$).

Example:

$$x^2+y^2-6x+9y-4=0$$

is a circle, centre at $(3, -4\cdot5)$ and

$$\text{radius} = \sqrt{\left(9+\frac{81}{4}+4\right)}$$

$$= 5\cdot77$$

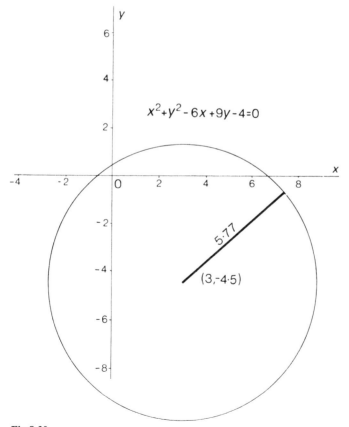

Fig 8.30

N.B. In polar co-ordinates, the equation of a circle can be very simple:

$$r = R$$

where R is the radius, and the centre is the origin of co-ordinates. The equation does not involve θ, as it is true for all values of θ.

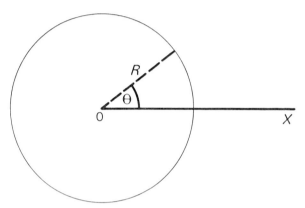

Fig 8.31

(3) $\dfrac{x^2}{A^2} + \dfrac{y^2}{B^2} = 1$

This represents an ellipse, centre the origin, with the lines of greatest and least breadth as the co-ordinate axes (Fig 8.32).

This curve has found applications in medical work; e.g. Fisher (1969) has used it as approximation to the shape of the lens capsule of the eye, and Whitney (1953) used it as an approximation to the cross-section of the human leg and arm. We have also seen it used as a representation of patient cross-section in radiotherapy—albeit not very convincingly in this case. It is also important in statistical work.

From Fig 8.32, we see that there are particular measurements of the ellipse corresponding to the parameters A and B; they are called the *semi-major axis* and *semi-minor axis* respectively. The major axis of the ellipse is therefore of length $2A$ and the minor axis $2B$.

There are two points on the major axis, which are known as the *foci* (singular: focus) of the ellipse. They are equidistant from the origin, and the distanc between them is

$$2Ae$$

where e is a parameter called the *eccentricity* of the ellipse, and defined by

$$e = \sqrt{(1 - B^2/A^2)}$$

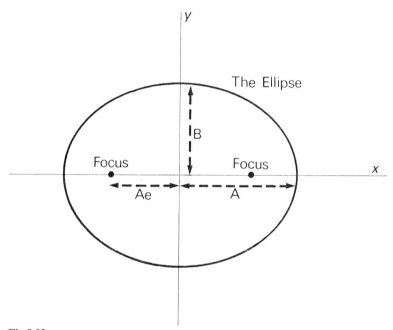

The Ellipse

Fig 8.32

It is a measure of the flattening of the ellipse; the larger e becomes, the smaller the ratio of B to A. We see that $e < 1$.

This quantity e has been used in describing the shapes of erythrocytes (*Documenta Geigy*, 6th Edition).

The circle is a special case of the ellipse for which $e = 0$.

The foci are important as a means of drawing an ellipse. One of the properties of the ellipse is that the sum of the distances of any point of it from the two foci is constant; this constant is actually $2A$, the length of the major axis. So to draw an ellipse of given major axis $2A$ and eccentricity e, set up two drawing pins at a distance $2Ae$ apart, join a thread of length $2A$ to them, and holding the thread taut use it as a drawing guide (Fig 8.33).

(N.B. To avoid having to tie the threads to the pins, make a loop of length $2A (1+e)$, loop it round the pins and use this as the guide.)

The conditions to be satisfied by the coefficients of the general equation (8.23) in order for it to represent an ellipse are rather more complicated than with a circle. They are listed in the Appendix along with the conditions for the other curves of the second degree.

N.B. The use of the symbol e for eccentricity is a mathematical convention; do not confuse it with $e = 2 \cdot 71828 \ldots$, the base of natural logarithms.

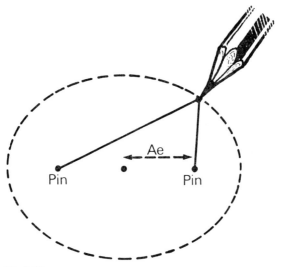

Fig 8.33

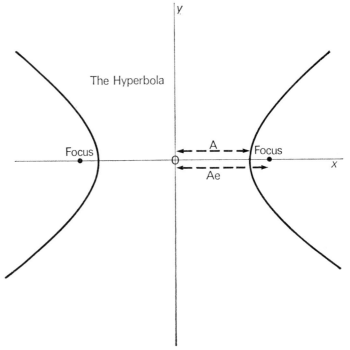

Fig 8.34

(4) $\dfrac{x^2}{A^2} - \dfrac{y^2}{B^2} = 1$

This is a *hyperbola*. Unlike the other curves represented by the second degree equation, it has two separate branches (Fig 8.34).

The parameter $2A$ corresponds to the minimum distance between the branches with the origin half way along; there is no line corresponding to the parameter B. As with the ellipse, two foci and an eccentricity are defined. The distance between the foci is again $2Ae$, but now

$$e = \sqrt{(1 + B^2/A^2)} > 1$$

To draw a hyperbola mechanically is a rather more awkward procedure than drawing an ellipse, and it is much simpler to use a desk calculator to compute values of pairs of points from the equation of the curve, along with a table of square roots if the machine does not have an automatic square root facility.

A particular type of hyperbola—the *rectangular hyperbola*—can have its equation expressed in the form $xy = c^2$, which leads to very easy plotting of variables related in this way—see Note (i) of Example 1, Section 8.10.2.

As with the ellipse, the conditions for the general equation (8.23) to represent a hyperbola are complicated (see Appendix, page 409).

(5) $y^2 = Kx$

This is a *parabola*, passing through the origin (Fig 8.35a and 8.35b).

It is symmetric about the x-axis, and is a single-branched curve defined only for positive or zero x if $K > 0$, and only for negative or zero x if $K < 0$.

This is the 'square root' curve if $K = 1$; to any value of x there then correspond the two values $y = \pm \sqrt{x}$.

The parabola has only one focus in the finite plane, at the point $(K/4, 0)$, though in purely theoretical terms, there is a second focus 'at infinity'. The focus has significance in the mechanical drawing of a parabola, and for other reasons, but as such drawing is even more awkward than with the hyperbola, we will not pursue the topic, except to remark on an interesting and useful property of the *parabolic mirror*, namely, that light rays parallel to the axis of such a mirror are reflected through the focus (Fig 8.36).

It is easiest to draw a parabola by plotting points. For positive x, y and K, the use of log/log paper leads to a straight line, since

$$\log y = \tfrac{1}{2} \log x + \tfrac{1}{2} \log K$$

The conditions for the general equation of the second degree to represent a parabola are given in the Appendix.

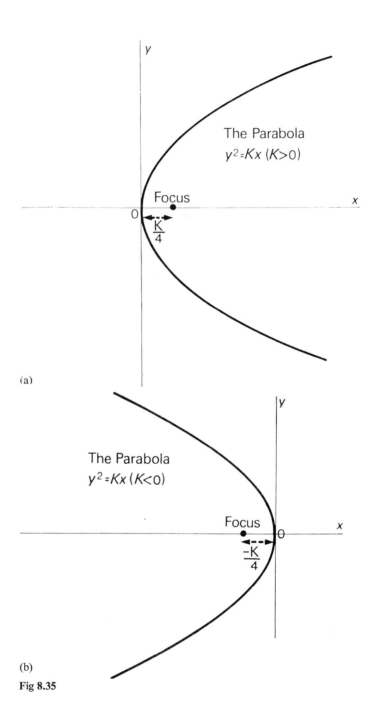

(a)

(b)

Fig 8.35

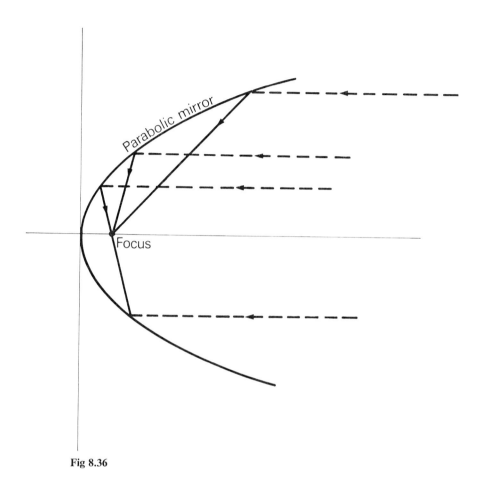

Fig 8.36

8.10.1.1

The curves (1)–(5) above can all be obtained as the boundaries of various planar cross-sections of a cone; for this reason they are called *conic sections*, or more briefly, *conics*. A great deal is known about their geometry, since they have been a subject for mathematical study since the time of the ancient Greek mathematicians. Our present discussion is not intended as other than a very brief introduction to the subject, and we will not now take it any further than relating a few more definitions, and dealing with points arising from these; for more detail the reader is referred to text-books on analytic geometry such as those mentioned in Section 8.5.

8.10.2   Asymptotes

Alone among the conic sections, the hyperbola provides a simple example of a useful geometrical concept: the *asymptote*.

In practical terms, an asymptote of a curve—when it exists, which is not always the case—provides a *straight line approximation to the long term behaviour* of the curve. Many curves and functions approach a linear form for high values of one or other variable, which then simplifies the mathematics involved.

Mathematically speaking, an asymptote of a curve is defined as a *line cutting the curve in two points 'at infinity'*; an alternative definition is that it touches or is *tangent to* the curve 'at infinity'. 'At infinity' in this context means that x and/or y are infinite.

(N.B. Not every curve which looks as though it should have an asymptote will in fact have one—e.g. a parabola has no asymptotes. Only mathematical investigation can decide in any particular case.)

Examples of asymptotes

Example 1:

Asymptotes of the hyperbola $\dfrac{x^2}{A^2} - \dfrac{y^2}{B^2} = 1$

An asymptote, if it exists, will be a straight line. If we take this to be of the form

$$y = mx + c$$

then we have to find m and c. The x co-ordinate of the point of intersection of this line with the hyperbola is found by substituting $y = mx + c$ into the equation of the hyperbola (since the co-ordinates of the point of intersection must satisfy both equations simultaneously). This gives

$$\frac{x^2}{A^2} - \frac{(mx+c)^2}{B^2} = 1$$

i.e. $(B^2 - m^2 A^2) x^2 - 2A^2 mcx - A^2 c^2 - A^2 B^2 = 0$ \hfill (8.26)

This is a quadratic in x, and there will be corresponding values of y; in other words, the straight line meets the hyperbola in *two* points. (This is a general result for all conics, since substitution of $y = mx + c$ in the general equation of the second degree (8.23) leads to a quadratic in x.) Now if the line $y = mx + c$ is to cut the hyperbola in two points 'at infinity', this means that the roots of (8.26) must both be infinite, or more precisely, must tend to infinity. It can be shown that *both the roots of a quadratic equation tend to infinity as the* *coefficients of x^2 and x simultaneously tend to zero.* Hence m and c for the asymptote must satisfy

$$B^2 - m^2 A^2 \to 0 \qquad \text{i.e.} \qquad m \to \pm B/A$$

$$2A^2 mc \to 0 \qquad \text{i.e.} \qquad c \to 0 \quad \text{(since } m \neq 0\text{)}$$

The asymptotes are therefore

$$y = \frac{B}{A} x$$

$$y = -\frac{B}{A} x$$

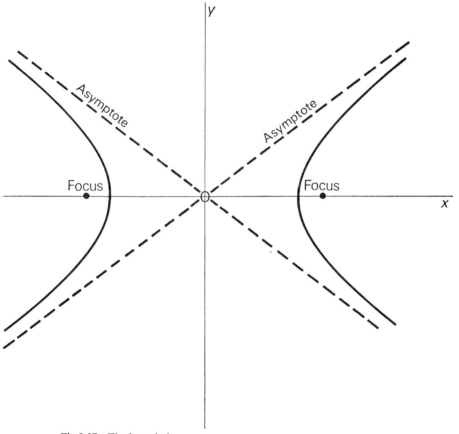

Fig 8.37 The hyperbola.

Notes:

(i) A hyperbola whose asymptotes are mutually perpendicular is called a *rectangular hyperbola* (more rarely an *equilateral hyperbola*). For such a hyperbola, $B = A$†. Now we can use the perpendicular asymptotes as an axis system; the transformation is a rotation through an angle $\theta = \arctan(B/A) = 45°$ (since $B/A = 1$) and the resulting equation is

$$xy = \frac{A^2}{2}$$

or writing $c = A/\sqrt{2}$

$$xy = c^2$$

a form used in an earlier example (Section 8.2).

This form represents a system in which the product of two variables is constant, a common practical situation.

In practice, such a relationship is probably more easily handled logarithmically:

$$\log x + \log y = 2 \log c \quad \text{(for } x, y > 0)$$

which if plotted on log/log paper will be a straight line, as with the parabola.

(ii) The use of the behaviour of the roots of the quadratic as the coefficients of x and $x^2 \to 0$ is a special case of a general technique for obtaining asymptotes of curves in general; see e.g. Frost (1960), Coolidge (1959), or Hilton (1932).

(iii) Both the equations $xy = c^2$ and $y^2 = Kx$ are particular cases of a general form which always plots for positive x, y and K as a straight line on log/log paper, namely

$$y^m = Kx^n \tag{8.27}$$

giving $m \log y = n \log x + \log K$

For a rectangular hyperbola, $m = 1$, $n = -1$; for a parabola, $m = 2$, $n = 1$. Curves of the form (8.27) are called *parabolic curves*.

Example 2

This is an example arising in a discussion by Forker (1967) on bile formation. The curve is

$$c = \frac{f^2 + Dx * (Aw/L) f}{(Aw/Ax) f + Dx * (Aw/L)} \tag{8.28}$$

---

† From the fact that the slopes are $\pm B/A$ and the condition for perpendicularity (Section 8.5.6).

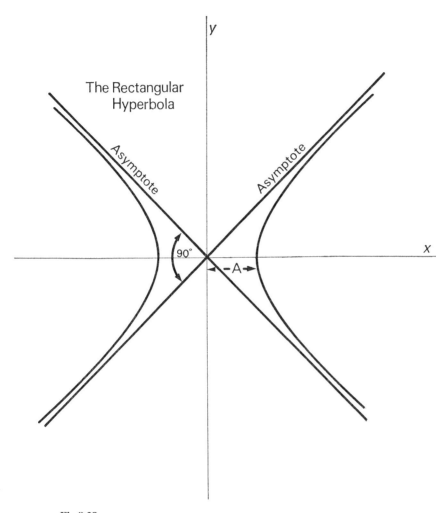

The Rectangular
Hyperbola

Asymptote

Asymptote

90°

←–A→

Fig 8.38

where **c** is the dependent variable and **f** the independent one; the other quantities are parameters. Although apparently complicated in form, it is in fact another hyperbola (cross-multiply (8.28) by $(Aw/Ax)\,\mathbf{f} + Dx * (Aw/L)$; this gives a second-degree curve involving the variables **c** and **f**. Then apply the criteria given in the Appendix).

If there is an asymptote, it will be of the form $\mathbf{c} = m\mathbf{f} + k$ and we have to determine the slope m and the intercept k. Substituting for **c** in (8.28) from

$\mathbf{c}=m\mathbf{f}+k$, we have for the $\mathbf{f}$ co-ordinate of the intersection point:

$$m\mathbf{f}+k=\frac{\mathbf{f}^2+Dx(Aw/L)\,\mathbf{f}}{(Aw/Ax)\,\mathbf{f}+Dx(Aw/L)}$$

i.e. $(m\mathbf{f}+k)\left[\dfrac{Aw}{Ax}\mathbf{f}+Dx\left(\dfrac{Aw}{L}\right)\right]=\mathbf{f}^2+Dx(Aw/L)\,\mathbf{f}$

i.e. $\mathbf{f}^2\left[m\dfrac{Aw}{Ax}-1\right]+\mathbf{f}\left[mDx\dfrac{Aw}{L}+k\dfrac{Aw}{Ax}-D\dfrac{Aw}{L}\right]+kDx\dfrac{Aw}{L}=0$

This is a quadratic in $\mathbf{f}$ and as before, for infinite roots we must have the coefficients of $\mathbf{f}^2$ and $\mathbf{f}$ simultaneously tending to zero; whence

$$m\frac{Aw}{Ax}-1\to0,\qquad\text{i.e.}\qquad m\to\frac{Ax}{Aw} \tag{8.29}$$

and $mDx\dfrac{Aw}{L}+k\dfrac{Aw}{Ax}-\dfrac{DxAw}{L}\to0$

i.e. $k\to\dfrac{Ax}{Aw}\left[\dfrac{DxAw}{L}-m\dfrac{DxAw}{L}\right]$

or $k\to Dx\dfrac{Ax}{L}\left[1-\dfrac{Ax}{Aw}\right]$ (from (8.29))

These are the formulae for m and k used by Forker. Fig 8.39 illustrates the result for the case $Aw/Ax=5$, $DxAw/L=12\cdot5$.†

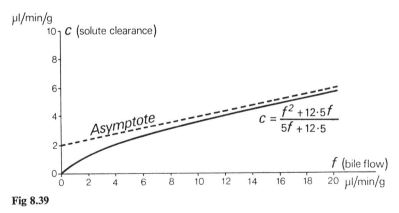

Fig 8.39

---

† We are very grateful to Dr. Forker for data and advice in this example.

8.10.3   *Equations of degree > 2*

There is no simple classification system for curves of degree > 2 other than by their degree. A further difficulty with such curves is that it may not be easy or even feasible to plot them in practice; e.g. finding pairs of co-ordinates on the curve.

$$x^5 + xy^4 + y^5 = 6 \qquad\qquad (8.30)$$

involves solving a quintic equation for y if x is given and similarly for x if y is given. As it can be shown that an explicit algebraic solution cannot in general be found for equations of degree > 4, an equation such as (8.30) has to be solved *numerically* (Chapter 11), with the five possible roots of the quintic equation to be located for each given value of x (or y).

One way round the difficulty in practice is to recognize that very frequently it is either an overall picture of the *shape* of the curve which is required, or else a detailed analysis of a small section of it. If the latter case, often mathematical analysis can answer questions of relevance, e.g. whether there is a *maximum* or *minimum* or *inflection point* (see Chapter 9) in the area of interest, or a point where the curve crosses the axes, etc. The larger problem of sketching an overall picture of the curve is the concern of the mathematical technique known as *curve-tracing*.

This latter subject is too extensive to be treated in the limited space available to us here. Readers with an interest or a problem in this area should read the delightful little book by Frost (1960), written with great courtesy towards the reader and with a fine set of drawings illustrating the methods.

8.11   Curves satisfying given conditions

Consider the general equation of the second degree

$$ax^2 + 2hxy + by^2 + 2gx + 2fy + c = 0 \qquad\qquad (8.31)$$

For any specific curve, numerical values have to be assigned to the parameters a, b, c, f, g, h. For instance, if we ask that the curve (8.31) should pass through the point (1, 5), this means that

$$a + 10h + 25b + 2g + 10f + c = 0$$

Since there are six unknown quantities here, it would appear that another five conditions, leading to five similar equations, are needed to determine a, b, c, f, g, and h uniquely. In fact, there are only five unknown quantities in (8.31), and not six, because if we divide across by any non-zero coefficient, we are left with five *ratios* of coefficients—e.g. if we divide across by a, say, the equation becomes

$$x^2 + 2\left(\frac{h}{a}\right)xy + \left(\frac{b}{a}\right)y^2 + 2\left(\frac{g}{a}\right)x + 2\left(\frac{f}{a}\right)y + \left(\frac{c}{a}\right) = 0.$$

From this we see that to be able to draw the conic (8.31), we must find the values of only *five* quantities, namely, five ratios of the six parameters a, b, c, f, g, h to one another.

This means that if we wish a given situation to be represented by some curve of the second degree—i.e. by a conic—then this can be done provided that not more than five conditions are imposed. For instance, it is always possible to find a curve of the second degree which passes through five points, or passes through four points and touches a given straight line. Each condition will lead to an equation between the coefficients, leading to five equations for the five coefficient ratios. However, specifying that the curve should be of a particular type—e.g. a circle—uses up some of the available conditions, and therefore reduces the number of additional constraints which can be imposed. For example, if we wish to use a circle in a problem, then since the general equation of a circle can be written as

$$ax^2 + ay^2 + 2gx + 2fy + c = 0$$

with three unknown coefficient ratios—g/a, f/a and c/a—it follows that only *three* conditions can be imposed on the curve in this case.

If fewer than the maximum number of possible conditions are imposed, there will be an unlimited number of curves of the given degree which will satisfy the conditions; in this case, further criteria are needed to decide which curve to use.

On the other hand, trying to impose more than the permissible maximum number of conditions is useless. For instance it is not possible to find a second degree curve passing through more than five points, though it could happen that such a curve chosen to pass through five given points also passes by coincidence through some other specified points. But to attempt to find, e.g. a parabola which passes exactly through ten or fifteen experimental points, simply because it is felt that a parabola would be a convenient form to use, is—except by luck—impossible. Even if the underlying physical situation was such that all the points *did* lie on a parabola, experimental and observer error would almost certainly prevent them as measured from doing so. What can be done is to find the curve of given form which passes most closely among the points; this is known as *curve fitting* (Section 11.7).

8.11.1   Conditions on nth degree curves

The result that five conditions are the maximum which can be imposed on a second-degree curve has the following generalization.

> A curve of degree n cannot in general *satisfy more than* $\frac{1}{2}n * (n+3)$ *conditions*   (8.32)

(see e.g. Coolidge (1932)).

The result (8.32) follows from a consideration of the maximum number of coefficients possible in an nth degree equation. Specific forms of nth degree curve may have fewer coefficients and therefore satisfy fewer conditions before being uniquely determined. For example, only two conditions can be imposed on a curve of the form $ax^5 + by^5 = 1$, since there are but two coefficients to be determined—a and b.

Similar considerations can be shown to apply to non-polynomial curves also.

8.12   Extension to three dimensions

Space does not permit us to treat the subject in any detail but the reader should note that our two-dimensional techniques can be enlarged to deal with three dimensions. For this we need *three* axes, usually called the x, y and z axes (Fig 8.40).

Analogously to two dimensions, these are normally taken to be mutually perpendicular. The co-ordinates of any point in space relative to these axes are the distances one has to go along or parallel to the x, y and z axes in order to arrive at the point; e.g. the point P in Fig 8.40 has co-ordinates $x=3$, $y=2$, $z=4$.

By a simple extension of two-dimensional notation, the point P would be referred to as the point $(3, 2, 4)$; and the general point is (x, y, z).

Our formulae and equations also generalize in a fairly straightforward way in three dimensions. For example, in two dimensions the distance between the points (x_1, y_1) and (x_2, y_2) is

$$\sqrt{\{(x_1-x_2)^2+(y_1-y_2)^2\}};$$

in three dimensions the distance between (x_1, y_1, z_1) and (x_2, y_2, z_2) is

$$\sqrt{\{(x_1-x_2)^2+(y_1-y_2)^2+(z_1-z_2)^2\}},$$

an obvious generalization (cf. Section 7.2.1).

Again, in two dimensions the path of a point which moves so as to keep a constant distance r from a fixed point is a circle, equation

$$x^2+y^2=r^2$$

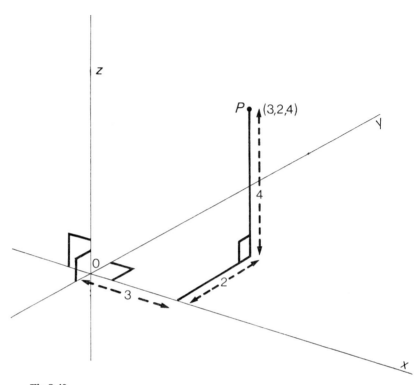

Fig 8.40

if the fixed point is taken as the origin; in three dimensions, the curve is replaced
by a *surface*, namely the *sphere* of radius r, and the equation of this is

$$x^2+y^2+z^2=r^2.$$

As before, the generalization is obvious.

The concepts of point and curve in two dimensions enlarge in three dimensions to include that of a *surface*. In two dimensions, a curve is described by
one equation—$f(x, y)=0$—and a point by two equations—either as $x=x_1$,
$y=y_1$ or as the intersection of two curves $f(x_1, y_1)=0$, $g(x_1, y_1)=0$. In three
dimensions, it is the *surface* which is defined by one equation, the curve by two
(representing the intersection of two surfaces) and the point by three equations
(representing the intersection of three surfaces). Such equations will usually
involve all three co-ordinate variables—cf. the equation of the sphere given
above.

The addition of an extra dimension introduces problems as well as analogies,
however; properties of three-dimensional structures are not always a clear

extension of two-dimensional ones. For further information the reader is advised to consult specialist texts such as Kindle (1950), Protter & Morrey (1966), and Sommerville (1943).

8.13   Matrix algebra and co-ordinate geometry

Although we have developed the idea of the subject using ordinary algebra, a very much more unified treatment is achieved by using matrix algebra for handling problems in co-ordinate geometry. Indeed, 'geometry' in N dimensions $(N > 3)$ is essentially a branch of matrix algebra (since the structures cannot be drawn), finding considerable application in statistics, in the solution of systems of algebraic and *differential* equations (Chapter 12), etc. As we progress—in concept at least—to more than three dimensions—i.e. to handling more than three variables—algebraic forms appear which have an analogy to points, lines, distances, and surfaces as with two- and three-dimensional geometry. For example, the equation of a line in two dimensions is $lx + my + n = 0$, and of a plane in three dimensions is $lx + my + nz + p = 0$. In four dimensions, the form $lx + my + nz + pw + q = 0$ is referred to as a four-dimensional *hyperplane*, while the row vector (x, y, z, w) is regarded as if it were a 'point' in the 'space' defined by four mutually 'perpendicular' axes.

The use of matrix algebra also facilitates the handling of co-ordinate transformations, especially in computer work. For example, we can write the general equation of the second degree

$$ax^2 + 2hxy + by^2 + 2gx + 2fy + c = 0$$

in two dimensions as

$$\mathbf{X}^T * \mathbf{A} * \mathbf{X} = 0 \tag{8.35}$$

where $\mathbf{X} = \begin{pmatrix} x \\ y \\ 1 \end{pmatrix}$

$\mathbf{X}^T$ is its transpose $(x, y, 1)$

and $\mathbf{A} = \begin{pmatrix} a & h & g \\ h & b & f \\ g & f & c \end{pmatrix}$

If we now carry out any form of linear transformation such that the old co-ordinates X are related to new co-ordinates X' by

$$\mathbf{X} = \mathbf{C} * \mathbf{X}'$$

where $\mathbf{X}' = \begin{pmatrix} x' \\ y' \\ 1 \end{pmatrix}$

and $\mathbf{C}$ is a 3 by 3 matrix of coefficients, the equation (8.35) becomes, in terms of the co-ordinates x', y':

$$(\mathbf{CX}')^{\mathrm{T}} * \mathbf{A} * (\mathbf{CX}') = 0$$

i.e. $(\mathbf{X}')^{\mathrm{T}} * [\mathbf{C}^{\mathrm{T}}\mathbf{AC}] * \mathbf{X}' = 0$ (cf. Section 7.7.3)   (8.36)

another second degree form. For example, if

$$\mathbf{C} = \begin{pmatrix} \cos \theta & -\sin \theta & 0 \\ \sin \theta & \cos \theta & 0 \\ 0 & 0 & 1 \end{pmatrix}$$

then (8.36) represents the form of the conic (8.35) referred to co-ordinate axes rotated through an angle θ relative to the co-ordinate axes used in (8.35) (cf. Section 8.6.3). The use of the formal procedures so characteristic of matrix algebra is of great assistance in computer manipulation of co-ordinate geometric problems or problems analogous to them.

Chapter 9
The Calculus

9.1   Introduction

The development of a branch of mathematics for handling varying rates of change and their cumulative effect has been vital in the study of dynamic systems. From the simple pendulum to rockets and satellites this branch of mathematics, the calculus, has demonstrated its power as an aid to understanding and technological development. There is hardly any field of modern science to which it has not contributed, and its techniques are being used, increasingly, in the study of the most complex dynamic systems such as the human body and social relationships. The functional relationships in dynamic systems are often described in terms of a rate of change of some measurement; for example, the rate of transfer of a compound across a semi-permeable membrane is proportional to the difference in concentration across the membrane. Many physical laws are relationships governing the rate of change of these rates of change; for example, velocity is the rate of change of distance, while acceleration is the rate of change of velocity, and one of the basic laws in physics states that acceleration is proportional to the applied force.

In this chapter we will illustrate our mathematics by considering variables changing in time, but it is essential to realize that the reasoning will apply equally well when we are studying relationships between any variables. Once we have reduced our reasoning to the handling of symbols, then that reasoning will apply to any real measurement which can be substituted for the symbols.

9.2   Rate of change and slope

9.2.1   *The straight line*

Discussion about the rate of change is particularly simple if the graph of the measure against time is a straight line. Figure 9.1 shows an empirical relationship between the maximum diameter of the legs of mice after an injection of tumour cells and the days since the injection; the full line is based on the paper by Hewitt & Blake (1968)

It is easily seen that the growth rate is constant, i.e. the increase in size from 10 to 15 days is the same as the increase from 15 to 20 days. The growth *rate* is obtained by dividing the growth over *any* time interval by the length of the time interval; for example, the diameter at 15 days is 13 mm and at 20 days is 18 mm and so the growth rate is given by

$$\frac{18 \text{ mm} - 13 \text{ mm}}{5 \text{ days}} = 1 \cdot 0 \text{ mm/day}$$

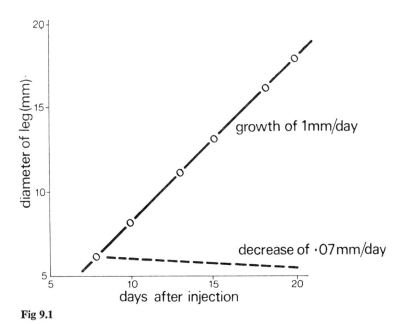

Fig 9.1

The calculation involves a subtraction and a division, and the units of the answer imply a division. We will formalize this concept by expressing it algebraically. Let the measure be a function of time denoted by $f(t)$, and let the time interval be from time t to time $t+\delta t$, that is the interval has length δt. Then the rate of increase of $f(t)$ is:

$$\frac{f(t+\delta t)-f(t)}{\delta t} \tag{9.1}$$

In the case of a straight line relationship, we have $f(t)=at+b$, where a and b are constants in time. Applying formula (9.1) gives

$$\text{The rate of increase of } (at+b)=\frac{a*(t+\delta t)+b-(a*t+b)}{\delta t}$$

$$=a$$

This calculation is also the process used to obtain the slope of a line (Section 3.10.3).

If in this example some treatment has prevented the transplanted tumour from establishing itself, we might observe a *decrease* with time, giving a line sloping in the opposite direction (the dotted line in Fig 9.1). If we apply the formula given above it can be seen that $f(t+\delta t)$ will always be less than $f(t)$ and so the rate of increase will be a negative number, and the line would be said to have negative slope. Figure 9.2 shows various lines and the slope or rate of change associated with them. Positive rates of change imply increases in the value of the function, and negative rates, decreases.

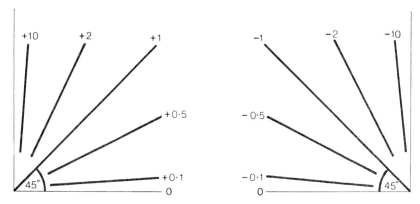

Numerical values of the slope of various lines

Fig 9.2

9.2.2   *Varying rates of change*

For a straight line relationship, the rate of change is constant and it does not matter which value of t or δt we choose, the calculation of formula (9.1) will always give the same answer. If the growth is not proceeding at a constant rate, however, we may get a smooth curve such as *ABCDE* in Fig 9.3.

With such a curve, the definition of slope at a point or the rate of change at an instant in time is not so obvious. However, it is possible to approximate the curve by a series of straight lines; as these lines become smaller and we take more of them so the approximation becomes more accurate until it is quite acceptable. In Fig 9.3 we very rapidly approach a good approximation to the curve, and no point on the curve is very far from its approximating straight lines, *AB*, *BC*, *CD*, and *DE*.

Each of these lines has an acceptable definition of slope or rate of change, so we may consider the slope or rate of change at a point on the curve as the corresponding calculation on the small straight line being used as an approximation to the curve at that point.

What we then do with the formula we have been using to calculate the rate of change, is to make the value δt become smaller and smaller, until this rate

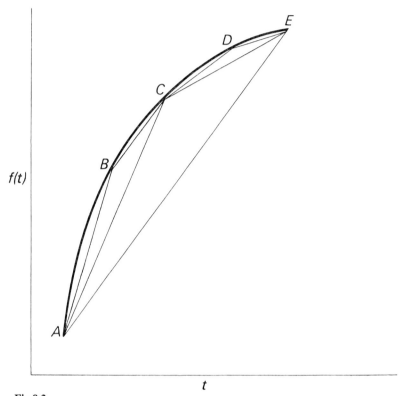

Fig 9.3

becomes acceptably constant. This corresponds to the *limiting process* described in Chapter 5. We can then mathematically define the rate of change by altering formula (9.1) to

$$\text{rate of change of } f(t) \text{ at time } t = \lim_{\delta t \to 0} \frac{f(t + \delta t) - f(t)}{\delta t} \qquad (9.2)$$

9.2.3   Changes other than in time

It is obvious that there is an analogy between slope and rate of change. Let us consider a relationship between other measures, for example, between the dose of a drug and its effect. When this is represented by a graph, with dose on the horizontal axis, and effect on the vertical axis, then the slope of the graph represents the change in effect for a unit change in dose. We describe this as the *rate of change of effect with respect to dose.* If the dose is denoted by the letter x, and the effect is a function of the dose denoted by $y(x)$ then we substitute x for t and y for f in formula (9.2) giving

$$\text{rate of change of } y(x) \text{ at dose } x = \lim_{\delta x \to 0} \frac{y(x + \delta x) - y(x)}{\delta x} \tag{9.3}$$

9.3   Notation

9.3.1   Rate of change; the derivative

A special notation and nomenclature is used to describe the limit formulae given in (9.2) and (9.3). The operation of obtaining the rate of change or the slope is called *differentiating* or *differentiation*, the resulting rate or slope is called the *derivative* or *differential coefficient*, though sometimes it is called the *first derivative* or *first differential coefficient*. The names of the variables can also be indicated, for example, the *derivative of f with respect to t*, or the *derivative with respect to dose*. There are a set of standard symbolic representations for the process of differentiation, and for the derivatives. The process with respect to t, i.e. obtaining the limit given in formula (9.2), is denoted by the symbol $\frac{d}{dt}$ (spoken as 'd by dt'). This is regarded as a single symbol, and it is sometimes replaced by the symbol D.

$$\frac{d}{dt} f(t) \text{ is usually written } \frac{df}{dt} \tag{9.4}$$

(spoken as 'd by dt of f' or 'df by dt') and, formally,

$$\frac{df}{dt} = \lim_{\delta t \to 0} \frac{f(t + \delta t) - f(t)}{\delta t}$$

Similarly

$$\frac{dy}{dx} = \lim_{\delta x \to 0} \frac{y(x + \delta x) - y(x)}{\delta x}$$

$\frac{df}{dt}, \frac{dy}{dx}$ are often written in one of the following ways:

$$f', f'(t), f^{(1)}(t), \dot{f} \tag{9.5}$$

(spoken as 'f dash', 'f dash t' 'f one', and 'f dot')

$$y', y'(x), y^{(1)}(x), \dot{y}$$

Where there is no mention of the variable which is being used as the base for differentiation, this has to be deduced from the context, though the use of a dot over the symbol normally indicates a differential coefficient with respect to time.

The derivative $\dfrac{df}{dt}$ is the rate of change of the function f at time t. It will generally have different values at different times. Therefore it is, itself, a function of t. The notation $f'(t)$ is a convenient one for handling the derivative, when there is no confusion over the independent variable being used as the basis for change. In this notation the value of $\dfrac{df}{dt}$ at $t=1$ would be written $f'(1)$. An alternative way of representing a value of the derivative at this point is $\left[\dfrac{df}{dt}\right]_{t=1}$. Similar notation can be used for derivatives at other values of t.

Examples:

We use this notation to describe two types of growth; see Fig. 9.4. The methods for deriving the formulae in the figures is dealt with in Chapter 12 and Section 9.5.2.

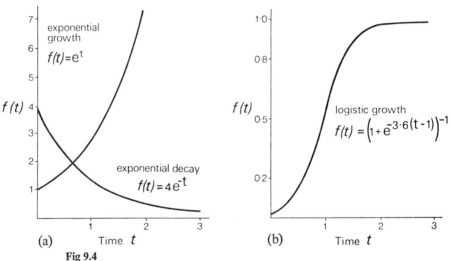

(a)   Time t

(b)   Time t

Fig 9.4

(i) Exponential (sometimes called logarithmic) growth is one in which the rate of growth is proportional to the size of the organism. If the size at time t is denoted by the function $f(t)$, this can be written

$$f'(t)=k*f(t)\quad(k\text{ is a constant in time})\tag{9.6}$$

This sort of growth would go on forever getting faster and faster if $k>0$, or slower and slower if $k<0$: e.g. Fig. 9.4(a) when $k=\pm1$.

(ii) Logistic growth is one in which the growth tends to a maximum limit and the growth rate slows down, in such a way that the value of k in formula (9.6) is proportional to the difference in size of the organism from its maximum size. This can be written

$$f'(t) = c * (M - f(t)) * f(t) \tag{9.7}$$

where M is the maximum size and c is constant in time; e.g. Fig 9.4b, where $c = 3 \cdot 6$ and $M = 1$.

9.4 Higher-order derivatives

The rate of change of $f'(t)$ may itself change as t changes, so we could evaluate the rate of change of the rate of change, i.e.

$$\frac{d}{dt}\left(\frac{df}{dt}\right) \quad \text{or} \quad (f'(t))'.$$

This is equivalent to applying the operation of differentiation twice in succession and the answer is called the *second derivative* or *second order derivative*. It is represented symbolically by one of the forms:

$$\frac{d^2}{dt^2}f(t), \ \frac{d^2f}{dt^2}, \ f'', \ f''(t), \ f^{(2)}(t), \ \ddot{f}, \ D^2(f(t)) \tag{9.8}$$

These are straightforward extensions to the notation given in (9.4) and (9.5). Care should be taken to distinguish the symbols

$$\frac{d^2f}{dt^2}$$

meaning the result of differentiating twice, i.e. the rate of change of the rate of change, from the symbol

$$\left(\frac{df}{dt}\right)^2$$

meaning the rate of change multiplied by itself. The notation may be continued in an obvious fashion to third-order derivatives, i.e. the rate of change of the rate of change of the rate of change; and so on to fourth, fifth and in general nth-order derivatives, with the notation

$$\frac{d^nf}{dt^n} \quad \text{or} \quad f^{(n)}(t) \quad \text{or} \quad D^n(f(t))$$

The dot or dash notations are rarely used above third-order derivatives, and are of course impossible when the order of the derivative is itself a variable.

Examples:

The notation is used to describe two types of oscillatory motion; see Fig 9.5.

(i) *Simple harmonic motion* is the movement which occurs when the force on a particle is proportional to its distance from the centre of oscillation and directed towards the centre. This results in the acceleration of the particle being proportional to this distance. If we write $f(t)$ as the distance from the centre of oscillation at time t, $f(t)$ will take positive values on one side of the centre of oscillational and negative values on the other, $f'(t)$ is then the rate of change of distance—i.e. velocity—and $f''(t)$ is the rate of change of velocity, i.e. the acceleration. Simple harmonic motion can be written as:

$$f''(t) = -k * f(t) \tag{9.9}$$

This motion describes an idealized vibration of a spring or the particles in a sound wave, and it would go on, back and forth forever; see Fig 9.5a.

(ii) In practice friction will slow the above process down, and *damped harmonic motion* introduces another force of deceleration which is proportional to the velocity, and can be written as:

$$f''(t) = -m * f'(t) - k * f(t) \tag{9.10}$$

The methods for finding the values of $f(t)$ from formulae of this type are dealt with in Chapter 12; also see Fig 9.5b and c.

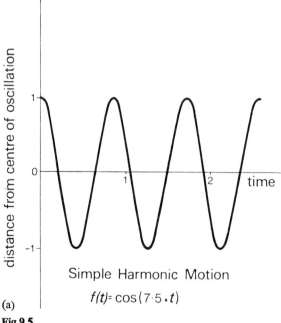

Simple Harmonic Motion

$f(t) = \cos(7 \cdot 5 * t)$

(a)

Fig 9.5

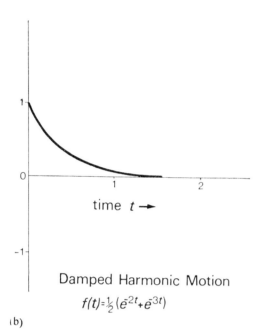

Damped Harmonic Motion
$$f(t) = \tfrac{1}{2}(\bar{e}^{2t} + \bar{e}^{3t})$$

(b)

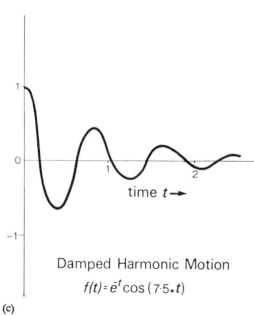

Damped Harmonic Motion
$$f(t) = \bar{e}^{t}\cos(7{\cdot}5_{*}t)$$

(c)

Fig 9.5

K

9.5   Calculation of the derivative

9.5.1   Common derivatives

The derivative of a function could be computed by a process of approximation, but these calculations are liable to error and can be lengthy. The derivatives of functions which have been expressed in algebraic form can be found by a combination of algebraic manipulation (Chapter 1) and application of the limiting process (Chapter 5). It is very tedious to go through all this mathematics each time we want a derivative, so the experienced mathematician knows by heart the derivatives of a large number of common functions, and is well practised in the rules for combining them. The formula for the derivative of an algebraic function can nearly always be found, and several computer programs have been written to perform this task automatically (Barton, Bourne & Fitch (1970)).

Table 9.1 gives a list of a few of the common derivatives; other derivatives are in the Appendix. In this Table the function is always differentiated with respect to the variable t and the letters k and n represent constants. The value of derivatives may be found by substituting the appropriate values for the variable and constants in the expression for $f'(t)$. For example, the rate of change of the function $6 * t^{-3}$ at time $t=2$ is obtained from the 2nd line of the Table, by substituting 6 for k, -3 for n, and 2 for t giving $6 * (-3) * 2^{-4}$ which is $-1 \cdot 125$.

Table 9.1 Derivatives of simple functions

The function is differentiated with respect to the variable t, and the letters k and n represent values which are constant.

Function	Derivative		
$f(t)$	$f'(t)$	$f'(t)$ when $k=1$ and $n=1$	
k	0	0	
$k * t^n$	$k * n * t^{(n-1)}$	1	
$\dfrac{k}{t^n}$	$\dfrac{k * (-n)}{t^{(n+1)}}$	$-\dfrac{1}{t^2}$	
$(t+k)^n$	$n * (t+k)^{n-1}$	1	
$k * \ln(t)$	$\dfrac{k}{t}$	$\dfrac{1}{t}$	
$\exp(k * t)$	$k * \exp(k * t)$	$\exp(t)$	$\exp(k * t)$ is e^{kt}
$\sin(k * t)$	$* \cos(k * t)$	$\cos(t)$	$k * t$ in radians
$\cos(k * t)$	$-k * \sin(k * t)$	$-\sin(t)$	$k * t$ in radians

The reasons why e and the functions exp, ln, sin, and cos occur so frequently in mathematical work can be seen by examining their derivatives.

Consider the derivative of the logarithm to base e, the so called natural logarithm.

$$\frac{d}{dt} \ln (t) = \frac{1}{t}$$

Now if we took logarithms to some other base, say base 10, we would have:

$$\log_{10} (t) = \log_{10} (e) * \log_e (t) = 0 \cdot 4343 * \ln (t)$$

So
$$\frac{d}{dt} \log_{10} (t) = \frac{d}{dt} (0 \cdot 4343 * \ln (t)) = \frac{0 \cdot 4343}{t}$$

This can be found from the fifth line of Table 9.1 by putting $k = 0 \cdot 4343$.

By taking natural logarithms we avoid having continually to allow for this constant $0 \cdot 4343$. For this reason logarithms are usually assumed to be to base e in algebraic work. Similar reasoning applies to the use of radians and not degrees to measure angles for the sine, cosine and other trigonometric functions.

The functions $\exp (k * t)$, $\sin (k * t)$, and $\cos (k * t)$ when differentiated a number of times, return to their original form or a simple multiple of it. This makes them very useful for describing relationships involving both the function and its derivatives. It can be seen that $\exp (k * t)$ satisfies the condition for exponential growth in formula (9.6) and Fig 9.4a, and $\sin (t * \sqrt{k})$ or $\cos (t * \sqrt{k})$ would satisfy the condition for simple harmonic motion given in formula (9.9). It is not surprising, therefore, that these three functions occur again and again in the study of dynamic systems, and have an importance far beyond the simple geometrical definitions of sine or cosine.

9.5.2   More complicated derivatives

The derivatives of more complicated algebraic expressions can be obtained by the application of a few simple rules. These rules, together with some examples are given in this section. They will only be of direct help when the reader is trying to differentiate an algebraic expression, and as with algebraic manipulation, the ease of handling these rules only comes with continual practice.

Throughout this section we will abbreviate $f(t)$ to f and introduce three more functions of t, denoted by u, v, and w. That is, the value of u, v, and w will vary as t varies; the other letters denote quantities unaffected by changes in t. It will be seen that the *derivative can be treated almost as if it were a fraction* df *divided by* dt.

This section may be omitted until needed

(i) If $f = u + v$

then $\dfrac{df}{dt} = \dfrac{du}{dt} + \dfrac{dv}{dt}$;

if $f = u - v$

then $\dfrac{df}{dt} = \dfrac{du}{dt} - \dfrac{dv}{dt}$

By repeated application of these two rules we can differentiate sums and differences term by term:

If $f = u + v - w$

then $\dfrac{df}{dt} = \dfrac{du}{dt} + \dfrac{dv}{dt} - \dfrac{dw}{dt}$ (9.11)

Example:

$$f = \sin(t) + t^2 - e^t$$

$$\frac{df}{dt} = \cos(t) + 2 * t - e^t$$

(ii) If $f = k * u$

then $\dfrac{df}{dt} = k * \dfrac{du}{dt}$;   (9.12)

Example:

$$f = \exp(-2t) + \exp(-3t)$$

$$\frac{df}{dt} = -2 * \exp(-2t) - 3 * \exp(-3t) \quad \text{(using rule (i) and Table 9.1)}$$

$$\frac{d^2f}{dt^2} = 4 * \exp(-2t) + 9 * \exp(-3t) \quad \text{(using rule ii)}$$

For this function,

$$\frac{d^2f}{dt^2} = -5\frac{df}{dt} - 6f$$

which is a particular example of the damped harmonic motion given in formula (9.10), and Fig 9.5(b). In this case the damping is so severe that the particle comes smoothly to rest and does not oscillate at all.

(iii) If $f = u * v$

then $$\frac{df}{dt} = u * \frac{dv}{dt} + \frac{du}{dt} * v$$

This may be extended to multiple products by repeated application of this rule:

If $f = u * v * w$

then $$\frac{df}{dt} = u * v * \frac{dw}{dt} + u * \frac{dv}{dt} * w + \frac{du}{dt} * v * w \qquad (9.13)$$

Example:

$f = \exp(-t) * \cos(7 \cdot 5 t)$ i.e. $u = \exp(-t) \quad v = \cos(7 \cdot 5 t)$

$$\frac{df}{dt} = -\exp(-t) * 7 \cdot 5 * \sin(7 \cdot 5 t) + (-1) * \exp(-t) * \cos(7 \cdot 5 t)$$

also $$\frac{d^2 f}{dt^2} = 15 * \exp(-t) * \sin(7 \cdot 5 t) - 55 \cdot 25 * \exp(-t) * \cos(7 \cdot 5 t)$$

Note $$\frac{d^2 f}{dt^2} = -2 \frac{df}{dt} - 57 \cdot 25 f$$

which is another example of damped harmonic motion given in formula (9.10) and Fig 9.5c. In this case the particle does oscillate, but the oscillations get smaller as the factor $\exp(-t)$ gets smaller.

(iv) If f is a function of the variable u, and the variable u is a function of t, then

$$\frac{df}{dt} = \frac{df}{du} * \frac{du}{dt} \qquad (9.14)$$

Example:

$$f = \frac{1}{1 + \exp\{-c(t-1)\}}$$

This may be written $f = u^{-1}$ where $u = 1 + \exp\{-c(t-1)\}$.
Applying (9.14) gives

$$\frac{df}{dt} = -[1 + \exp\{-c(t-1)\}]^{-2} * [-c \exp\{-c(t-1)\}] \qquad (9.15)$$

Note that (9.15) may be written in the form

$$\frac{df}{dt} = c * (1-f) * f$$

This section may be omitted until needed

which is the particular case of the logistic growth curve given in formula (9.7) and Fig 9.4b when the maximum size $M=1$ and $c=3.6$

The rule in this and (iii) above enables us to differentiate $f=\dfrac{u}{v}$ by writing this as $f=u * v^{-1}$. The result is

$$\frac{df}{dt} = -u * v^{-2} * \frac{dv}{dt} + v^{-1} * \frac{du}{dt}$$

This is usually written in the form

$$\frac{d}{dt}(u/v) = \left(v * \frac{du}{dt} - u * \frac{dv}{dt}\right) \Big/ v^2 \qquad (9.16)$$

(v) If f is a function of u, and u is a function of v, and v is a function of t then formula (9.14) can be extended to:

$$\frac{df}{dt} = \frac{df}{du} * \frac{du}{dv} * \frac{dv}{dt} \qquad (9.17)$$

and similarly for more complicated expressions.

This is the way derivatives of complicated expressions can be obtained by differentiating successively smaller parts and multiplying the answers together.

Example:

$$f = \ln\{\sin(k * t^2 + 1)\}$$

First consider everything in the log bracket as a variable u, so that $f = \ln(u)$, $u = \sin(k * t^2 + 1)$

$\dfrac{df}{du}$: differentiating $\ln(u)$ gives $\dfrac{1}{u} = \dfrac{1}{\sin(k * t^2 + 1)}$

Consider everything in the sine bracket as v so that $u = \sin(v)$, $v = k * t^2 + 1$.

$\dfrac{du}{dv}$: differentiating $\sin(v)$ gives $\cos(v) = \cos(k * t^2 + 1)$

Now $v = k * t^2 + 1$ which can be easily differentiated with respect to t:

$$\frac{dv}{dt} = \frac{d}{dt}(k * t^2 + 1) = 2 * k * t$$

Multiplying all these together will give $\dfrac{df}{dt}$:

$$\frac{df}{dt} = \frac{2 * k * t * \cos(k * t^2 + 1)}{\sin(k * t^2 + 1)}$$

With practice such differentials can be written straight down.

(vi) Differentiating both sides of an equality will maintain the equality, i.e. if $f=u$ then $\dfrac{df}{dt}=\dfrac{du}{dt}$. This is particularly useful when the function is defined implicitly.

Example:

Consider the function $y(x)$ defined by the equation

$$x^2+y^2+2gx+2fy+c=0 \tag{9.18}$$

This is the general equation of a circle as given in formula (8.25) and its slope at any point is given by $\dfrac{dy}{dx}$. It is possible to manipulate this function to give y as a function of x, but it is easier to differentiate both sides of the $=$ sign. To do this we will have to use the rule given in (9.14) to find the differential of y^2 with respect to x.

$$\frac{d}{dx}(y^2)=\left(\frac{d}{dy}(y^2)\right)*\frac{dy}{dx}=2y\frac{dy}{dx}$$

Differentiating equation (9.18) with respect to x (regarding f, g and c as constant), gives:

$$2x+2y\frac{dy}{dx}+2g+2f\frac{dy}{dx}+0=0$$

Rearranging the terms gives:

$$2(y+f)\frac{dy}{dx}=-2(x+g)$$

and so
$$\frac{dy}{dx}=-\frac{x+g}{y+f} \tag{9.19}$$

This gives the slope of a circle described by the equation (8.25).

9.6   Shape of a curve

9.6.1   Maxima and minima

The slope of a curve and the rate of change of the slope have an important role to play in describing the shape of a curve. The points at which a curve changes direction are useful guides to drawing the curve, and they often correspond to points of physical interest such as minimum error, or maximum displacement.

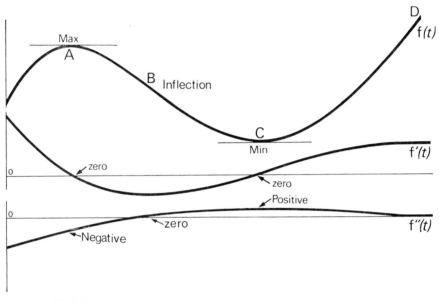

Fig 9.6

Figure 9.6 shows the plot of a function $f(t)$ and its first two derivatives. The peaks and troughs of the curve A and C are approximated by short horizontal lines and so the slope is zero at these points, i.e. $f'(t)=0$. These points are called *maxima* and *minima*, *stationary points* or *turning points*. They do not represent absolute maxima and minima, for as we can see A is only the maximum value of the function in a local region and is exceeded for large values of t at the points beyond D. For this reason the points at which $f'(t)=0$ are often called *local maxima or minima*. It is easy to distinguish maxima (i.e. points like A) from minima (i.e. points like C).

For a maximum the slope has a positive value on the left of the point, and a negative value on the right of the point; the slope decreases as t increases, i.e. $f''(t)<0$. At a minimum the reverse is true. This may be put formally as:
At a maximum

$$\frac{df}{dt}=0 \quad \text{and} \quad \frac{d^2f}{dt^2}<0. \tag{9.20}$$

At a minimum

$$\frac{df}{dt}=0 \quad \text{and} \quad \frac{d^2f}{dt}>0. \tag{9.21}$$

If both $\frac{df}{dt}$ and $\frac{d^2f}{dt^2}$ are zero the curve must be investigated further.

Example:

Consider a problem which can arise in the analysis of paired measurements $(x_1, y_1), (x_2, y_2) \ldots (x_n, y_n)$, when the underlying relationship is believed to be: 'y is proportional to x' (i.e. $y=a*x$, the equation of a straight line through the origin of co-ordinates). The problem comes in estimating the value of a when there is random error in the measurement of y. One method of tackling this is to choose the value of a such that

$$S=\sum_{i=1}^{n}(y_i-ax_i)^2$$

is a minimum; this is called the *least squares* technique. S is regarded as a function of a, that is, a is the variable we are going to alter until we find a minimum value of S. Now at the minimum

$$\frac{dS}{da}=0 \quad \text{and} \quad \frac{d^2S}{da}>0;$$

differentiating

$$\sum_{i=1}^{n}(y_i-ax_i)^2$$

with respect to a gives:

$$\frac{dS}{da}=\sum_{i=1}^{n}2(y_i-ax_i)*(-x_i)=-2\sum y_i x_i+2a\sum x_i^2$$

$$\frac{d^2S}{da^2}=2\sum_{i=1}^{n}x_i^2$$

The condition for dS/da to be zero is that

$$a=\left(\sum_{i=1}^{n}x_i y_i\right)\bigg/\left(\sum_{i=1}^{n}x_i^2\right) \tag{9.22}$$

So that for any known set of values for x_i and y_i it is possible to compute a from formula (9.22). To satisfy ourselves that this is the value of a that minimizes the value of S, we can either examine the value of S for values of a both sides of the computed minimum, or evaluate d^2S/da^2 at the turning point. We observe that d^2S/da^2 is the sum of values which are the squares of numbers, and so must be positive, which establishes the value of S as a minimum for this value of a.

9.6.2   The computation of maxima and minima

There is a trick which is sometimes useful for handling the turning points of functions which are the product of a large number of terms. It is applicable to that part of the function which is *greater than zero*. The method is to differentiate the logarithm of the function rather than the function itself. The turning point of the logarithm will also be the turning point of the function. This is used in genetics and statistics with the method of maximum likelihood; very often the logarithm of the likelihood is much easier to handle than the likelihood itself.

Example:

To find the value of x which maximizes $x^4(1-x)^3$.

Let $\quad f = \ln\{x^4(1-x)^3\}$

then $\quad f = 4\ln(x) + 3\ln(1-x)$

$$\frac{df}{dx} = \frac{4}{x} - \frac{3}{1-x}$$

When $x = \dfrac{4}{7}$ then $\dfrac{df}{dx}$ is zero and the function has a turning point which easily can be shown to be a maximum of $x^4(1-x)^3$.

9.6.3   Points of inflection

The point B on Fig 9.6 shows a point where the curve is beginning to bend from one direction to another. At this point the value of $f''(t)$ *is zero*, the curve is comparatively straight and the point is called a *point of inflection*. If $f'''(t)$ is also zero the curve must be investigated further. It is difficult to accurately locate the point of inflection just from looking at a graph, however it is very easy to draw the straight line approximation through the point of inflection and Wise (1966) used this fact to devise a simple method for estimating cardiac output from lines drawn through the two points of inflection of a dye dilution curve.

9.6.4   Discontinuities

The definitions of differentials must be used with some caution. To be useful $\frac{df}{dt}$ should take the same value however we choose our small approximating straight lines. Consider Fig 9.7, however. We see that the slope at point B, i.e. the bottom of a wedge, is undefined—we may regard it as the slope of AB or the slope of BC.

Another problem is illustrated by the discontinuity DE; although the slope is defined, i.e. zero, either side of DE, for an interval straddling DE any attempt find the limit of $\delta f/\delta t$ as $\delta t \to 0$ will lead to an undefined result.

The function is said to be *not differentiable* at these points or to have singularities. One should be aware that the process of differentiation does not apply at these points, but in practice we may usually ignore them by an intelligent look at the actual physical situation being represented; sometimes the discontinuities will represent points at which correspondence between the mathematical model and the physical system it is supposed to represent breaks down.

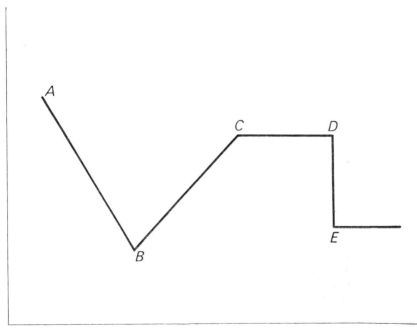

Discontinuities of slope

Fig 9.7

9.6.5   Relative positions of maxima and minima

There are a number of mathematical laws concerning the order of occurrence of maxima and minima of a *continuous* function. These rules can all be seen intuitively by examining a curve such as Fig 9.6 and can be proved formally for continuous functions with continuous derivatives:

(i) If $f(t)$ has the same value for two different values of t, t_1, and t_2, then there is at least one maximum or minimum (i.e. $f'(t)=0$) somewhere in the interval $[t_1, t_2]$.

(ii) There can be any number of minima between any two maxima, similarly there can be any number of maxima between any two minima. In particular, there must be one minimum between neighbouring maxima and one maximum between neighbouring minima.

(iii) There must be a point of inflection between a maximum and a minimum.

9.7   Functions of more than one variable

So far, we have considered functions of a single variable. However, a function may depend on more than one variable. The behaviour of the rate of change of such functions is usually investigated by examining the effect of changing one variable at a time.

9.7.1   Notation

The differential of a function of several variables with respect to one of the variables only is called a *partial derivative* and the symbol ∂ is used to replace the letter d in the notation for the derivative.

Example:

$$f=x^2+y^2-xy-3y \tag{9.23}$$

$$\frac{\partial f}{\partial x}=2x-y \qquad \text{i.e. regarding } y \text{ as constant}$$

$$\frac{\partial f}{\partial y}=2y-x-3 \qquad \text{i.e. regarding } x \text{ as constant}$$

Functions of two variables can be regarded as defining a surface in three dimensions (see Section 8.12), and in this case the partial derivative corresponds to the
slope of the surface in the direction of the changing variable. The notation may
be extended to higher-order partial derivatives in the same fashion as for functions of a single variable.

$$\frac{\partial}{\partial x}\left(\frac{\partial f}{\partial x}\right) \text{ is written } \frac{\partial^2 f}{\partial x^2}, \quad \frac{\partial}{\partial y}\left(\frac{\partial f}{\partial y}\right) \text{ is written } \frac{\partial^2 f}{\partial y^2}$$

and $\quad \dfrac{\partial}{\partial x}\left(\dfrac{\partial f}{\partial y}\right)$ is written $\dfrac{\partial^2 f}{\partial x \partial y}$

The expression

$$\frac{\partial^2 f}{\partial x^2}+\frac{\partial^2 f}{\partial y^2}+\frac{\partial^2 f}{\partial z^2}$$

which is known as *del squared f* and denoted by the symbol $\nabla^2 f$, is the basis of
the physical laws governing flow and electric potential.

Example:

In the theory of diffusion, if f represents the concentration of a solute at points
defined by the co-ordinates (x, y, z) at time t, then f will satisfy the relationship

$$\frac{\partial f}{\partial t} = D * \nabla^2 f$$

The constant D is known as the *diffusion coefficient*.

9.7.2   Turning points for functions of several variables

The turning points for functions of several variables are given by the simultaneous solution of the equations obtained by putting each of the partial derivatives
equal to zero. In the example given in (9.23) $\dfrac{\partial f}{\partial x}$ and $\dfrac{\partial f}{\partial y}$ are zero when $x=1$ and
$y=2$. This is therefore a turning point of that function. If we regard the function
as defining a surface there are a larger number of different types of turning
point than on a curve. For a true minimum, i.e. the bottom of a bowl, the surface
must be minimal from whichever direction it is approached and so both $\dfrac{\partial^2 f}{\partial x^2}$
and $\dfrac{\partial^2 f}{\partial y^2}$ must be greater than zero (or less than zero for a true maximum or

mountain peak). These conditions are not sufficient to determine a maximum or minimum, for if

$$\left(\frac{\partial^2 f}{\partial x \partial y}\right)^2 > \frac{\partial^2 f}{\partial x^2} * \frac{\partial^2 f}{\partial y^2}$$

the point will be a *saddle point*, i.e. a crest in a valley. It is usually most convenient to examine the exact nature of the turning point by computing values around the point, or perhaps the context of the problem only permits the existence of a minimum (or maximum).

Example:

If we consider an extension of the example given at the end of Section 9.6.1 and let our relationship be $y = b + ax$, i.e. a straight line not constrained through the origin, and try to find values of a and b which minimize

$$S = \sum_{i=1}^{n} (y_i - b - ax_i)^2$$

then

$$\frac{\partial S}{\partial a} = \sum_{i=1}^{n} 2(y_i - b - ax_i)(-x_i) = -2\sum x_i y_i + 2b\sum x_i + 2a\sum x_i^2$$

and

$$\frac{\partial S}{\partial b} = \sum_{i=1}^{n} 2(y_i - b - ax_i)(-1) = -2\sum y_i + 2\sum b + 2a\sum x_i$$

$\frac{\partial S}{\partial a} = 0$ and $\frac{\partial S}{\partial b} = 0$ for S to be minimum and so we get a pair of simultaneous

equations for a and b which can be rearranged as

$$b\sum x_i + a\sum x_i^2 = \sum x_i y_i$$
$$nb + a\sum x_i = \sum y_i \quad \text{(note } \sum_{i=1}^{n} b = nb)$$

The solutions of these equations are:

$$a = \frac{n\sum x_i y_i - (\sum x_i)(\sum y_i)}{n\sum x_i^2 - (\sum x_i)^2}$$

$$b = \frac{\sum y_i - a\sum x_i}{n}$$

which is a least squares solution for fitting a straight line to a set of points (the regression line).

The presence in a text of a number of partial derivatives, all equated to zero, probably indicates an attempt to minimize, or maximize, some function.

Although it may be possible to obtain the algebraic expressions for the derivatives, it is not always possible to solve the resulting equations by algebraic manipulation. When this happens some form of numerical solution has to be attempted by the methods discussed in Chapter 11.

Computer programs are available for hunting for minimum (or maximum) by a process of trial and error. These programs have to be given a starting point, that is an initial guess of the answers to the variables. They then automatically evaluate the function at surrounding points and if they successfully reduce the function, or increase it for a maximum, they record the new point and proceed with the search from that point. They function rather like a blind man might trying to find his way up or down a mountain. Some of these programs, e.g. Bell & Pike (1966), do not require the derivative of the function to be given and are therefore very easy to use provided we make a reasonably good guess at the starting point.

9.8   The indefinite integral

9.8.1   Notation

We have shown in the preceding sections of this chapter how to obtain the rate of change of various functions. We often require to perform the inverse operation, i.e. given the laws governing the rate of change of a function we wish to find the function. The function of t whose rate of change with respect to increasing t is $f(t)$ is called the *indefinite integral of f with respect to t* and is denoted by the symbol:

$$\int f(t)\,dt \quad \text{or} \quad \int f dt$$

The word 'indefinite', which is often omitted, is used to contrast this operation with a related operation known as the 'definite integral' which is considered in Section 9.9. We must emphasize that the use of the term 'indefinite' does not imply any vagueness or lack of definition. The process of obtaining the integral is called *integration*, and the function f is called the *integrand*.

Example

We can see from Table 9.1 that the rate of change of $\ln(t)$ with respect to t is given by the calculation of $1/t$, therefore the integral of $1/t$ with respect to t is $\ln(t)$. The two equations

$$\frac{d}{dt}\ln(t)=\frac{1}{t} \quad \text{and} \quad \int \frac{1}{t}\,dt=\ln(t)$$

are two different ways of expressing the same thing, and the derivatives given in Table 9.1 and the Appendix can be used as a list of integrals by looking for the function in the column headed $f'(t)$ and finding the answer in the column headed $f(t)$.

9.8.2   Arbitrary constant

We have:

$$\frac{\mathrm{d}}{\mathrm{d}t}(e^t)=e^t, \quad \text{and} \quad \frac{\mathrm{d}}{\mathrm{d}t}(e^t+6)=e^t \quad \text{and} \quad \frac{\mathrm{d}}{\mathrm{d}t}(e^t-91\cdot45)=e^t;$$

all these may be deduced from the formula (9.11) and Table 9.1. This means that

$$\int e^t\mathrm{d}t=e^t, \quad \text{or} \quad e^t+6, \quad \text{or} \quad e^t-91\cdot45$$

In general we can add or subtract any arbitrary constant from the integral and still have a valid answer. This constant is important in practical work and is discussed further in Chapter 12, but it is usually omitted in simple statements of the integral, and the reader assumes its presence without being told.

9.8.3   Repeated integration

The indefinite integral will generally be a function of the variable t and could itself be integrated again; this is equivalent to finding a function whose second derivative gives the desired answer. These are called *double integrals* and the notation

$$\int\int f\mathrm{d}t\mathrm{d}t$$

is used. The notation may be extended in an obvious way to third, fourth, or higher-order integrals. When the number of integrations is large, this is written

$$\int \ldots \int f\,\mathrm{d}t \ldots \mathrm{d}t$$

which is much more cumbersome and less explicit than the notation for the derivative.

Example:

$$I=\int\int t^2\,\mathrm{d}t\,\mathrm{d}t=\int\left(\int t^2\,\mathrm{d}t\right)\mathrm{d}t$$

Integrating the part in the bracket we note that

$$\frac{\mathrm{d}}{\mathrm{d}t}(t^3/3)=t^2$$

so $\qquad I = \int (t^3/3 + C)\, \mathrm{d}t$

where C is the arbitrary constant. By similar reasoning applied to $t^3/3 + C$

$\qquad I = t^4/12 + Ct + D$

where both C and D are arbitrary constants.

(Note $\quad \dfrac{\mathrm{d}^2 I}{\mathrm{d}t^2} = t^2$)

The repeated integral sign is most frequently used for functions of several variables. For example, the symbols

$$\int\!\!\int g(x, y)\, \mathrm{d}x\, \mathrm{d}y$$

means that g is a variable which depends on both x and y, that first g has been integrated with respect to the variable x, regarding y as constant then the answer has been integrated with respect to y.

9.8.4   *Evaluation of the indefinite integral*

Fortunately the evaluation of the indefinite integral is largely left to mathematicians. Unlike the derivative, the integral often presents great problems algebraically, and the algebraic expressions of the integral cannot be found for many important functions. For example,

$$\frac{1}{\sqrt{(2\pi)}} \exp\left(-\tfrac{1}{2}t^2\right)$$

is the *normal probability function* and its integral is frequently required; but it has to be evaluated and tabled by complicated numerical methods, as its algebraic form cannot be found. There are extensive tables of integrals such as the normal probability integral which occur so frequently as to be regarded as implicit functions in much the same way as the square root is regarded as a function; see e.g. Abramowitz & Stegun (1965).

For the general handling of integrals the reader is referred to any elementary text on Calculus—e.g. Schaff (1963) or Courant (1934). We give three simple rules:

(i) From the definition just given, the integral of the derivative is the original function plus an arbitrary constant c. This can be expressed symbolically in a number of ways, e.g.

$$\int f'(t)\, \mathrm{d}t = f(t) + c \quad \text{or} \quad \int \frac{\mathrm{d}f}{\mathrm{d}t}\, \mathrm{d}t = f + c \quad \text{or} \quad \int \frac{\mathrm{d}y}{\mathrm{d}x}\, \mathrm{d}x = y + c \qquad (9.24)$$

(ii) From the second line in Table 9.1 we can see that if the function of t is equal to t itself then the derivative is 1.

$\int 1 \, dt$ is written as $\int dt$ so we say:

$\int dt = t + c$, or using other letters instead of t:

$$\int dx = x + c, \quad \int dy = y + c, \quad \int df = f + c, \quad \text{and so on.} \tag{9.25}$$

By comparing (9.24) and (9.25) it can be seen that the symbols df and dt can be treated as if they were simple variables and the symbols $\dfrac{df}{dt} \, dt$ treated as if it were the product $\dfrac{df}{dt} * dt$. Generally the integral $\int f(t) \, dt$ can be treated as if the term being integrated was the product $f(t) * dt$. Similar remarks apply to x, y, dx, dy, etc.

(iii) We stated in Section 9.5.2 that sums and differences can be differentiated term by term; similarly so sums and differences can be integrated term by term. For example:

$$\int (t^2 + t) \, dt = \frac{t^3}{3} + \frac{t^2}{2} + c$$

In practice there is an element of inspired guesswork to put the algebra in a suitable form. Maynard Smith (1968) recalls his attempts to find $\int x \tan (x) \, dx$ before it occurred to him to try the methods we are about to discuss.

9.9   The definite integral

9.9.1   The area under a curve

Let CD be a portion of the curve representing the value of $f(t)$ plotted as a graph against t, with the value of $f(t)$ on the vertical axis and the value of t on the horizontal axis—see Fig 9.8. Let the extreme positions on the t axis be A and B where the value of t at A is a and the value of t at B is b.

To find the area under the curve, i.e. the area of $ABCD$ we may divide the figure into thin vertical strips. Although it is not essential we shall assume that all these strips have equal width and denote this width by δt. To find the area of one of the strips we multiply the width of the strip by its height. This is an approximation that does not take account of the slope at the top of the curve, but, if the strips are very narrow, it will be a good approximation. The height

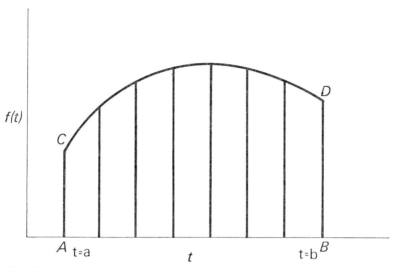

Fig 9.8

of the strip is the value of $f(t)$ at some point in the strip, so its area is a term of the form: $f(t) * \delta t$. We obtain the whole area by summing the contribution from each of the strips as t goes from the value a to the value b, and we denote this sum by the symbols

$$\sum_{t=a}^{b} f(t) * \delta t.$$

We can improve the accuracy of this approximation by dividing AB into a greater number of smaller intervals, and consequently diminishing the size of δt. What we are doing mathematically is to consider the limit of

$$\sum_{t=a}^{b} f(t) * \delta t$$

as δt tends to zero.

9.9.2   *Notation*

The symbol

$$\int_{a}^{b} f(t)\, \mathrm{d}t$$

is used to denote this limit as δt tends to zero,

i.e. $\displaystyle\int_{a}^{b} f(t)\, \mathrm{d}t = \lim_{\delta t \to 0} \sum_{t=a}^{b} f(t) * \delta t$ (9.26)

This symbol is called the *definite integral of f with respect to t between the limits a and b*, (the word definite is often omitted) and the process of obtaining the sum given in (9.26) is called integration between limits.

The connection between the definite integral and the indefinite integral already considered will be shown in Section 9.10, for the use of the same symbol for both suggests that the concepts are analogous.

9.9.3   Calculation of the area

The reader may demonstrate that the formula (9.26) does represent area by drawing, e.g. a semicircle of radius 5 cm on millimetre graph paper (Fig 9.9). If we divide the figure into four strips each 2·5 cm wide and take the height at the midpoint of each strip as $f(t)$,

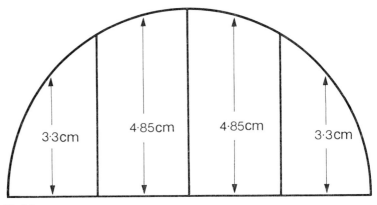

3·3cm   4·85cm   4·85cm   3·3cm

Fig 9.9

we get for the calculation of area:

$$\text{area} = 3\cdot3 * 2\cdot5 + 4\cdot85 * 2\cdot5 + 4\cdot85 * 2\cdot5 + 3\cdot3 * 2\cdot5 = 40\cdot75 \text{ sq cm}$$

If we divide the semicircle into ten strips each of width 1 cm we will get

$$\text{area} = 2\cdot2 + 3\cdot6 + 4\cdot35 + 4\cdot8 + 5\cdot0 + 5\cdot0 + 4\cdot8 + 4\cdot35 + 3\cdot6 + 2\cdot2$$

$$= 39\cdot9 \text{ sq cm}$$

The process can be continued and the results will eventually approach a limiting value of 39·3 sq cm. More elaborate methods of calculating the area under a curve from the heights of a number of its ordinates are given in Section 9.12 but they work on the same principle.

It can be seen that the definite integral could be computed for curves with discontinuities provided we select the edges of strips to coincide with the discontinuities so that there is not a discontinuity within any of the strips.

9.9.4 The integral and the average

If we have a function varying in time with values $f(t)$ at time t and we want its average value over the period of say 10 to 20 min we may divide the interval into ten 1-min intervals and evaluate f at the mid-point of each interval; the average is then

$$\frac{f(10\cdot5)+f(11\cdot5)+f(12\cdot5)+\ldots+f(19\cdot5)}{10}$$

We may get a more accurate average by dividing the interval into twenty $\frac{1}{2}$-min intervals and evaluating

$$\frac{f(10\cdot25)+f(10\cdot75)+f(11\cdot25)+\ldots+f(19\cdot75)}{20}$$

Algebraically if we take intervals of width δt there will be $(20-10)/\delta t$ of them and the average will be given by

$$\frac{\Sigma f(t)}{(20-10)/\delta t}=\frac{\Sigma f(t)*\delta t}{20-10}$$

where the function $f(t)$ is calculated at the mid-points of the intervals between $t=10$ and $t=20$.

For a continuous function we may let δt tend to zero and the average is then expressible as the definite integral

$$\frac{\int_{10}^{20}f(t)\,dt}{20-10}$$

So the average value of a function is the area under the graph of the function divided by the range of time (or independent variable) which the area covers.

9.9.5 Other interpretations

The definite integral is expressed algebraically as the sum of a very large number of very small terms of the form $f(t)*\delta t$, so the ideas and notation will obviously apply to any other concept which can be expressed in this fashion. For example, the specific heat of a body is the heat required to raise the temperature of unit mass of the body 1°C. The specific heat of water changes with temperature, so if we wish to find the heat required to raise a gram of water from 0°C to 4°C we will have to approximate it by supposing the specific heat, instead of changing continuously, changes in small steps. Let us divide the interval 0°C to 4°C into a number of small intervals equal to $\delta\theta°C$ and suppose the specific heat during each small interval remains constant; as it is a function of temperature let us denote its value by $f(\theta)$. The heat required to take the temperature of the water from $\theta°C$ through the small increase $\delta\theta$ is just specific heat times temperature rise, i.e. $f(\theta) * \delta\theta$. We obtain the heat required for the whole rise from 0° to 4° by adding all these, i.e.

$$\sum_{t=0}^{4} f(\theta) * \delta\theta$$

is approximately equal to the heat required. As with the area under a curve we get a more and more accurate result by imagining the interval divided into smaller and smaller steps, and we may say as before that the heat required is the limit of this sum as δt tends to zero, i.e.

$$\int_0^4 f(\theta) \, d\theta$$

We may find the value of this integral by plotting the values of specific heat against temperature and finding the area under the curve.

Again, if we denote the rate of excretion of a biochemical compound by the symbol $f'(t)$, and if this rate of excretion is constant then the total amount of compound excreted between 10 and 20 min after a test injection would just be the product of the rate of excretion and the time interval. However, the rate of excretion is affected by the injection and will change with time, i.e. $f'(t)$ changes with time, and so the total amount of compound excreted between 10 and 20 min after the meal will have to be obtained by dividing the time interval 10 to 20 min into very small time intervals denoted by δt. The total amount secreted will now be

$$\sum_{t=10}^{20} f'(t) * \delta t.$$

If we take the time intervals smaller and smaller to obtain a more accurate answer we can again denote the amount of compound excreted by the definite integral

$$\int_{10}^{20} f'(t) \, dt \qquad\qquad (9.27)$$

We may find the amount of compound excreted by finding the area under the graph of rate of excretion against time.

9.10   Connection between the definite and indefinite integral

In the last example we chose the symbols $f'(t)$ to represent the rate of excretion. If we represent the total amount of compound excreted by time t as $f(t)$, then the rate of increase in this amount is the rate of excretion, and is denoted by $f'(t)$. The amount excreted between 10 and 20 min is the difference between the total amount excreted by 10 min and the total amount excreted by 20 min, which can be written symbolically as

$$f(20)-f(10). \tag{9.28}$$

Formulae (9.27) and (9.28) are two ways of representing the same thing and so

$$\int_{10}^{20} f'(t)\, dt = f(20)-f(10) \tag{9.29}$$

That is, *if we can find the function, $f(t)$ whose derivative is the known rate of change $f'(t)$, then we can evaluate the definite integral by obtaining the values of this function at either end of the range.*

N.B. A difference such as $f(20)-f(10)$ is sometimes written as

$$\left[f(t) \right]_{t=10}^{t=20}$$

or as $\quad \left[f(t) \right]_{10}^{20}$

Example:

If the rate of excretion during the period could be obtained by evaluating $0{\cdot}01\,\exp\,(-0{\cdot}01t)$ then this is $f'(t)$. To calculate the total amount excreted we could try to find the function $f(t)$ which when differentiated gave $0{\cdot}01\,\exp\,(-0{\cdot}01t)$. By reference to Table 9.1 this is $-\exp\,(-0{\cdot}01t)$. Replacing $f(t)$ by $\exp(-0{\cdot}01t)$ in formula (9.29), gives the total amount excreted as

$$\int_{10}^{20} 0{\cdot}01\,\exp\,(-0{\cdot}01t)\, dt = \left[-\exp\,(-0{\cdot}01 * t) \right]_{10}^{20}$$
$$= -\exp\,(-0{\cdot}01 * 20) + \exp\,(-0{\cdot}01 * 10)$$
$$= 0{\cdot}086$$

The process of finding the function which when differentiated gives the function being integrated, is the same as the process of obtaining the indefinite integral given in Section 9.8. Providing the function being integrated has an algebraic expression for its *indefinite* integral, then the *definite* integral can be evaluated by taking the difference between the two values of the *indefinite* integral at either end of the range of integration (ignoring the arbitrary constant). This technique will only be of use when the functions can be represented by simple algebraic expressions and unless the function is a very simple combination of terms of the sort given in Table 9.1 the resulting mathematics may be very difficult or even impossible. It is unlikely to be of use for functions defined by an empirical set of observations.

9.11   Negative areas

If we follow the calculations of area for curves which can have negative values, we will see that it is possible to get a negative answer. Figure 9.10 shows a curve which can take negative and positive values. In the shaded area between the points B and C the values of the function represented by this curve are negative so that when we form the sum of the terms $f(t) * \delta t$ the answer will be negative. In the unshaded area the answer is positive, so the definite integral

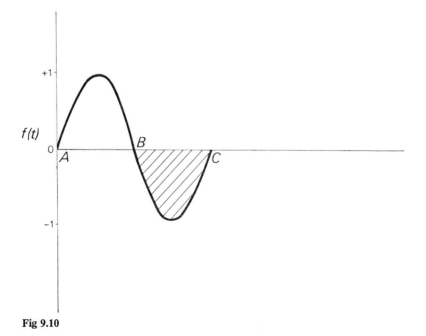

Fig 9.10

as defined in (9.26) will regard contributions to the total area from parts of the curve below the t axis as negative. This means that we must take care when calculating areas to make sure the signs are correct for the problem. In Fig 9.10 the shaded area and the unshaded area would cancel each other out giving the total area under the curve as zero. This would be acceptable if we were using the area to represent the average value of $f(t)$ but not acceptable if we were actually concerned with the physical area under a curve of this shape. In the latter case we would integrate the function separately for the shaded and unshaded regions and add the absolute values of the two areas.

The outer limits between which the sum is being formed are called the *limits of integration*. Normally the top limit will be larger than the bottom one; if the order is reversed this reverses the sign of the integral, and is equivalent to regarding the δt term of (9.26) as negative. A combination of negative values of $f(t)$ and decreasing values of t, i.e. negative values of δt, will give a positive contribution to the area.

9.12   Integration by numerical methods

The technique for evaluating the integral by numerical methods (numerical quadrature) consists of dividing the range of integration into a number of small intervals and approximating the area under the curve in that interval. Essentially we consider an approximation

$$\int_a^b f(t)\, dt = \sum_{j=1}^{n} w_j * f(t_j)$$

that is, a weighted sum of the function evaluated at n different points along the curve between $t=a$ and $t=b$. The choice of the weights w_j and the positions of t_j are controlled by attempts to achieve the maximum accuracy for a given number of intervals. Various schemes have been proposed based on approximating the function within each small interval by a polynomial.

Examples:

(i) $f(t) = a + bt$

These are called *first-order formulae* and are equivalent to regarding the function as a straight line within each strip. They require the value of the function at two points in each interval.

(ii) $f(t) = a + bt + ct^2$.

These are called *second-order formulae* and require the value of the function at three points per interval.

(iii) $f(t) = a + bt + ct^2 + dt^3$.

These are called *third-order formulae* and require the value of the function at four points per interval.

Generally it is inadvisable to use high-order quadrature formulae unless the high-order differential coefficients can be studied.

There are two main types of integration formulae:

(i) *Newton–Cotes formulae* based on equidistant values of t.
(ii) *the Gauss formulae* where there are special rules for the spacing of t.

The Gauss formulae tend to be the more accurate and more efficient, the Newton–Cotes formulae simpler to compute.

These formulae are given in the Appendix and each is followed by the error term which is a function of the second or fourth differential of $f(t)$ evaluated at t somewhere in the interval $[a, b]$.

The most popular formula is the 2nd order Newton–Cotes formula, usually called *Simpson's Rule*. The interval $[a, b]$ is divided into n equal intervals (n must be even) and the function evaluated at the end of each interval. The formula is:

$$h = (b-a)/n$$

$$\text{area} \doteq \frac{h}{3} \{ f(t_0) + 4f(t_1) + 2f(t_2) + 4f(t_3) + \ldots + 2f(t_{n-2}) + 4f(t_{n-1}) + f(t_n) \}$$

(9.30)

where $t_0 = a$, $t_1 = a+h$, $t_2 = a+2h$, $\ldots t_n = b$

Example:

Consider the semi-circle in Fig 9.9 (Section 9.9.3) divided into four strips width $2 \cdot 5$ cm. The heights of the end points are 0, $4 \cdot 35$, 5, $4 \cdot 35$ and 0.

Simpson's Rule (9.30) gives the area as:

$$\frac{2 \cdot 5}{3} (0 + 4 * 4 \cdot 35 + 2 * 5 + 4 * 4 \cdot 35 + 0) = 37 \cdot 3$$

These strips are very wide for an accurate integral but the answer is still correct to within about 5%. The reader may also notice that these higher-order formulae are not necessarily more accurate than the mid-point method described in Section 9.9.3. Further details are given in Ralston & Wilf (1960).

9.13   Volumes

We have considered the integral by analogy with area under a curve as the limit of $\sum f * \delta t$ when δt tends to zero. If we were considering volume under a surface then the height of the surface may be considered constant over a very small *area*. The height may be represented by a function $z = f(x, y)$ (see Section 8.12) and the small elements of area over which it is considered constant are rectangles with side lengths δx and δy (Fig 9.11).

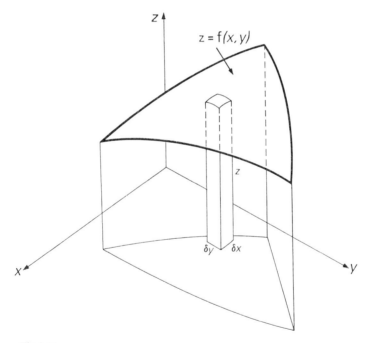

Fig 9.11

The volume of this small thin pencil with height z and base δx by δy is $z * \delta x * \delta y$, and so the total volume of the solid is $\sum z * \delta x * \delta y$, where we take the sum over all small areas under the surface. As δx and δy tend to zero this leads to another form of the integral which corresponds to a double limit and is written:

$$\iint_{\substack{\text{area in the} \\ x, y \text{ plane}}} z \, dx \, dy = \lim_{\substack{\delta x \to 0 \\ \delta y \to 0}} \sum z * \delta x * \delta y \qquad (9.31)$$

This is a *double integral*; it clearly applies to any summation that can be expressed in the form (9.31), and there is an obvious extension of this notation to limits of the form

$$\lim_{\delta x \to 0} \lim_{\delta y \to 0} \lim_{\delta z \to 0} \sum f * \delta x * \delta y * \delta z = \iiint_{\substack{\text{volume in } x,\, y,\, z \\ \text{space}}} f \, dx \, dy \, dz$$

These integrals are the definite integral versions of repeated integration considered in Section 9.8.3.

For regular solids, e.g. cones etc., it is usually easier to consider the solid as made of a number of very thin parallel discs, depth δz, and form the sum

$$\text{Volume} = \sum A \, \delta z$$

where A is the area of the disc. In the limit this becomes $\int A \, dz$, which is often easier to handle than the multiple integral.

Example:

To find the volume of a segment of a sphere cut off by a plane as in Fig 9.12:

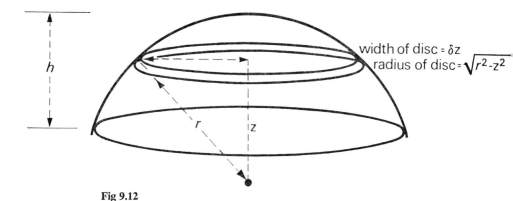

width of disc $= \delta z$
radius of disc $= \sqrt{r^2 - z^2}$

Fig 9.12

Let the radius of the sphere be r and the depth of the segment be h. Then the volume can be considered as composed of a very large number of thin discs distance z from the centre, with z varying from $r - h$ to r. The radius of a disc distance z from the centre is $\sqrt{(r^2 - z^2)}$ and its area is therefore $\pi(r^2 - z^2)$ (area of a circle $= \pi * \text{radius}^2$).

The volume of the segment is

$$\int_{r-h}^{r} \pi(r^2 - z^2) \, dz$$

which is $[\pi(r^2z-z^3/3)]$ evaluated at $z=r$, minus $[\pi(r^2z-z^3/3)]$ evaluated at $z=r-h$

(cf. Section 9.10)

$$= \pi(r^3-r^3/3) - \pi(r^2(r-h)-(r-h)^3/3)$$

which simplifies to

$$\pi h^2(r-h/3).$$

For further details of the techniques and applications of multiple integration the reader is referred to Schaff (1963) or Courant (1934).

Chapter 10
Series

10.1   Introduction

This Chapter deals with functions which are represented by the sum of a number of terms. As an example of a problem giving rise to such a function, consider a compartment of fluid with an input and an excretion. Suppose the flow of fluid through the compartment is so arranged that if a small volume of tracer dye, which mixes completely with the liquid, is injected into the compartment, then at the end of the first hour after this injection, the amount of dye present is half the original, at the end of the second hour the amount remaining is half that at the end of the first hour—i.e., one quarter of the original amount; and so on. The relationship between the amount of dye excreted and the amount remaining can be set out as follows:

Time (Hours)	Proportion remaining	Total proportion excreted	
0	1	0	
1	$\frac{1}{2}$	$\frac{1}{2}$	$= 0\cdot5$
2	$\frac{1}{4}$	$\frac{1}{2}+\frac{1}{4}$	$= 0\cdot75$
3	$\frac{1}{8}$	$\frac{1}{2}+\frac{1}{4}+\frac{1}{8}$	$= 0\cdot875$
4	$\frac{1}{16}$	$\frac{1}{2}+\frac{1}{4}+\frac{1}{8}+\frac{1}{16}$	$= 0\cdot9375$
.	.	.	.
n	$\dfrac{1}{2^n}$	$\displaystyle\sum_{i=1}^{n}\frac{1}{2^i}$	

We note that at any time the overall total proportion of dye excreted plus dye retained remains constant at 1; that is,

$$\frac{1}{2^n}+\sum_{i=1}^{n}\frac{1}{2^i}=1$$

From this, we have:

$$\sum_{i=1}^{n}\frac{1}{2^i}=1-\frac{1}{2^n} \qquad (10.1)$$

i.e. the proportion of dye excreted after n hours, which $=\displaystyle\sum_{i=1}^{n}\frac{1}{2^i}$, can also be represented by $1-\dfrac{1}{2^n}$ which therefore gives the value of the sum $\displaystyle\sum_{i=1}^{n}\frac{1}{2^i}$.

As time progresses (i.e. $n\to\infty$) the above process involves a larger and larger series of additions, but as $n\to\infty$, $1-\dfrac{1}{2^n}\to1$ (see Section 5.8), and so we conclude that

$$\tfrac{1}{2}+\tfrac{1}{4}+\tfrac{1}{8}+\tfrac{1}{16}+\ldots \text{ etc.} \to 1 \qquad (10.2)$$

Physically speaking, this simply means that the proportion of dye excreted tends to 1 as time goes on; this is not a very startling conclusion, but arising out of this problem has come the purely mathematical result (10.2) which can be useful in other contexts.

10.2   Series

An expression such as $\frac{1}{2}+\frac{1}{4}+\frac{1}{8}+\frac{1}{16}+\ldots$ is an example of a *series*. Generally speaking, a series is simply a sum of terms, but with the essential feature that each term is related to the preceding term or terms in some mathematically defined way—e.g. in the example (10.2) the rule is that each term is half the preceding term. The terms in a series may be positive or negative, numerical or algebraic. A series may have an unlimited number of terms, in which case it is called an *infinite series*, or a finite number of terms, when it is called a *finite series*. We see from (10.2) that it is possible for an *infinite* series to have a *finite* sum (or more precisely, to have a finite *limit*). This is not always the case, however; for it to happen, there are various conditions necessary which broadly speaking amount to the requirement that successive terms in the series decrease at a fast enough rate. A finite series, on the other hand, will normally have a computable sum.

Infinite series can arise in two ways: they can be the natural representation of a physical process (the series given in (10.2) is an example of the classical 'half-life' approach which is used in problems involving the transfer or degradation of biochemical compounds in the body), or they can be a useful mathematical tool for handling more difficult functions. It can be proved for example that:

$$1+\frac{1}{2}+\frac{1}{3}+\frac{1}{4}+\frac{1}{5}+\frac{1}{6}+\frac{1}{7}\ldots \text{etc.} \rightarrow \infty \tag{10.3}$$

$$1-\frac{1}{2}+\frac{1}{3}-\frac{1}{4}+\frac{1}{5}-\frac{1}{6}+\frac{1}{7}\ldots \text{etc.} \rightarrow \ln(2) \tag{10.4}$$

$$1-\frac{1}{3}+\frac{1}{5}-\frac{1}{7}+\frac{1}{9}-\frac{1}{11}+\frac{1}{13}\ldots \text{etc.} \rightarrow \frac{\pi}{4} \tag{10.5}$$

$$1+\frac{1}{2^2}+\frac{1}{3^2}+\frac{1}{4^2}+\frac{1}{5^2}+\frac{1}{6^2}+\frac{1}{7^2}\ldots \text{etc.} \rightarrow \frac{\pi^2}{6} \tag{10.6}$$

$$1+\frac{1}{1*2}+\frac{1}{1*2*3}+\frac{1}{1*2*3*4}\ldots \text{etc.} \rightarrow e \tag{10.7}$$

Relationships such as (10.5)–(10.7) obviously provide a practical means of computing values of numbers such as π and e to any desired accuracy. It is perhaps reasonable to suppose from such examples that if complicated functions could be expressed in the form of a series then they too could be computed or handled more easily. As we shall see, Taylor's formula (Section 10.4) gives a means of doing just this. Series are particularly useful for computation on digital computers, since the relationship of any one term to the preceding ones can usually be programmed in a simple repetitive loop.

Series are also of very great interest to mathematicians; for example π could be regarded as an inconvenient constant necessary for evaluating the circumferences and areas of circles, but when we consider in (10.5) and (10.6) the different and rhythmic arrangement of numbers which also lead to this same strange constant it is clearly more than just a geometrical accident. Mathematicians have considered in great detail the conditions under which infinite series have a finite limit, and why, for example series such as

$$1 + \frac{1}{2^{1\cdot001}} + \frac{1}{3^{1\cdot001}} + \frac{1}{4^{1\cdot001}} + \frac{1}{5^{1\cdot001}} + \frac{1}{6^{1\cdot001}} \cdots \text{etc.} \tag{10.8}$$

or the series (10.4) have finite limits while a series such as (10.3) has not. We do not intend to go into these conditions in any detail, as the reasoning employed requires quite a sophisticated level of mathematical thought. In practice many series are handled with only a cursory investigation into the conditions for them to have a finite limit, or *converge* as it is called. This disregard can sometimes cause errors; if we were computing (10.3), for example, after a few thousand terms had been added to the series we might be convinced that we had a fairly good approximation to the correct answer, and be quite wrong. For this reason we have included the error term in both the series used for simplifying the calculations of functions (Sections 10.4 and 10.5) and this should normally be examined to see that it is sufficiently small. In using a series as a representation of an actual physical process the conditions of the process usually dictate that it will have a finite sum. Simple rules which determine in some cases whether an infinite series has a finite sum are given in the last section of this chapter (Section 10.7).

10.3   Sums of some special series

10.3.1   *Geometric series*

In the example given in formula (10.2), we note that each term of this series is a constant multiple, i.e. $\frac{1}{2}$, of the preceding term. A similar but more general

L

series can be obtained by replacing the $\frac{1}{2}$ by an unassigned value, say x, and considering

$$1+x+x^2+x^3+x^4+x^5+x^6+\ldots \text{ etc.}$$

Such a series is called a *geometric series* or *geometric progression*. To find a formula for the sum of the first n terms of this series, we write the sum of the first n terms as S_n; this is a common general notation when handling series. We note that if we multiply S_n by the values of x the effect is to move the series on one place:

$$S_n = 1 + x + x^2 + x^3 + x^4 + \ldots + x^n$$

$$xS_n = \qquad x + x^2 + x^3 + x^4 + \ldots + x^n + x^{n+1}$$

and therefore

$$S_n = x * S_n + 1 - x^{n+1}$$

This equation can be arranged to give

$$(1-x) * S_n = 1 - x^{n+1}$$

i.e.
$$S_n = \frac{1 - x^{n+1}}{1 - x} \tag{10.9}$$

If x is fractional and $n \to \infty$, then S_n tends to the finite limit $1/(1-x)$. The limiting process is given in Section 5.9.2.

Thus $\qquad 1 + x^2 + x^3 + x^4 + x^5 + x^6 + \ldots \to \dfrac{1}{1-x} \tag{10.10}$

if $\qquad -1 < x < 1$

10.3.2   Arithmetic series

Another important series is the *arithmetic series* or *arithmetic progression* in which each term differs by a fixed amount from the preceding term.

Examples:

$$1 + 3 + 5 + 7 + 9 + \ldots \text{ (common difference} = 2)$$

$$5 + 1 - 3 - 7 - \ldots \text{ (common difference} = -4)$$

In general if **f** is the first term of the series and **l** the nth (or last) term, the sum of the first n terms is given by

$$S_n = \frac{n * (f+l)}{2}$$ (10.11)

Examples:

$$2+4+6+8+10 = (2+10) * \frac{5}{2} = 30$$

$$1+2+3+4 \ldots +100 = (1+100) * \frac{100}{2} = 5050$$

The proof of the result (10.11) can be established by rewriting the series backwards under the original series and adding up the two series; e.g.

$$2+ \ 4+ \ 6+ \ 8+10$$
$$10+ \ 8+ \ 6+ \ 4+ \ 2$$
$$\overline{}$$
$$12+12+12+12+12 = 60$$

Thus twice the sum of the series equals 60, so the series equals 30. The general formula (10.11) can be established in the same way.

Note that an infinite arithmetic series will *not* have a finite sum.

10.4   Taylor's formula

Taylor's formula (or *Taylor's series*) provides a means of expressing a function of x as a series of powers of x. It is applicable to functions for which we can find the derivatives. Let the function be $f(x)$, and denote its first, second, third, ... etc., derivatives by $f^{(1)}(x), f^{(2)}(x), f^{(3)}(x), \ldots$ etc. Taylor's formula provides the *series expansion*, as it is called, of the function at a point distance x from a reference value R on the assumption that the values at R of the function and its derivatives are known. The series is:

$$f(R+x) = a_0 + a_1 * x + a_2 * x^2 + \ldots + a_n * x^n + \text{'remainder'}$$ (10.12)

where $a_0 = f(R)$ $a_1 = \frac{f^{(1)}(R)}{1!}$ $a_2 = \frac{f^{(2)}(R)}{2!}$ $a_3 = \frac{f^{(3)}(R)}{3!}$

and generally

$$a_n = \frac{f^{(n)}(R)}{n!}$$

and the 'remainder'

$$= \frac{x^{n+1}}{(n+1)!} * f^{(n+1)}(R+\theta * x), \qquad 0 \leqslant \theta \leqslant 1 \qquad (10.13)$$

The value of θ is unspecified. The notation implies that $f^{(n+1)}$ is evaluated somewhere in the interval $(R, R+x)$. Remember that

$$n! = n * (n-1) * (n-2) * \ldots * 3 * 2 * 1 \qquad \text{(Section 4.2.3)}.$$

If we examine this formula in detail, we can see that $f(R+x)$ is expressed as a series of powers of x up to the power x^n; we say '$f(R+x)$ has been *expanded* as an nth order power series (or Taylor's series) *around the point R*'. In the main part of the series x only appears in powers of x, i.e. $x, x^2, x^3 \ldots x^n$, the derivatives of $f(x)$ being replaced by their actual values at $x=R$. The remainder, however contains the term $f^{(n+1)}(R+\theta * x)$ that is, the $(n+1)$th derivative evaluated somewhere in the interval $(R, R+x)$. In practice it will not be known exactly where in the interval, but this indeterminacy is generally unimportant. To be of any practical use the remainder term given in (10.13) must become sufficiently small for fairly small values of n, i.e. after a small number of terms in the expansion. This often implies that the value of x is fractional. The Taylor's series expansion of all the common functions has been investigated, and from this the range of x for which the expansions are practical has been determined.

In the particular case $R=0$, Taylor's series takes on a simpler form known as *Maclaurin's formula* (or *Maclaurin's series*):

$$f(x) = f(0) + \frac{x * f^{(1)}(0)}{1!} + \frac{x^2 * f^{(2)}(0)}{2!} + \ldots \frac{x^{(n)} * f^{(n)}(0)}{n!} + \text{remainder}$$

$$(10.14)$$

where the remainder

$$= \frac{x^{n+1}}{(n+1)!} * f^{(n+1)}(\theta x) \qquad 0 \leqslant \theta \leqslant 1 \qquad (10.15)$$

This expands $f(x)$ around the point 0.

It can be seen that all those functions with fairly simple derivatives, discussed in Chapter 9, will have a fairly simple power series expansions, and to illustrate this we will examine the function $\sin(x)$, i.e. $f(x) = \sin(x)$. If x is measured in radians the derivatives of $\sin(x)$ are given by

$$f^{(1)}(x) = \cos(x), \quad f^{(2)}(x) = -\sin(x), \quad f^{(3)}(x) = -\cos(x),$$

and $\qquad f^{(4)}(x) = \sin(x)$

and so $\quad f(0) = 1, \quad f^{(1)}(0) = 0, \quad f^{(2)}(0) = -1. \quad f^{(3)}(0) = 0 \quad \text{and} \quad f^{(4)}(0) = 1$

Applying Maclaurin's formula gives

$$\sin(x) = x - \frac{x^3}{3!} + \frac{x^5}{5!} - \frac{x^7}{7!} + \text{etc.} \tag{10.16}$$

Examples:

(i) To find the sine of $0 \cdot 3$ radians, (approximately 17°).

We shall use the series given in (10.16), approximating the answer by the first two terms only.

$$\sin(x) = 0 \cdot 3 - \frac{(0 \cdot 3)^3}{3 * 2} = 0 \cdot 2955$$

The accuracy of this approximation can be judged by examining the remainder term in Maclaurin's formula.

$$\text{The remainder} = \frac{x^4}{(n+1)!} \sin(\theta x) \qquad 0 \leqslant \theta \leqslant 1$$

But $\sin(\theta x)$ must be less than 1 whatever the value of θx, and so the remainder must be less than $(0 \cdot 3)^4/4!$ i.e. less than $0 \cdot 00034$.

(ii) Again, consider the expansion of $\ln(1-x)$ by Taylor's series.

$f(R+x)$ is $\ln(1-x)$ and so $f(R)$ is $\ln(1)$ which is 0.

$f^{(1)}(R+x)$ is $\dfrac{-1}{(1-x)}$ and so $f^{(1)}(R)$ is -1

$f^{(2)}(R+x)$ is $\dfrac{-1}{(1-x)^2}$ and so $f^{(2)}(R)$ is -1

If we continue to differentiate the function of x and put $x=0$ we get

$$f^{(n)}(R) = -[(n-1)!]$$

and so the Taylor's series for the logarithm to base e is given by

$$\ln(1-x) = -x - \frac{x^2}{2} - \frac{x^3}{3} - \text{etc.} \tag{10.17}$$

Note that this series is only valid for x in the range $-1 \leqslant x < 1$.

Example:

King (1969) used this Taylor's series expansion of the logarithm to handle

$$P = \frac{V}{2At} \ln\left(\frac{C_0}{C_0 - 2C_2}\right) \tag{10.18}$$

in the case when C_2/C_0 had values of about $0 \cdot 05$.

Let us write x for the value of C_2/C_0:

$$P = \frac{V}{2At} \ln \left(\frac{1}{1 - 2C_2/C_0} \right) = -\frac{V}{2At} \ln (1 - 2x)$$

As a simple approximation use the first two terms of the Taylor's series expansion instead of $\ln (1 - 2x)$.

$$P = -\frac{V}{2At} \left(-2x - \frac{(2x)^2}{2} \right) = \frac{V}{At} (1 + x) \, x$$

The error in using this approximation to the logarithm can be judged by examining the remainder term in the series.

$$\frac{(2x)^3}{3(1 - 2\theta x)^3} \qquad 0 \leqslant \theta \leqslant 1$$

This must lie between $8x^3/(3(1 - 2x)^3)$ and $8x^3/3$, i.e. between $0 \cdot 00033$ and $0 \cdot 00045$ when x is $0 \cdot 05$.

The approximation is quite good for small values of x. In practice the smallness of x would be related to the acceptable error of taking the first few terms of the series. Often the smallness is part of the nature of the problem, as for instance when one is measuring very small changes in hormone concentration. In statistical work a 'small measurement error' is often assumed and so one can use a Taylor's series approximation to obtain expressions for mean and standard deviation of complicated functions of variables subject to measurement error.

Examining formula (10.12) again we see that it is possible to provide a polynomial approximation to a function by successively higher-order power series:

$$f(R + x) = f(R) + f^{(1)}(R) * x \tag{10.19}$$

$$f(R + x) = f(R) + f^{(1)}(R) * x + \frac{f^{(2)}(R)}{2!} * x^2 \tag{10.20}$$

$$f(R + x) = f(R) + f^{(1)}(R) * x + \frac{f^{(2)}(R)}{2!} * x^2 + \frac{f^{(3)}(R)}{3!} * x^3 \tag{10.21}$$

Formula (10.19) is an expression linear in x (Section 3.10). Its graph is a straight line, and represents therefore a straight line approximation to the graph of $f(R + x)$. Formula (10.20) is a second degree polynomial approximation; its graph is parabolic in shape (Section 8.10), and so on.

A function which can be represented by a power series in the neighbourhood of the point R is called *analytic* at R.

10.5   Fourier series and frequency analysis

The Taylor and Maclaurin formulae show the way in which a function can be expressed as a weighted sum of terms in x, x^2, x^3 ... with the weights depending on the values of the derivatives of the function. The *Fourier Series* provides a means of expanding a function as a weighted sum of sine or cosine terms. In this section we will use t for the variable, as Fourier series most often find their application in the analysis of functions of time.

Consider first a periodic function $f(t)$, of period 2π, as in Fig 10.1.

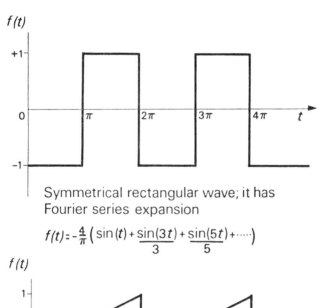

Symmetrical rectangular wave; it has Fourier series expansion

$$f(t) = -\frac{4}{\pi}\left(\sin(t) + \frac{\sin(3t)}{3} + \frac{\sin(5t)}{5} + \cdots\right)$$

Saw-tooth wave; it has Fourier series expansion

$$f(t) = \frac{1}{2} - \frac{1}{\pi}\left(\sin t + \frac{\sin(2t)}{2} + \frac{\sin(3t)}{3} + \frac{\sin(4t)}{4} + \cdots\right)$$

Two simple examples of functions with period 2π

Fig 10.1

The Fourier series expansion of $f(t)$ is

$$f(t)=a_0+a_1*\sin(p_1+t)+a_2*\sin(p_2+2*t)+a_3*\sin(p_3+3*t)$$
$$+\ldots+a_n*\sin(p_n+n*t)+\text{remainder}$$
$$(10.22)$$

where the a's and p's are given by expressions involving definite integrals of the forms

$$\frac{1}{\pi}\int_0^{2\pi}f(t)*\sin(n*t)\,dt \quad \text{and} \quad \frac{1}{\pi}\int_0^{2\pi}f(t)*\cos(n*t)\,dt$$

and the remainder is a more complicated expression of similar type. The full details of these quantities are given in the Appendix, page 421†.

If we examine the formula (10.22), we see that its value depends on the weighted sum of a number of sine functions. It shows the way in which a periodic function can be built up or constructed by taking sine waves—e.g. pure tones or pure alternating current oscillations—and adding them together, suitably weighted. The coefficients a_0, a_1, a_2, ... etc. correspond to the 'amplitudes' of the sine waves; the quantities p_1, p_2, p_3, ... etc. correspond to a shift along the scale of t and are called *phases*. Now the sine function is periodic (Section 6.9), and the series (10.22) corresponds to a sum of sine waves of smaller and smaller periods, i.e. increasing frequency (Section 6.17). In fact the whole series for $f(t)$ is periodic, of period 2π, because

$$a_1*\sin(p_1+t)=a_1*\sin(p_1+(t+2*\pi))$$
$$a_2*\sin(p_2+2t)=a_2*\sin(p_2+2*(t+2*\pi))$$

and so on for all terms of the expansion.

Thus both $f(t)$ and its Fourier series expansion have the same period, as we would expect if they were to be equivalent.

If the period of $f(t)$ is other than $2*\pi$, say T, then the expansion is a sum of terms such as

$$a_n\sin\left(p_n+\frac{2*\pi*n*t}{T}\right);$$

the period of such a term is T/n and its frequency is n/T.

If the function $f(t)$ is not periodic then we may still consider a Fourier Series expansion for it over a finite interval $(0, T)$, by constructing a periodic function which is $f(t)$ in $(0, T)$ but which goes on to repeat itself outside this interval (see Fig 10.2).

† In many texts the first term is written as $\frac{1}{2}a$.

N.B. In this case the series may not truly represent the function at the boundary points $t=0$, $t=T$.

The coefficients of the Fourier expansion depend on integrals of the function, which contrasts with the Taylor series expansion where the coefficients depend on the differentials. The integral is more easily calculated for observed empirical functions, and for functions with discontinuities, while the differential is more easily handled in the case of algebraically defined continuous functions. Hence

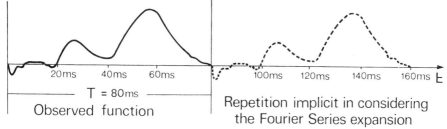

T = 80ms

Observed function

Repetition implicit in considering
the Fourier Series expansion

Fig 10.2 Somatosensory evoked response to ulnar nerve stimulus

Fourier and Taylor's expansions tend to be applied in corresponding situations. A further contrast is that the Taylor's series coefficients depend on the value of a derivative at a point, whilst the Fourier coefficients depend on the value of $f(t)$ throughout its range.

There are two important variations on the representation of the Fourier series given in formula (10.22).

$f(t)$ can be expressed as the sum of sine and cosine terms instead of just sine terms, thus:

$$f(t) = a_0 + b_1 * \sin(t) + b_2 \sin(2 * t) + b_3 \sin(3 * t) + \ldots$$
$$+ c_1 * \cos(t) + c_2 \cos(2 * t) + c_3 \cos(3 * t) + \ldots \quad (10.23)$$

Notice that the sine and cosine terms now contain only simple multiples of t (if the period of the function was T and not 2π they would contain only simple multiples of $2\pi t/T$). The phase terms p of formula (10.22) have been absorbed into the relationship between the b and c coefficients. The two expressions (10.22) and (10.23) are completely equivalent, the values of the a's, b's, c's and p's being related by the following rules:

$$a_1 = \sqrt{(b_1^2 + c_1^2)}, \quad a_2 = \sqrt{(b_2^2 + c_2^2)}, \quad a_3 = \sqrt{(b_3^2 + c_3^2)}, \quad \text{etc.}$$

and p_1 is the angle whose tangent is $\dfrac{c_1}{b_1}$,

p_2 is the angle whose tangent is $\dfrac{c_2}{b_2}$,

etc.

The phases p_1, p_2, p_3, etc. are often referred to as the *phase angles*. The form of the Fourier series given in (10.23) is the easier one to handle particularly for applications involving the algebraic manipulation of the series.

The Fourier series expansion is also applicable to functions which are observed at a finite number of discrete points. This is essentially the discrete analogue of the series, replacing the integral sign $\int$ by the summation sign $\sum$.

If we observe the function $f(t)$ at an odd number of points, say the $2N+1$ times t_0, t_1, t_2, t_3, $\ldots t_{2N}$, where the times are regularly spaced in the interval 0 to 2π so that

$$t_r = \frac{2 * \pi * r}{2N+1}$$

then $f(t)$ can be expanded as

$$f(t_r) = \alpha_0 + \sum_{p=1}^{N} (\alpha_p * \sin (p * t_r) + \beta_p * \cos (p * t_r)) \tag{10.24}$$

There are $2N+1$ coefficients in this expansion: α_0, α_1, α_2, $\ldots \alpha_N$ and β_1, β_2, $\beta_3 \ldots \beta_N$ and there are $2N+1$ known values of the function, and so the values of α_0, α_1, $\alpha_2 \ldots \alpha_N$ and β_1, $\beta_2 \ldots \beta_N$ can be determined. The values for the α's and β's for this form of the expansion are given in the Appendix, page 422.

We may notice that the $2N+1$ points defining the function $f(t)$ can be transformed by the formula (10.24) into a set of α's and β's ($2N+1$ in all). Both sets of numbers define the *same* function, but they represent two different ways of presenting it. If we present the values of $f(t_0)$, $f(t_1)$, $f(t_2)$, $f(t_3)$, etc. we present the observed measurements. If however we present the values of α_0, α_1, $\alpha_2 \ldots$ etc. and β_1, β_2, $\beta_3 \ldots$ etc. then we represent the function in a manner related to a set of frequencies and phases, and we sometimes talk of presenting the function 'in the frequency domain'. This technique has been used to examine pictures obtained in radioisotope scans, in the hope that features of abnormal scans may show patterns in the α or β terms which are not obvious in the ordinary pictures (Rosenfeld, A. (1969), Todd-Pokropek, A. E. (1969)). Similar techniques are applied to neurological waveforms. The techniques are also used for examining a long series of temperature measurements for diurnal, monthly and other rhythms; in this application the meaning and reason for obtaining a 'frequency representation' of the observations is perhaps more obvious. For mathematical details of the Fourier series see Davis (1963), Ross (1964), or texts dealing with specialised applications.

N.B. The computation of the coefficients in the formula (10.23) appears to be a simple set of summations. However, the process can be greatly increased in speed by using a technique which has been called the 'fast Fourier transform' and improvements of computing speeds by factors of $n/\log_2 (n)$ are possible, where n is the number of coefficients computed. For further information on this see Singleton (1968), or Cooley & Tukey (1965).

The Fourier series expansion is also important in considering the theoretical behaviour of instruments for electrical measurement.

10.6   Fourier and Taylor's series: general comments

In using the Fourier or Taylor expansion any value of the variable x gives a unique computable value of the function and these expansions are only applicable to single valued functions. Reference to books on numerical analysis will show that there are many alternative series which can be used for calculating the standard mathematical functions and constants and often one of these will be preferred in practice because it needs less computing time to achieve the same accuracy.

As given, Taylor's and Fourier's series apply to functions of a single variable, but there are analogous expansions for functions of more than one variable. For details consult, e.g., Korn & Korn (1961) under the headings: 'multiple (or multidimensional) Taylor and Fourier series'.

10.7   Conditions for a finite limit

10.7.1   Simple tests

We noted that the series (10.3) does not have a finite limit while (10.4) does. There are several theorems for helping to find out if a series does tend to finite limit or *converge* as it is called. We give three of them here. In these theorems we shall refer to the 'absolute value' of a term in the series meaning the value ignoring the sign, e.g. both $1 \cdot 5$ and $-1 \cdot 5$ have absolute value $1 \cdot 5$.

(i) *The sum of an infinite series of terms will have a finite limit if:*

The terms in the series satisfy all three conditions:

1. They alternate in sign, i.e. $+, -, +, -,$ or $-, +, -, +.$

2. They decrease in absolute value.

3. They tend to zero as the number of terms increases.

E.g. $1 - \frac{1}{2} + \frac{1}{3} - \frac{1}{4} + \frac{1}{5} - \ldots$ etc. will have a finite limit.

N.B. This gives *no* information about series which do not satisfy the conditions.

(ii) *The sum of an infinite series will have a finite limit if:*

The absolute value of each term is less than a corresponding term in a series that is known to have a finite limit.

E.g. $1 + \dfrac{1}{2^2+1} + \dfrac{1}{3^2+1} + \dfrac{1}{4^2+1} + \ldots$ etc.

will have a finite limit by comparison with (10.6), the second term being less than the term $1/2^2$, the third less than $1/3^2$ etc.

In this context it is useful to know a series which only just manages to have a finite limit such as:

$$1 + \frac{1}{2^k} + \frac{1}{3^k} + \frac{1}{4^k} + \frac{1}{5^k} + \ldots + \text{etc.}\quad\text{for any } k > 1$$

or $$1 + \frac{1}{2 * \ln(2)} + \frac{1}{3 * \ln(3)} + \frac{1}{4 * \ln(4)} + \ldots + \text{etc.,}$$

both of which have finite limits.

(iii) *The sum of an infinite series will have a finite limit if:*

The limit of the absolute value of the quotient of any **term** divided by the preceding term is less than 1.
E.g. consider the series

$$1 + 2 * x^2 + 3 * x^3 + 4 * x^4 + \ldots + \text{etc.}$$

The nth term is $n * x^n$, the $(n-1)$th term is $(n-1) * x^{n-1}$

and therefore the nth term divided by the $(n-1)$th term gives

$$\frac{n}{n-1} * |x|$$

in absolute value.
The limit as

$$n \to \infty \text{ of } \frac{n}{n-1} * |x| \text{ is } |x|$$

and so the series will converge if $|x|$ is less than 1.

Note that in this test we have to consider the limit of the ratio when $n \to \infty$ and this limit has to be *less* than 1. If the limit is greater than 1 then the series will not converge. If the limit equals 1 then further tests must be done—many of these may be found in e.g. Ferrar (1938) or Hyslop (1950), but the reader is cautioned that applying these tests can be a very tricky mathematical process.

10.7.2   Validity of Fourier and Taylor's series

It will be seen that we have not clearly stated the conditions for which Taylor's or Fourier series expansions are valid, i.e. we have always assumed that the remainder term tends to zero as n tends to infinity, while in practice we probably would not wish n to be very large. We are likely to want not more than five or six terms for the Taylor series, or perhaps a hundred frequencies for the Fourier series.

There are theorems concerning the conditions under which these series will converge to a limit and the reader is referred to, e.g. Protter & Morrey (1964) or James & James (1968), for more details than we have given. In a practical application we would also be concerned with the *speed* of convergence—i.e. the rate at which the remainder term tends to zero as we increase the number of terms—and how to tell how near the limit we are; these points are covered in texts on Numerical Analysis. In particular there are a variety of other polynomial approximations—notably *Chebychev* and similar *orthogonal polynomials* (Section 11.7.2)—which converge faster and are less liable to error than the Taylor series. The reader is also referred to Hastings (1955), who gives an empirical approach to the problem of approximation in a very readable way and includes a number of examples of *rational function* approximations.

Chapter 11
Computational Methods and Curve Fitting

11.1   Introduction

In practice, it may be very difficult to find the value of some variable satisfying a complicated relationship. Indeed, the reader may already have formed the opinion that in mathematical work, it is not usually possible to find values for a variable by purely algebraic manipulation, unless one is lucky enough to have a 'text book' situation. For example, if we have

$$(x-a) * (x-b) * (x-c) * (x-d) = 0 \tag{11.1}$$

then a, b, c, or d are values of x which make this equation true, and they are in fact the only such values. We say that $x = a, b, c,$ or d are 'solutions' of (11.1) or that a, b, c and d are 'roots' of (11.1) (cf. Section 1.10).

Again, consider

$$x^4 - 10x^3 + 35x^2 - 50x + 24 = 0 \tag{11.2}$$

This factorizes to

$$(x-1) * (x-2) * (x-3) * (x-4) = 0$$

i.e. $x=1$, $x=2$, $x=3$, and $x=4$ are roots of (11.2)

But (11.2) is very obviously an artificial example; the authors knew the answers before they constructed the equation. In practice an equation such as

$$x^4 - 19 \cdot 15x^3 + 16 \cdot 1x^2 + 0 \cdot 03x + 6 \cdot 12 = 0 \tag{11.3}$$

may present itself; how do we find its roots?

Alternatively, we may have a theoretical model of some physiological situation—a common example is the two-compartment model of tracer kinetics, which gives rise to an equation of the form

$$y_1 \exp(-x_1 t) + y_2 \exp(-x_2 t) = f \tag{11.4}$$

in which x_1, x_2, y_1 and y_2 are the unknown variables and t and f are known values, f being the observed concentration of tracer at time t. It will require four sets of observations at different times to determine the four unknowns x_1, x_2, y_1 and y_2, but the method of solution is not obvious, and what would happen if the observations were subject to error?

In this Chapter we introduce some of the techniques for dealing with these practical situations. We will also consider to what extent these processes can be automated, thus removing the intuitive mathematical approach to problems of this type. We shall see that it is of great advantage to have a rough idea of the answers, and this is often available from experiments conducted on the physical situation we are modelling.

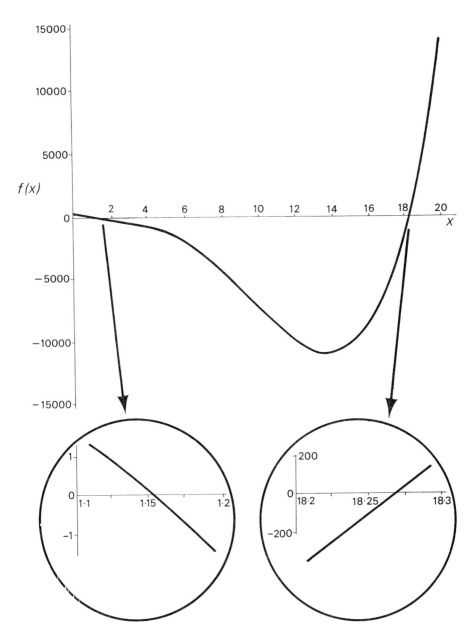

Fig 11·1   Graphical method of finding the roots of $f(x)=0$. The function plotted is

$$f(x)=x^4-19\cdot15x^3+16\cdot1x^2+0\cdot03x+6\cdot12$$

The insets show parts of this function near the roots redrawn on a larger scale to give a more accurate location of the value of x for which $f(x)=0$.

11.2   Graphical methods for solving equations

11.2.1   Graph plotting

Let us consider the roots of an equation $f(x)=0$, such as equation (11.3). We could compute the values of $f(x)$ for various values of x and draw a graph of $f(x)$ against x (Fig 11.1). From such a graph we can find the values of x at which $f(x)=0$, i.e. $x \doteqdot 1 \cdot 15$ or $18 \cdot 27$ in Fig 11.1.

In this example there is a conflict between the scale required to keep the curve on the graph and that needed to achieve the desired accuracy, but the graphical method is simple and it gives us a bonus by showing the behaviour of $f(x)$ over a range of the variable x. Various techniques for the graphing of functions have been discussed in the previous chapters, particularly in Chapters 2, 3, 8, and 9. If we want to be sure that we have covered all the relevant roots of $f(x)=0$, we can get help by examining the limiting conditions of $f(x)$ when $x \to \pm \infty$ or $x \to 0$ (Chapter 5) and seeing how well the outer limits of our graph conform to these. Of greater difficulty is detecting whether we have considered a small enough interval of x to detect any very sharp kinks in the curve, but this is a problem which exists in most of the methods for finding the roots of $f(x)=0$.

Although simple, the graphical method has its disadvantages. We may need a solution of $f(x)=0$ as part of a larger computation, and it may not be convenient to interrupt the computation to examine visually the graph of $f(x)$ every time a root is needed. It is also apparent that there is a lot of unnecessary computation in finding graphically the values of x for which $f(x)=0$. Again, when we consider functions of two variables, the process of drawing the functions becomes more difficult and we noted in the chapter on co-ordinate geometry that it is useful to discuss the characteristics of drawings in terms of functions and numbers, which is the exact reverse of the graphical method.

11.2.2   Curve stripping

This is a technique applicable to complicated expressions where *part* of the graph of the expression is dominated by one *part* of the expression, with the remaining terms contributing very little to the value of the function in that region of the graph.

Consider for example the function:

$$f = 0 \cdot 8 \exp(-0 \cdot 2t) + 0 \cdot 3 \exp(-0 \cdot 04t)$$

The values of this expression are given in Table 11.1.

We see that the value of the function at higher values of t is dominated by the second term $0 \cdot 3 \exp(-0 \cdot 04t)$ and receives little contribution from the first

Table 11.1. Contributions from each term of
$f = 0 \cdot 8 \exp(-0 \cdot 2t) + 0 \cdot 3 \exp(-0 \cdot 04t)$

| t | f | Contributions to f from | |
		$0 \cdot 8 \exp(-0 \cdot 2t)$	$0 \cdot 3 \exp(-0 \cdot 04t)$
1	0·943222	0·654985	0·288237
2	0·813191	0·536256	0·276935
3	0·705125	0·439049	0·266076
4	0·615106	0·359463	0·255643
5	0·539923	0·294304	0·245619
10	0·309364	0·108268	0·201096
15	0·204473	0·039830	0·164643
20	0·149451	0·014652	0·134799
25	0·115754	0·005390	0·110364
30	0·092341	0·001983	0·090358

term $0 \cdot 8 \exp(-0 \cdot 2t)$. So for large values of t we may use the approximation

$$f \doteqdot 0 \cdot 3 \exp(-0 \cdot 04t)$$

This is a simple power law relationship; the variable t is in the index of e and we have shown in Chapter 4 that if we plot $0 \cdot 3 \exp(-0 \cdot 04t)$ on a logarithmic scale and t on a linear scale then the graph will be a straight line where this approximation holds. The line represents the curve

$$\ln(f) = \ln(0 \cdot 3) - 0 \cdot 04t$$

The general situation is where we only have observed values of f and t and wish from these to find values of x_1, x_2, y_1 and y_2 satisfying

$$f = y_1 \exp(-x_1 t) + y_2 \exp(-x_2 t)$$

If we know that one of the x's, say x_2, is much smaller than the other, then for higher values of t, f will be approximately equal to $y_2 \exp(-x_2 t)$ and we can proceed as follows:

(i) *Plot a graph* of f against t on log/linear graph paper. Since for higher values of t, $f \doteqdot y_2 \exp(-x_2 t)$, we have $\ln(f) \doteqdot \ln(y_2) - x_2 t$, i.e. the graph is approximately a straight line in this region and so we can:

(ii) *Draw a straight line along the curve for 'high' values of t.* The slope of this line gives the value of $-x_2$ (Section 4.3.13) and the intercept of the line with the f axis gives the value of y_2. For lower values of

t the line diverges from the observed curve of f against t because the term $y_1 \exp(-x_1 t)$ becomes increasingly effective. However the value of f deduced from this line represents the contribution from the second term in the equation (11.4) and so:

(iii) *The contribution from the term $y_2 \exp(-x_2 t)$ can be computed for lower values of t and subtracted from the observed value of f; i.e. the curve is 'stripped' of the second term.* The result of this subtraction should give a curve of the form $f = y_1 \exp(-x_1 t)$ which when plotted logarithmically is a straight line whose slope gives $-x_1$ and whose intercept with the f axis is y_1. Failure to find a straight line at this point would indicate that the data did not conform to the shape $f = y_1 \exp(-x_1 t) + y_2 \exp(-x_2 t)$ (often referred to as a *double exponential* curve).

Example:

The example given in Fig 11.2 is taken from a paper by Wilkinson *et al* (1969). Radioactive Xenon was used as a marker to study the regional blood flow in

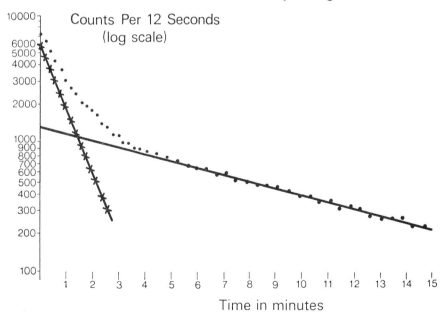

Fig 11·2   A [133]Xenon clearance curve, plotted logarithmically against time, represented by the upper series of dots. The clearance of [133]Xenon from the white matter is represented by the shallow exponential, and its clearance from the grey matter is represented by the steep exponential. (Reproduced by permission of the authors and the Editor, *J. Neurol. Neurosurg. Psychiat.*)

the normal cerebral hemisphere. The count rate of radioactivity from the Xenon was observed for a period of 15 min during which it gradually cleared from the hemisphere. Observations are seen to conform very well to a double exponential formula as we get two straight lines on a logarithmic scale after stripping the curve. Wilkinson and his co-workers interpreted the two lines, each representing one of the terms in the double exponential, as the clearances from the white matter and from the grey matter respectively.

The actual calculations proceed as follows:

Having drawn the shallow line we may work out its formula, i.e. the values of y_2 and x_2 in $y_2 \exp(-x_2 t)$, and this is done by the methods outlined in Section 4.3.12 and 4.3.13. The line cuts the $t=0$ axis at a value of 1275 and so $y_2 = 1275$. The half-life can be found from this line as the time at which the line passes through $1275/2$, i.e. $637 \cdot 5$; this can be read from the graph and is about 6 min. Thus $1275 \exp(-x_2 * 6) = 637 \cdot 5$; taking logarithms to base e, we have

$$-x_2 * 6 = \ln\left(\frac{637 \cdot 5}{1275}\right) = \ln\left(\frac{1}{2}\right) = -0 \cdot 6932 \quad \text{and so} \quad x_2 \doteqdot 0 \cdot 12$$

The shallow line therefore represents the term $1275 \exp(-0 \cdot 12t)$.

For values of t between 0 and 3, the value of the contribution of this term is read off the shallow line and subtracted from the observed points. Alternatively the value of $1275 \exp(-0 \cdot 12t)$ can be calculated and subtracted from the observed points.

The new points are plotted and are observed to lie on a somewhat steeper line (indicated by crosses in Fig 11.2). Its value at $t=0$ is 6000 and so $y_1 = 6000$. With a line as steep as this it is advisable to look at a range somewhat larger than the half-life and we examine the time this line takes to reduce to a tenth of the original value, i.e. 600. This occurs at time $t=2$ min approximately and so:

$$-x_1 * 2 = \ln\left(\frac{600}{6000}\right) = \ln\left(\frac{1}{10}\right) = -2 \cdot 30$$

$$x_1 \doteqdot -1 \cdot 15$$

The steep curve therefore represents the term $6000 \exp(-1 \cdot 15t)$. Hence the Xenon clearance curve is approximately represented by

$$f = 6000 \exp(-1 \cdot 15t) + 1275 \exp(-0 \cdot 12t)$$

where t is the time in minutes, and f is the observed activity in counts per 12 sec.

This illustrates how the technique of curve stripping can be used, even where there are measurement errors in the observations, provided the straight lines can be drawn to fit the observed points as closely as possible.

Although easy to implement, it must be admitted that curve stripping suffers from all the disadvantages of graphical methods mentioned in Section 11.2.1, and in addition leaves great scope for personal manipulation of the stripping line. For instance it can be seen in the above example that we are using the first straight line to extrapolate values of f at a considerable distance away from the fitted line, and so quite small errors on the slope of the line will be very much magnified when stripping the second term from the equation (Section 3.10.3). But it remains a popular technique, possibly because the alternatives employ quite sophisticated mathematics (Worsley & Lax, 1962).

Curve stripping may be applied to other functions in which the unknown parameters in separate terms can be deduced from the shape and position of different parts of the curve.

11.3   Iterative solution of equations

In cases where graphical solutions are not desirable or feasible, other methods have to be used. One approach is to use *iterative* methods, so called because they involve the repetition of a process over and over again, each time obtaining a better approximation to the answer. We will illustrate two such techniques, one known as the *method of bisection*, and the other based on the Taylor series (Section 10.4).

11.3.1   *The method of bisection*

We will illustrate this method with reference to equation (11.3).

For convenience we will call the left hand side of (11.3) $f(x)$, i.e.

$$f(x) = x^4 - 19 \cdot 15x^3 + 16 \cdot 1x^2 + 0 \cdot 03x + 6 \cdot 12$$

and we wish to find a value of x which makes $f(x)$ equal to zero. We proceed as follows:

(i) *Start with a guess*, say $x=0$ (though it may be possible to make a better one).

(ii) *Compute $f(x)$ at the guess*: $f(0)=6 \cdot 12$ and is larger than zero.

(iii) *Try another value of x*, say $x=1$.

$f(1) = 1 - 19 \cdot 15 + 16 \cdot 1 + 0 \cdot 03 + 6 \cdot 12 = 4 \cdot 1$.

$f(1)$ is still larger than zero but it is closer to zero than the value of $f(x)$ at $x=0$, i.e. $6 \cdot 12$, so we try yet another value of x, moving in the same direction, say $x=2$.

$f(2) = -66 \cdot 62$

$f(x)$ is now less than zero; we have gone too far, since we want $f(x)$ to equal zero. Because $f(1)>0$ and $f(2)<0$ then if $f(x)$ is continuous, as it is here, there is at least one root between $x=1$ and $x=2$ (Section 5.10).

(iv) *Try a value of x half way between those giving positive and negative values, $x=1\cdot5$.*

$f(x) = -17\cdot17875$

This is still negative, so the root lies between $x=1$ and $x=1\cdot5$. Therefore we try half way between these, i.e. $x=1\cdot25$ and so on, repeating the process from (iv) as many times as is necessary to get the desired accuracy; the results are given in Table 11.2.

Table 11.2. Solution of $f(x) = 0$ by the method of bisection.
The function $f(x)$ is the polynomial $x^4-19\cdot15\,x^3+16\cdot1\,x^2+0\cdot03\,x+6\cdot12$. Successive values of x are taken half way between the last values in the x_1 and x_2 columns.

Values of x		
When $f(x)>0$	When $f(x)<0$	Value of $f(x)$
x_1	x_2	
$1\cdot0$		$+\ 4\cdot100$
	$2\cdot0$	$-66\cdot620$
	$1\cdot5$	$-17\cdot179$
	$1\cdot25$	$-3\cdot647$
$1\cdot125$		$+0\cdot866$
	$1\cdot1875$	$-1\cdot220$
	$1\cdot15625$	$-0\cdot136$
$1\cdot14063$		$+0\cdot375$
$1\cdot14844$		$+0\cdot122$
	$1\cdot15234$	$-0\cdot062$
$1\cdot15039$		$+0\cdot058$
$1\cdot15137$		$+0\cdot026$
$1\cdot15186$		$+0\cdot010$

The equation $x^4-19\cdot15\,x^3+16\cdot1\,x^2+0\cdot03\,x+6\cdot12 = 0$, therefore has a root somewhere between $1\cdot15186$ and $1\cdot15234$—cf. Section 11.2.1.

The *iteration* is the repetition of step (iv).

In general terms the process is started by finding two values of x, say x_1, and x_2, such that $f(x_1)$ and $f(x_2)$ are of opposite sign. Next form $x_3=(x_1+x_2)/2$ and find the sign of $f(x_3)$. Then use x_3 to replace x_1 or x_2, whichever has $f(x)$

of the same sign as $f(x_3)$, and repeat the process with the new values of x_1 and x_2 and so on until the desired accuracy is obtained. At any stage, the difference between the two guessed values is called the *step-size*. In our example the initial guess was zero and the initial step-size, 1. The 'desired accuracy' is the point at which two successive guesses differ by less than some pre-determined amount of numerical magnitude. In Table 11.2 the answer was accepted when successive guesses for x differed by less than $0 \cdot 0005$.

The rule is simple enough to automate and its only restriction is that $f(x)$ should be continuous; however, it requires the user to supply a first guess, the desired accuracy of the answer and the initial step-size in x to search for the two values of x either side of a root. If—as with (11.3)—the equation has more than one root, the first guess and step size will be important in determining onto just which root of $f(x)$ the process will converge.

11.3.2   Iterative solutions based on Taylor's series

Let us consider finding a root of $f(x)=0$ by taking x_1 as a first guess and assuming it differs from the true root by δx_1, i.e. $f(x_1+\delta x_1)=0$. With a Taylor's series expansion of $f(x)$ about x_1 we have:

$$f(x_1+\delta x_1)=f(x_1)+f'(x_1) * \delta x_1+\text{remainder}=0$$

Optimistically ignoring the remainder, we get

$$0=f(x_1)+f'(x_1) * \delta x_1$$

i.e.
$$\delta x_1=\frac{-f(x_1)}{f'(x_1)} \tag{11.5}$$

so we can take as our next guesses: $x_2=x_1+\delta x_1$, $x_3=x_2+\delta x_2$ and so on, repeating (11.5) in the form:

$$\delta x_n=\frac{-f(x_n)}{f'(x_n)}$$

i.e.
$$x_{n+1}=x_n+\delta x_n=x_n-\frac{f(x_n)}{f'(x_n)} \tag{11.6}$$

which gives us a rule for obtaining a next guess (x_{n+1}) from the current one (x_n).

Example:

$$f(x)=x^2-3=0 \quad \text{(i.e. find the square root of 3)}$$

then $f'(x)=2x$

and so $x_{n+1}=x_n-\dfrac{x_n^2-3}{2x_n}$

Let us take $x_1=2$, this being the nearest guess we can reasonably make.

Then $x_2=2-\dfrac{2^2-3}{2*2}=1\cdot75$

$x_3=1\cdot75-\dfrac{(1\cdot75)^2-3}{2*1\cdot75}=1\cdot73214$

$x_4=1\cdot73214-0\cdot00009=1\cdot73205,$ etc.

which converges quite quickly to $\sqrt{3}$.

This technique is often used for finding square roots on desk calculators.

The process just described is usually called *Newton's method* and needs to have specified beforehand a first guess, the formula for the first derivative, and the desired accuracy for terminating the process.

If the formula for the derivative is not known it can be approximated from two successive estimates of $f(x)$. Thus in formula (11.6) we could replace $f'(x_n)$ by

$$\dfrac{f(x_n)-f(x_{n-1})}{x_n-x_{n-1}}$$

giving the iterative formula

$$x_{n+1}=x_n-\dfrac{(x_n-x_{n-1})*f(x_n)}{f(x_n)-f(x_{n-1})} \tag{11.7}$$

or $$x_{n+1}=\dfrac{x_{n-1}*f(x_n)-x_n*f(x_{n-1})}{f(x_n)-f(x_{n-1})} \tag{11.8}$$

This is an attractive method to the non-mathematician as, to start, it requires only two guesses (x_1 and x_2) and the desired accuracy for terminating the process. It will run into trouble if at any stage before terminating $f(x_n)=f(x_{n-1})$.

N.B. One difficulty which can arise when using Newton's or similar methods is that it is possible for the process to step outside the range of x for which the function is a valid model of the physical situation, and to home on to meaningless roots, e.g. negative doses of a drug. This has to be watched for.

Improved speed of convergence with this technique is sometimes obtained by taking the Taylor's series expansion up to the third term which gives a quadratic in x. For this process (usually called the Modified Newton method) one needs to give a first guess, formulae for the first *and second* derivatives, and the desired accuracy for terminating the process. The arithmetic can be quite formidable and liable to error with this method as against the relative simplicity of the

Newton formula, and the latter is often preferred even though the convergence may be slower. Note that the Newton method can itself run into difficulties if $f'(x_n)$ becomes zero or very small at any stage.

11.4   Solving simultaneous linear equations

In this section we shall consider by means of a very small example the solution of simultaneous equations by *Gaussian elimination* or *pivotal condensation*, as it is also known. Consider:

$$x_1 - 3x_2 + x_3 = 5 \qquad\qquad\qquad (11.9)$$

$$2x_1 + 4x_2 - 4x_3 = 1 \qquad\qquad\qquad (11.10)$$

$$3x_1 + 14x_2 + 5x_3 = 6 \qquad\qquad\qquad (11.11)$$

The technique for solving the equations (11.9)–(11.11) can be illustrated as follows:

(i) *Take the top left hand coefficient as 'pivot', i.e. that of variable x_1 in equation (11.9).*

Add or subtract an appropriate multiple of the first equation from the other equations so as to eliminate the 'pivotal variable'—at this stage, x_1:

$$x_1 - 3x_2 + x_3 = 5$$

$0 + 10x_2 - 6x_3 = -9$ (equation (11.10) minus twice equation

(11.9))   (11.12)

$0 + 23x_2 + 2x_3 = -9$ (equation (11.11) minus 3 $*$ equation

(11.9))   (11.13)

That is, we have removed x_1 from all but the first equation.

(ii) *We now ignore the first equation and work with the bottom two 'reduced' equations. Take the top left hand coefficient of the reduced equations as pivot, i.e. the coefficient of variable x_2 in equation (11.12) and repeat the process:*

$$10x_2 - 6x_3 = -9$$

$0 + 15 \cdot 8x_3 = -11 \cdot 7$ (equation (11.13) $- 2 \cdot 3 *$ equation (11.12))

(11.14)

Notice that the last equation is now solvable for x_3, i.e.

$$x_3 = \frac{11 \cdot 7}{15 \cdot 8} = 0 \cdot 7405.$$

(iii) *Find the value of the last variable from the last equation, substitute the value in the next to last equation and find the value of the next to last variable and so on:*

from (11.14) $x_3 = \dfrac{11 \cdot 7}{15 \cdot 8} = 0 \cdot 7405$

from (11.12) $10x_2 - 6x_3 = -9,$

and so $x_2 = \dfrac{6 * 0 \cdot 7405 - 9}{10} = -0 \cdot 4557$

from (11.9) $x_1 - 3x_2 + x_3 = 5$

and so $x_1 = 3 * (-0 \cdot 4557) - 0 \cdot 7405 + 5$

$= 2 \cdot 8924$

This final procedure (iii) is known as *back substitution*.

If we have n equations, pivotal condensation can be shown to involve approximately $n^2/2$ divisions and approximately $n^3/3$ multiplications and subtractions.

The accuracy of the process can be improved by ensuring that the multiplication factors in the reduction process are always less than 1. This can be done by rearranging the equations and variables after each step to have the numerically largest coefficient in the top left hand pivotal position.

In matrix notation the equations (11.9)–(11.11) could be written

$$\mathbf{A} * \mathbf{x} = \mathbf{b} \quad \text{where} \quad \mathbf{A} = \begin{pmatrix} 1 & -3 & 1 \\ 2 & 4 & -4 \\ 3 & 14 & 5 \end{pmatrix}, \quad \mathbf{b} = \begin{pmatrix} 5 \\ 1 \\ 6 \end{pmatrix} \quad \text{and} \quad \mathbf{x} = \begin{pmatrix} x_1 \\ x_2 \\ x_3 \end{pmatrix}$$

A is called the *matrix of coefficients in this case.*

The solution is given formally by $\mathbf{x} = \mathbf{A}^{-1} * \mathbf{b}$, which may be directly expressible in this notation using a suitable computer program. Some computer programming languages now permit us to specify our problems in matrix notation, or alternatively there are special subroutines for handling matrices and equations. The solution of simultaneous linear equations is usually obtained by these techniques, because the computations often involve a very large number of multiplications and divisions, or access to very large blocks of data. Various programming schemes have been evolved to reduce either storage requirements, computer time, or inaccuracies due to round-off errors.

11.5   Unsolvable simultaneous equations

If the matrix of coefficients is *ill-conditioned* or *singular* (Section 7.10) we will find when using pivotal condensation that at some point the pivot is very small or zero and the computational process begins to break down. Consider the equations:

$$x_1 - 3x_2 + x_3 = 5$$
$$2x_1 + 4x_2 - 4x_3 = 1 \qquad\qquad (11.15)$$
$$5x_1 + 5x_2 - 7x_3 = 7$$

By pivotal condensation this gives:

$$x_1 - 3x_2 + x_3 = 5$$
$$0 + 10x_2 - 6x_3 = -9$$
$$0 + 20x_2 - 12x_3 = -18$$

If we or our program and computer mechanically follow the next stage of the reduction process we will get $0 * x_3 = 0$ and be unable to find a specific value for x_3. This is because equations (11.15) have an unlimited number of possible solutions. The third equation is only the sum of the first equation and twice the second and adds no additional information to the first two equations, i.e. the equations are not *independent* (Section 1.10.1). In fact

$$x_2 = \frac{6x_3 - 9}{10}$$

$$x_1 = \frac{8x_3 + 23}{10}$$

are solutions for *any* value of x_3. With any set of linear simultaneous equations, a singular matrix of coefficients indicates that the equations are not independent. This in turn means, as we have seen, that pivotal condensation will not give a unique answer in this case, and neither will any other procedure. In practice, due to round off errors in the computation some zeroes will not be exactly zero, and a computer program may produce an answer of some sort. At the present time it is very difficult to use purely numerical techniques for detecting dependence among a set of equations and users of computer programs generally have to supply their own criteria for detecting that the equations are going to give trouble. If the matrices are ill-conditioned rather than singular then very small changes in the numerical values of the elements can lead to very large changes in the answers—see e.g. Fox & Mayers (1968).

11.6   Non-linear simultaneous equations

We quite often need to solve simultaneous equations which are not linear in $x_1, x_2 \ldots$ etc.

As an example consider the problem of finding a value for x_1 and x_2 which will simultaneously satisfy two simple double exponential equations:

$$\exp (x_1) + \exp (x_2) = 0 \cdot 5$$
$$\exp (2x_1) + \exp (2x_2) = 0 \cdot 2 \tag{11.16}$$

A procedure for solving these is:

(i) *Take a guess at the solutions, say X_1, X_2,*

e.g. $X_1 = -1$ and $X_2 = -2$

Let the difference between the guess and the true value be denoted by δX

i.e. $x_1 = X_1 + \delta X_1$ and $x_2 = X_2 + \delta X_2$

The terms $\exp (x)$ and $\exp (2x)$ may be expanded in a Taylor's series giving:

$$\exp (X + \delta X) = \exp (X) + \exp (X) * \delta X + \text{remainder terms}$$

and $\exp \{2(X + \delta X)\} = \exp (2X) + 2 \exp (2X) * \delta X + \text{remainder terms}$

As our estimates of the true values become more accurate so the remainder terms which contain δX^2 and higher powers will become smaller.

(ii) *Ignore the remainder terms and replace the terms in equations (11.16) by the corresponding first two terms from the Taylor series;* since X_1 and X_2 are known the equations (11.16) may be rearranged as a set of equations for δX_1 and δX_2. (The process is analogous to that given in Section 11.3.2.) These equations are linear in the δX's and can be solved by the method of the previous section.

$$\exp (X_1) * \delta X_1 + \exp (X_2) * \delta X_2 = 0 \cdot 5 - \exp (X_1) - \exp (X_2)$$
$$2 \exp (2X_1) * \delta X_1 + 2 \exp (2X_2) * \delta X_2 = 0 \cdot 2 - \exp(2X_1) - \exp(2X_2) \tag{11.17}$$

(iii) *We substitute our guessed values for X_1 and X_2 in the equations (11.17) and solve the equations for δX_1 and δX_2. This gives the values*

$$\delta X_1 = 0 \cdot 27598 \quad \text{and} \quad \delta X_2 = -0 \cdot 02375$$

(iv) *Take the next guess for X_1 as $X_1+\delta X_1$ and for X_2 as $X_2+\delta X_2$*, i.e.

$$X_1 = -0\cdot72402 \quad \text{and} \quad X_2 = -2\cdot02375$$

and repeat the process from (iii)

The estimates will eventually converge giving values of

$$x_1 = -0\cdot81272 \quad \text{and} \quad x_2 = -2\cdot87616$$

after about six iterations.

With all iterative processes the convergence for any example has to be examined on its merits, and it is best to check that the answers are correct by substituting them back into the original equations.

11.7   Curve fitting: least squares

We now consider briefly the effect of measurement error on the drawing of curves. The topic is more thoroughly covered in statistical texts such as Sprent (1969).

Let us consider a simple polynomial function of variable x

$$y = f(x) = a_3 x^3 + a_2 x^2 + a_1 x + a_0 \tag{11.18}$$

We observe values y corresponding to various known values of x, and wish from these results to determine the coefficients a_3, a_2, a_1 and a_0 (note at this stage that it is the *constants* of the equation which are the unknowns).

If we make four sets of observations on the values of x and y, say: $x=1$ gives $y=5$, $x=2$ gives $y=7$, $x=3$ gives $y=8$ and $x=4$ gives $y=6$; then we will have four simultaneous equations in the four unknowns a_3, a_2, a_1, and a_0. These are

$$6 = 4^3 a_3 + 4^2 a_2 + 4a_1 + a_0$$
$$8 = 3^3 a_3 + 3^2 a_2 + 3a_1 + a_0$$
$$7 = 2^3 a_3 + 2^2 a_2 + 2a_1 + a_0$$
$$5 = 1^3 a_3 + 1^2 a_2 + 1a_1 + a_0$$

that is

$$6 = 64a_3 + 16a_2 + 4a_1 + a_0$$
$$8 = 27a_3 + 9a_2 + 3a_1 + a_0$$
$$7 = 8a_3 + 4a_2 + 2a_1 + a_0$$
$$5 = a_3 + a_2 + a_1 + a_0$$

These equations are solvable for a_3, a_2, a_1 and a_0. The values in this example
are $a_3 = -1/3$, $a_2 = 3/2$, $a_1 = -1/6$,   and $a_0 = 4$.

We see that a function of the form given in (11.18) has been found, i.e.

$$y = -x^3/3 + 3x^2/2 - x/6 + 4$$

which passes through the four observed points. Similarly a function with n unknown constants can be exactly determined when n points on the graph of the function are known (Section 8.11).

If there are less than four points then the constants of the equation (11.18) are not uniquely determined, but if there are more than four pairs of observations available, i.e. more than four equations, the question arises: which four should we take? In theory it should not matter which four are used, for if (11.18) was a completely accurate model of our observations then any four pairs of readings should give the same values for a_3, a_2, a_1 and a_0. In medicine it is rarely—if ever—so straightforward owing to measurement error and inadequacy of the model used in describing the physical situation, and we would get different values of a_3, a_2, a_1 and a_0 with different sets of four readings.

The solution to such problems is to find a curve which passes among the points 'as closely as possible'. There are various ways in which the concept 'as closely as possible' can be defined mathematically, but a very popular method is the *least squares* technique, which is defined as follows:

Suppose we have n pairs of readings (x_1, y_1), $(x_2, y_2) \ldots (x_n, y_n)$, and we wish to pass a curve of the form $y = f(x)$ as closely as possible in some sense among them (this is usually referred to as *fitting* the curve $y = f(x)$ to the points). We form

$$S = \sum_{i=1}^{n} \{y_i - f(x_i)\}^2$$

i.e. $$S = \sum_{i=1}^{n} \{\text{observed value } y_i - \text{computed value } f(x_i)\}^2$$

and attempt to adjust the coefficients of $f(x)$ so as to make S a *minimum*.

In the previous example, where $f(x) = a_3x^3 + a_2x^2 + a_1x + a_0$, we have

$$S = \sum_{i=1}^{n} (y_i - a_3x_i^3 - a_2x_i^2 - a_1x_i - a_0)^2$$

and we minimize S with respect to the parameters a_3, a_2, a_1 and a_0 of the function being fitted. It must be emphasized that there is no unique 'mathematical correctness' for this method; it is simply a reasonable criterion which in certain situations corresponds to optimum curves.

11.7.1   The normal equations

Applying this technique to equation (11.18) with n pairs of readings (x_i, y_i), $i = 1, 2, 3 \ldots n$, we have

$$S = \sum_{i=1}^{n} (y_i - a_3 x_i^3 - a_2 x_i^2 - a_1 x_i - a_0)^2$$

To minimize this with respect to a_3, a_2, a_1, a_0, we apply the rule of Section 9.7.2:

$$\frac{\partial S}{\partial a_3} = 0 \quad \text{i.e.} \quad \sum_{i=1}^{n} -2x_i^3(y_i - a_3 x_i^3 - a_2 x_i^2 - a_1 x_i - a_0) = 0$$

$$\frac{\partial S}{\partial a_2} = 0 \quad \text{i.e.} \quad \sum_{i=1}^{n} -2x_i^2(y_i - a_3 x_i^3 - a_2 x_i^3 - a_1 x_i - a_0) = 0$$

and similarly for $\dfrac{\partial S}{\partial a_1}$ and $\dfrac{\partial S}{\partial a_0}$. This gives a stationary point of S.

After collecting together terms in a_3, a_2, a_1 and a_0, we have to solve a set of four simultaneous linear equations to obtain the values.

These equations have a particular patterned structure, which is made up of the different combinations of terms in equation (11.18) in a particular way. The equations are known as the *normal equations* and are given in (11.19). The $\sum$ symbol represents the summation for all n points $(x_1, y_1), (x_2, y_2), \ldots (x_n, y_n)$. We have expressed the normal equations in a way which most clearly shows their structure; a term such as $\sum x_i^3 x_i^2$ is, of course, the same as $\sum x_i^5$:

$$a_3 \sum x_i^3 x_i^3 + a_2 \sum x_i^3 x_i^2 + a_1 \sum x_i^3 x_i + a_0 \sum x_i^3 = \sum x_i^3 y_i$$
$$a_3 \sum x_i^2 x_i^3 + a_2 \sum x_i^2 x_i^2 + a_1 \sum x_i^2 x_i + a_0 \sum x_i^2 = \sum x_i^2 y_i$$
$$a_3 \sum x_i x_i^3 + a_2 \sum x_i x_i^2 + a_1 \sum x_i x_i + a_0 \sum x_i = \sum x_i y_i$$
$$a_3 \sum x_i \quad + a_2 \sum x_i \quad + a_1 \sum x_i \quad + a_0 n \quad = \sum y_i$$

(11.19)

As all the values of x_i and y_i are known from the observations, the values of all the $\sum$'s can be calculated; this then gives four equations from which the four unknowns a_3, a_2, a_1 and a_0 can be found. It can be shown that these do in fact minimise S.

11.7.2   The use of orthogonal functions

The form of the normal equations (11.19) is related to the equation of the curve we are trying to fit in a very simple way. The curve is a combination of terms in x^3, x^2, x and a constant. The coefficients of the a's are the sums of products obtained by pairing the x^3, x^2, x and 1 in all possible ways. There is however, a difficulty with the normal equations—they can be tedious to calculate and also subject to considerable round-off error. This error may be quite unacceptable when trying to fit polynomials of higher than fourth or fifth order. Various extensions of the basic technique just given have therefore been devised to simplify the arithmetic and reduce the problems of round-off error; they also enlarge the ideas to the fitting of non-polynomial functions.

To see the sort of approach, consider the following variation on the example just given. In

$$f(x) = a_3 x^3 + a_2 x^2 + a_1 x + a_0$$

suppose we replace the terms x^3, x^2, and x by some other functions of x. Let us call them $P_3(x)$, $P_2(x)$ and $P_1(x)$ respectively—note that they are not necessarily polynomial functions of x. If we now apply the same procedure as before to the function

$$f(x) = a_3 P_3(x) + a_2 P_2(x) + a_1 P_1(x) + a_0$$

i.e. try to fit this new function to the data by least squares—we will get normal equations similar in form to (11.19) but with terms such as $\sum P_3(x_i) P_3(x_i)$ and $\sum P_3(x_i) P_2(x_i)$ instead of terms such as $\sum x_i^3 x_i^3$ and $\sum x_i^3 x_i^2$. The general structure of the equations remains the same, however.

There are special families of functions for which the calculations are greatly simplified. These functions have the property that:

$$\sum_{i=1}^{n} P_j(x_i) P_k(x_i) = 0 \quad \text{for} \quad j \neq k.$$

In the context of our particular example, this means that

$$\sum P_3(x_i) P_2(x_i) = 0, \quad \sum P_2(x_i) P_1(x_i) = 0 \quad \text{and} \quad \sum P_3(x_i) P_1(x_i) = 0$$

$$(11.21)$$

Functions with this property are called *orthogonal functions*. If we add the restriction that:

$$\sum P_3(x_i) = 0, \quad \sum P_2(x_i) = 0 \quad \text{and} \quad \sum P_1(x_i) = 0$$

then the normal equations reduce to the four very simple equations:

$$a_3 = \sum y_i P_3(x_i) / \sum \{P_3(x_i)\}^2, \qquad a_2 = \sum y_i P_2(x_i) / \sum \{P_2(x_i)\}^2,$$

$$a_1 = \sum y_i P_1(x_i) / \sum \{P_1(x_i)\}^2 \quad \text{and} \quad a_0 = (\sum y_i)/n$$

The use of orthogonal functions greatly simplifies the calculations, and reduces the errors due to round-off in the solution of the normal equations. Table 11.3 shows an arrangement of *polynomials* which are orthogonal when the observed values of x are 1, 2, 3, 4, and 5.

Table 11.3. An example of orthogonal polynomials

	Values of x, $P_1(x)$, etc.				
x	1	2	3	4	5
$P_1(x) = x-3$	-2	-1	0	1	2
$P_2(x) = x^2-6x+7$	2	-1	-2	-1	2
$P_3(x) = \frac{1}{6}(5x^3-45x^2+118x-84)$	-1	2	0	-2	1

E.g.: $\sum\limits_{i=1}^{5} P_1(x_i)\, P_2(x_i) = -2*2+(-1)*(-1)+0*(-2)+1*(-1)+2*2 = 0.$

Further formulae may be found in Owen (1962) & Kendall (1961).

The property of orthogonality as defined in this section can be generalized to more than three functions, and is very useful in other contexts. Many of the named mathematical families of functions are orthogonal, e.g. Legendre polynomials and Bessel functions. Furthermore, replacing the summation sign in equations (11.21) by an integral sign enables us to extend the idea to the situation where the data represented by x is a continuous rather than discrete variable. With this extension we find that, for example, $\sin x$ and $\cos x$ are orthogonal for x extending over the range 0 to π, since

$$\int_0^\pi \sin x \cos x \, \mathrm{d}x = 0$$

11.7.3   Change of dependent variable

A point to note about the least squares technique is that the answers depend on the way we express the dependent variable. For example we could consider y as a proportion of x and equation (11.18) would become

$$\frac{y}{x} = a_3 x^2 + a_2 x + a_1 + \frac{a_0}{x}$$

If we now minimize

$$S = \sum \left(\frac{y_i}{x_i} - a_3 x_i^2 - a_2 x_i - a_1 - \frac{a_0}{x_i}\right)^2$$

we will get a different set of normal equations from (11.19) and different values for a_3, a_2, a_1 and a_0. So we see that we must be quite clear as to what we are

M

minimizing to obtain the constants in the equation. In situations where the normal equations are not linear in a_3, a_2, etc., the techniques of Section 11.6 can be applied, the main disadvantage being more elaborate computation.

11.8   Choice of function for curve fitting

One is often faced with the problem of choosing a suitable function to represent a set of observations, or points on a graph. In medical work we may wish to use mathematical methods such as curve fitting but may not have an accurate mathematical model of the process involved. If we wish to estimate numerical values of a function of x between observed points, this can be most easily handled by finding some algebraic expression which adequately fits the observed points and does not give obviously false answers in between them. The mathematician can only *suggest* certain functions as suitable, and indicate that some functions are easier to handle than others, but care is always needed. One point to watch is that functions sometimes start off as an adequate description of a process based on the data and conditions at a particular time and place, but perhaps months or years later, as the conditions gradually change they no longer provide reasonable answers.

The first choice of the mathematician is usually some form of polynomial. In theory most functions could be described by a Taylor's series expansion and thus as a polynomial. But since an nth degree polynomial can have $n-1$ turning points whereas functions observed in medicine can be fairly smooth without any ripples, it follows that polynomials must be used with some caution. However, they are very easy to handle mathematically, which provides a compensating advantage, and provided the observed points are spread fairly evenly over the range of values, polynomials seem to perform quite well.

Another technique for curve fitting is to manipulate the observations by trying intuitive functions of them to see if the data can be transformed to lie close to the mathematician's delight of $y = mx + c$, a straight line. It is quite standard practice to try plotting the logarithms of the observations and on a surprising number of occasions this yields straight line relationships.

The reader is referred to the useful little book by Hastings (1947) for details of practical techniques for finding suitable functions when fitting data.

Chapter 12
Differential Equations

12.1   Introduction

Up until now, the relationships with which we have been dealing have had one characteristic in common: between dependent and independent variable there has been an explicit or implicit connection involving both of them directly.

However, physical phenomena are not often observable in this direct way. Our knowledge of the universe more commonly comes from observations of the *changes* in the systems being observed, and especially from determinations of the *rates* at which these changes take place.

We have already seen that the mathematical tool for handling rates of change is the differential calculus. Its use in the mathematical description or modelling of natural processes leads to a type of equation quite unlike those which we have met in previous chapters: the *differential equation.*

The differential equation approach has been enormously successful in physics, chemistry, engineering and indeed in all branches of science to which it has been applied. A great corpus of knowledge and expertise concerning these equations has been built up over the past two centuries or so, and it is probably true to say that the theory and application of differential equations constitutes one of the most important branches of applied mathematics. In medicine, differential equations have been used to describe, e.g. the flow and diffusion of dissolved substances across a semi-permeable membrane, population growth, the decay of specific activity of injected substances, the dynamics of blood circulation, etc. etc. Although the mathematical systems describing biological phenomena are frequently too complex to be handled without simplification, even these simplified models help to indicate new lines of thought, and are often surprisingly good approximation to reality.

To see how such equations can arise, let us consider a simple example. It will serve to illustrate some of the limitations as well as some of the advantages of the use of the differential calculus in describing physical situations.

12.2   The population growth problem

Suppose we have a population whose size varies with time. It may be a human population, or a population of bacteria or cells in a culture, or a population of ions in a gas, to take some possibilities covered by the example.

Let the size of the population at time t be denoted by $p(t)$, say. So, for example, the population at time $t=7$ is represented by $p(7)$, at time $100\cdot4$ by $p(100\cdot4)$, and so on. For this general treatment, it is unnecessary to specify the units in which p and t are measured. The question posed is: given $p(0)$, the size of the population at some starting time, which can be taken as zero without loss of generality, what is the size of the population at time t?

To answer this question, we need to know the laws governing reproduction and/or death in the population. The simplest situation is one in which a constant average birthrate (or death rate, which can be regarded as a negative birthrate) per member of the population is envisaged. Suppose this rate is k births per individual per unit time—so that the average increase per unit time for the whole population at time t is $k * p(t)$.

In this case, if the population at time t is $p(t)$, then T units of time later—i.e. at time $t+T$, the population will be

$$p(t)+k * T * p(t)$$

i.e. $$(1+kT) * p(t) \qquad (12.1)$$

—*provided that T is small enough to ensure that the new members of the population have not themselves contributed to the actual growth.* Let us suppose that T is the interval between reproductions, which also equals that between birth and first reproduction and is the same for each member of the population.

Now by the definition of $p(t)$, the population at time $(t+T)$ is $p(t+T)$. Whence from equation (12.1), we have

$$p(t+T)=[1+kT] * p(t) \qquad (12.2)$$

If we now assume that the reproduction process continues as before for another T units of time, then we will have, by the same reasoning,

$$p(t+2T)=(1+kT) * p(t+T)$$
$$=(1+kT) * (1+kT) * p(t)$$
$$=(1+kT)^2 * p(t) \qquad (12.3)$$

Similarly, a further T units later we will have

$$p(t+3T)=(1+kT) * p(t+2T)=(1+kT)^3 * p(t) \qquad (12.4)$$

In general, at time $t+nT$, we will have

$$p(t+nT)=(1+kT)^n * p(t) \qquad (12.5)$$

If we are counting from time zero, then $t=0$, and (12.5) becomes

$$p(nT)=(1+kT)^n * p(0) \qquad (12.6)$$

This is a 'compound interest' growth law, and from it we can determine the increase in population over any time interval nT from time zero.

Note that the value of $p(0)$ has to be known, as well as that of n, k and T, before $p(nT)$ can be found. We will here distinguish between $p(0)$, meaning in effect the point on the graph of $p(t)$ at which $t=0$, and the known numerical value of $p(t)$ for $t=0$, which we will denote by p_0. We have therefore $p(0)=p_0$, $p(nT)=(1+kT)^n * p_0$.

Example:

If $T=1$ second, and $k=0\cdot1$ births/individual/second, then a population of size 1000 at time $t=0$ would be of size

$$p(60)=(1+0\cdot1)^{60} * 1000 \doteqdot 304,500$$

at the end of 1 min. Here $n=60$, $p_0=1000$

Now in practice, there are some difficulties with this approach. Quite apart from the question as to whether unrestricted population growth is meaningful, the supposition that the maturation time, T, is a constant in time and the same for each member of the population is likely to be unrealistic. It is far more likely that T varies from one member of the population to another, so that the population increases, not by discrete steps of $k * p(t)$, but as a more or less continuous process over any time interval.

This leads us to consider a different approach which can be used if $k * p(t)$ —and therefore, after a suitable time period, $p(t)$ also—is large enough. Just how large 'large enough' has to be is a nice point; we will see the sort of consideration which has to be taken into account, but there is no hard-and-fast rule.

We reason as follows: the smallest increase which can take place in the population as a whole is the addition of one individual. Now, on the definitions above, the population increases by $k * p(t)$ over the interval $(t, t+1)$—provided that we choose our time units small enough to ensure that the new members do not themselves have time to contribute. Thus the average time for a unit increase will be $1/[k * p(t)]$.

If $k * p(t)$ is very large, then $1/[k * p(t)]$ is very small. Let us now suppose that $k * p(t)$ is so large that *to all intents and purposes we can safely take it that some change in $p(t)$ will take place in any measurable time interval, no matter how small.* This is an idealization, but not perhaps as great a strain on our credulity as our previous assumptions about T. What we are doing, in fact, is idealizing $p(t)$ into a continuous function of t, and for many biological situations, this is a reasonable assumption.

Let us now consider the change in the population over an interval $[t, t+\delta t]$. As before, we have

$$p(t+\delta t)=p(t)+k * \delta t * p(t)$$

but this is now an approximation, valid only if δt is small enough. This gives us

$$\frac{p(t+\delta t)-p(t)}{\delta t}=k * p(t) \tag{12.7}$$

As δt gets smaller, we see that the left-hand side of (12.7) approximates to $dp(t)/dt$ (Section 9.3.1), the *instantaneous* rate of change of $p(t)$. If we actually take things to the limit and let $\delta t \to 0$, (12.7) becomes

$$\frac{d}{dt}p(t)=k * p(t) \tag{12.8}$$

as the relationship *defining* $p(t)$.

This is a new kind of equation, and not one which immediately enables us to calculate $p(t)$, as we could with (12.6) above. It defines $p(t)$ by the rule that at any time, the instantaneous rate of change of $p(t)$ is proportional to the value of $p(t)$ at that time. It is an example of a *differential equation*, or more precisely, of an *ordinary differential equation*. To solve it, we have either to find a function of t obeying the relation (12.8) for all t for which the equation is defined, or else somehow use the information given by (12.8) to compute $p(t)$ for given values of t.

The quantity $dp(t)/dt$—or dp/dt for brevity—is the instantaneous rate of change of $p(t)$. In Nature, truly instantaneous changes do not occur—such changes would involve infinite rates of change—but what *do* occur are changes over very small time intervals or over very small distances, either at the molecular level or when we consider the behaviour of systems made up of a large number of active sub-units. In theory, we could describe (mathematically) such systems by considering the behaviour of each individual element and its interactions with all the others. In practice, to attempt to describe, e.g. the behaviour of a gas or solution by seeking to chart the behaviour of each individual molecule is an impossibility, and we must use some form of aggregate treatment of the system as a whole, as we did above. Almost invariably in such cases, we are led to formulate differential equations of one kind or another, and in spite of the idealizations and assumptions which are usually found to be needed in doing so, the solutions to these equations are found to be very good approximations to reality, although often the additional refinement of statistical considerations is needed as well.

The results (12.8) and (12.6) are not as disconnected as might be thought at first sight. From (12.6),

$$p(nT)=(1+kT)^n * p_0$$

If we write nT as t, this becomes

$$p(t)=\left(1+\frac{kt}{n}\right)^n * p_0$$

Now if t is taken to be some finite time interval measured from zero, then it follows from the relation $t=nT$ that if T is very small, n must be correspondingly large. In the limit, as $T \to 0$, $n \to \infty$ in such a way as to ensure nT continues to equal t.

Let $T \to 0$, or correspondingly $n \to \infty$. Then

$$p(t) = \lim_{n \to \infty} \left(1 + \frac{kt}{n}\right)^n * p_0$$

i.e. $p(t) = p_0 \exp(kt)$ (12.9)

from the definition of $\exp(kt)$ (Section 5.14). Thus, for small T and fixed $t=nT$, it appears that (12.6) is approximated by $p(t) = p_0 \exp(kt)$.

Differentiating both sides of the equation (12.9) with respect to t, we obtain

$$\frac{dp(t)}{dt} = \frac{d}{dt}\{p_0 \exp(kt)\} = p_0 k \exp(kt)$$

$$= k * p_0 \exp(kt)$$ (12.10)

and since $p(t) = p_0 \exp(kt)$, we have from (12.10)

$$\frac{dp(t)}{dt} = k * p(t)$$

which is equation (12.8).

We see therefore that where we can consider changes to be possible in very small time intervals, both the 'compound interest' and the instantaneous rate of change approaches seem to lead us to the same differential equation for $p(t)$. However, at first sight there would appear to be an important difference between them, as follows:

If $p(t) = \alpha \exp(kt)$, where α is *any* constant, then

$$\frac{dp(t)}{dt} = \alpha k \exp(kt) = k\alpha \exp(kt) = k * p(t)$$

In other words, *any* function of the form $\alpha \exp(kt)$ is a solution of (12.8), where α can take any value we please. Equation (12.8), therefore, appears to have an unlimited number of solutions, of which $p_0 \exp(kt)$ is only one. Why should this be, and are any of the other possible solutions valid?

The answer is that in considering $\alpha \exp(kt)$ as a solution of (12.8), we must take into account the condition that at time $t=0$, the population is of size p_0, which has to be known. If $p(t) = \alpha \exp(kt)$, then this has to be true for $t=0$. Whence

$$p_0 = \alpha \exp(k * 0) = \alpha$$

and therefore α can have only one value, i.e. p_0, if *all* the conditions of the problem are to be satisfied, Thus the two approaches do in fact coincide, giving $p(t) = p_0 \exp(kt)$ as the solution of equation (12.8) in this particular case.

12.3   The definition of a differential equation

So far, we have used the terms 'differential equation' and 'ordinary differential equation' without formal definition, simply citing a particular example. We have also talked rather vaguely of the 'solution' of a differential equation. We now define our terms more precisely.

Any equation involving derivatives (i.e. differential coefficients) is called a *differential equation*. If no partial derivatives (Section 9.7) occur in it, it is called an *ordinary differential equation*, as distinct from an equation including partial derivatives, which would be called a *partial differential equation*. Partial differential equations are outside the scope of a book such as this, and the reader who seeks information on them is referred to the appropriate text books (e.g. Ross (1964)). Such equations are really the province of the professional mathematician, and research workers who find themselves faced with a partial differential equation would do well to seek expert guidance unless they are very sure of their abilities in this field. To be truthful, the same can be said of ordinary differential equations as well, but certain biological situations of considerable importance can be described by relatively simple ordinary differential equations, and studying these will enable the reader to gain a toe-hold in this subject. It is not our intention to give him more than this.

Examples:

$$\frac{dp}{dt} - k * p = 0$$

$$\frac{d^2 y}{da^2} - \sin(x) * \frac{dy}{dx} + y^2 = \exp(x)$$

These are *ordinary* differential equations, while

$$\frac{\partial^2 \phi}{\partial x^2} + \frac{\partial^2 \phi}{\partial y^2} = 0$$

is a very famous partial differential equation known as *Laplace's equation in two dimensions*.

12.4   The solution of a differential equation

A function is said to be a *solution* of a differential equation if its substitution as the dependent variable in the equation results in a relationship which is true for all values of the independent variable, i.e. the equation becomes an identity. Other ways of putting this are to say that such a function *satisfies* the equation, or that it is an *integral* of the equation. Solving a differential equation is sometimes referred to as *integrating* the equation.

(Rather more strictly, if the identity holds only over a *range* of values of the independent variable, the function is said to be a solution of the equation *over the given range*.)

To illustrate this:

Consider the function $y=x^3$. Then $dy/dx=3x^2$. Also $x=y^{1/3}$, $x^2=y^{2/3}$, and so

$$\frac{dy}{dx}=3y^{2/3} \quad \text{for all and any } x.$$

In other words, by virtue of the relationship between the function y and its derivative,

$$y=x^3$$

is a *solution* of the equation

$$\frac{dy}{dx}=3y^{2/3} \tag{12.11}$$

for all x, since substituting x^3 for y in (12.11) results in an identity.

Similarly, since for all t

$$\frac{d^2}{dt^2}(\sin \omega t)+\omega^2 * \sin \omega t=0$$

identically, then

$$y=\sin \omega t$$

is a solution of

$$\frac{d^2y}{dt^2}+\omega^2y=0 \tag{12.12}$$

for all t.

Note that $A * \sin \omega t$ is also a solution of (12.12) for any constant value A. This brings out a point already met with, namely, that without additional constraints, a differential equation does not have a unique solution. But there is more to equation (12.12) than this, because the function

$$y = B * \cos \omega t \qquad (B \text{ a constant})$$

is also a solution. So in this case, not only is there a set of possible solutions based on sin ωt, but also a set based on cos ωt. We will return to this point later.

12.5   The nature of solutions

We see from the previous section and from our population growth example that certain aspects of the differential equation approach must be kept in mind when attempting to apply this technique in practice. In the first place, such equations and their solutions represent a mathematical abstraction, an approximation to reality, when applied to the solution or modelling of physical situations. Secondly, any given differential equation has an unlimited number of possible solutions, and the correct one in any given circumstances has to be picked out by considering the *boundary conditions*, as they are called, of the problem. In our population growth example, we saw that the boundary condition was that $p(t)$ should have a known value p_0 at $t = 0$.

This example was a particularly simple one, with simple boundary conditions, but differential equations can be extremely difficult to handle, and in fact it is more the exception than the rule to be able to find a known mathematical function or combination of known functions satisfying a real-life equation. If we *can* find such a solution, it is said to be in *closed form*; where we cannot do so, then a new function is *defined* by the equation, and for computational or manipulative purposes we have to approximate to the solution in some way.

The reader will no doubt realize that the process is self-generating. Once a new function has been defined, it can be regarded as 'known' and added to the list of functions which can be used to express the solutions of other equations in closed form—though of course, this is of little use until the properties of the new 'known' function have been excavated from its defining equation. Conversely, all 'known' functions—e.g. those discovered by Bessel, Legendre, etc.— were once 'new' (though not necessarily defined by differential equations). And sometimes, even when a function or solution can be expressed in closed form, it may be sufficiently useful or individualistic in its properties to be worth regarding as a function in its own right—e.g. the *Chebyshev polynomials* which are used so much in approximation work.

Closed-form and other mathematical solutions, however, although very useful for theoretical work, are sometimes a mixed blessing when it comes to using them. It can happen that obtaining such solutions is tedious and time-consuming, and may require the introduction of simplifying assumptions which 'dilute the scientific significance of the equations' in Ledley's (1965) striking phrase. In addition, the resulting expressions may be computationally and mathematically very awkward to handle.

For this reason, many techniques for the mathematical approximation and for the *numerical solution* of differential equations have been developed (Section 12.12). The latter are designed to compute the value of the solution for various values of the independent variable so that the graph of the solution can be drawn for the particular situation specified by the equation and its boundary conditions.

However, both theoretical and numerical solutions have their place, and since a greater insight into the underlying processes is obtained from the generality of mathematical results—when these are possible—it is worth while considering some aspects of the theory.

12.6   Order and degree

First, some definitions.

The *order* of a differential equation is defined as that of the highest-order derivative (Section 9.3.2) which occurs in it. Thus, for example, our equation

$$\frac{\mathrm{d}p(t)}{\mathrm{d}t} = k * p(t)$$

is an example of a *first-order* equation, since the derivative of highest order in it, i.e. $\mathrm{d}p(t)$, is of order 1. Again, the equations

$$\frac{\mathrm{d}^2 y}{\mathrm{d}x^2} = kx^3$$

$$\frac{\mathrm{d}^2 p}{\mathrm{d}t^2} - 3 \sin (t+1) * \frac{\mathrm{d}p}{\mathrm{d}t} - t = 0$$

are *second-order* equations. The greater part of the situations met with in practice are covered by either first- or second-order equations; and many of those of higher order can be reduced to systems of such equations.

The *degree* of a differential equation is the largest power of the highest-order derivative in the equation. For example,

$$\frac{\mathrm{d}^2 y}{\mathrm{d}x^2} + y * \left(\frac{\mathrm{d}y}{\mathrm{d}x}\right)^3 + x = 0$$

is of *second* order (the highest-ordered derivative being $\mathrm{d}^2 y / \mathrm{d}x^2$) and *first* degree (since d^2y/dx^2 is of power 1); but the equation

$$\left(\frac{d^2y}{dx^2}\right)^3 + \frac{dy}{dx} + x = 0$$

is of *second* order and *third* degree.

A differential equation in which the *dependent* variable and every derivative involved is to the first degree only, and in which no products or quotients of the dependent variable and/or its derivatives occur, is said to be *linear*. Linear differential equations have special properties which make them easier to handle than *non-linear* differential equations; these latter are defined quite literally, i.e. as not being linear. Of the previous examples,

$$\frac{dp}{dt} = k * p$$

$$\frac{d^2p}{dt^2} - 3 \sin (t+1) * \frac{dp}{dt} - t = 0$$

and $$\frac{d^2y}{dx^2} = kx^3$$

are all linear differential equations, while

$$\frac{d^2y}{dx^2} + y * \left(\frac{dy}{dx}\right)^3 + x = 0$$

and $$\left(\frac{d^2y}{dx^2}\right)^3 + \frac{dy}{dx} + x = 0$$

are non-linear. So is

$$\frac{d^2y}{dx^2} + y * \frac{dy}{dx} + 2y = 0$$

because of the term $y * dy/dx$.

12.7   Nature of solutions (*continued*)

Consider the linear equation

$$\frac{dy}{dx} = x \tag{12.13}$$

A solution of this is $y = \frac{1}{2}x^2$. But $y = \frac{1}{2}x^2 + 7$ also satisfies (12.13), since

$$\frac{d}{dx}(\tfrac{1}{2}x^2 + 7) = x$$

In fact, $y=\frac{1}{2}x^2+C$, where C is *any* constant, satisfies (12.13). Again, the equation

$$\frac{d^2y}{dx^2}+\frac{1}{x^2}=0 \qquad (x>0) \tag{12.14}$$

is satisfied by

$$y=\ln(x)+Ax+B$$

where A and B are constants, for any values of A and B. For example, if $y=\ln(x)+2x-7$ ($A=2$, $B=-7$), then

$$\frac{dy}{dx}=\frac{1}{x}+2$$

$$\frac{d^2y}{dx^2}=-\frac{1}{x^2}$$

i.e. $\qquad\qquad \dfrac{d^2y}{dx^2}+\dfrac{1}{x^2}=0$

and we obtain a similar result no matter what values we give to A and B.

The constants A, B and C occurring in (12.13) and (12.14) are examples of what are called *essential arbitrary constants*. They are *constants* in the sense that they are not functions of x or y, the variables of the equations, and *arbitrary* in that no matter what values we choose for them, the resulting functions are still solutions of our equations. The term *essential* implies that they cannot be replaced by a smaller number of arbitrary constants while still preserving a solution. To illustrate the point, consider the two functions

$$y=c_1x+\frac{c_2}{x}$$

and $\qquad y=(c_1+c_2)x$

In the first of these, c_1 and c_2 are *essentially* arbitrary. We cannot replace them by one arbitrary constant without losing one of the terms in x. In the second one, however, we could write $c_3=c_1+c_2$ and then have

$$y=c_3x$$

which is just as general as $y=(c_1+c_2)x$; in other words, giving two arbitrary values to c_1 and c_2 amounts to giving one arbitrary value to c_3. In this case, c_1 and c_2 are *not* essential.

As there is nothing to be gained by dealing with non-essential constants, we will take it as understood from now on that the term 'arbitrary constants'— or *constants of integration* as they are also known—implies that essential constants only are involved (unless otherwise stated).

We notice that the *first*-order equation (12.13) has a solution involving one arbitrary constant, and the *second*-order equation (12.14) a solution with *two* such constants. These are examples of a general rule that, subject to certain wide-ranging conditions, *an ordinary differential equation of order n has a solution involving n arbitrary constants,* such a solution being known as the *general solution* of the equation. Conversely, any solution containing *n* (essentially) arbitrary constants *is* the general solution.

Any solution obtained by giving specific values to the arbitrary constants is known as a *particular* solution. In any given application, it will be particular solutions which will be of interest, and the values to be given to the arbitrary constants will be determined by the boundary conditions of the problem.

12.8   Graphical interpretation of solutions: the role of the arbitrary constants

12.8.1   First-order equations

Consider again the first-order equation

$$\frac{dy}{dx} = x \tag{12.15}$$

The general solution of this is

$$y = \tfrac{1}{2}x^2 + C \tag{12.16}$$

For any given value of C, we may plot the graph of the function defined by (12.16), and different values of C will result in different curves (Fig 12.1).

In fact, (12.16) defines a *family* of curves all of the same shape but distinguished from one another by different values of C—which we see in this light as a parameter (Section 3.11) rather than a constant. Since C is the only parameter involved, the set of curves defined by (12.16) is called a *one-parameter family* of curves, and in this particular context, they are the *integral curves* of the equation (12.15).

Now through any given point in the plane, there passes one and only one curve of the family, corresponding to a given value of C. For example, the curve through the point (2, 6) is $y = \tfrac{1}{2}x^2 + 4$, as shown in Fig 12.1. The value of C for the specific curve passing through a given point (x_0, y_0) is obtained by substituting x_0 and y_0 for x and y respectively in (12.16); e.g. in the case of the point (2, 6) we have

$$6 = \tfrac{1}{2} * 2^2 + C$$

an equation for C, with solution $C = 4$, which confirms that the particular curve

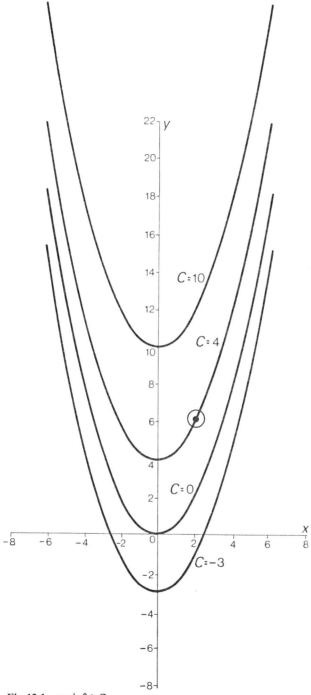

Fig 12.1 $y = \frac{1}{2}x^2 + C$

of the family which passes through the point (2, 6) is indeed

$$y=\tfrac{1}{2}x^2+4.$$

Giving a particular value to the arbitrary constant C thus amounts to picking out a particular curve of the family (12.16) and conversely, picking out the particular curve of the family which passes through a given point is equivalent to giving a specific value to the arbitrary constant C. We can thus determine a particular solution of (12.15) passing through a specific point, or in algebraic terms, *we can ask for the particular solution of equation (12.15) such that $y=y_0$ when $x=x_0$.* We proceed as follows:

$$y_0=\tfrac{1}{2}x_0^2+C,$$

whence $C=y_0-\tfrac{1}{2}x_0^2$

giving $y=\tfrac{1}{2}x^2+y_0-\tfrac{1}{2}x_0^2$ (12.17)

We can therefore determine the solution satisfying our condition that $y=y_0$ when $x=x_0$ for any pair of values x_0, y_0. Note that imposing this condition fixes the value of the arbitrary constant for given x_0 and y_0.

12.8.2   Second-order equations

The solution of a second-order equation will contain two arbitrary constants. This defines a *two-parameter* family of integral curves. In this case there are two different kinds of constraint or boundary conditions possible when defining particular solutions:

(1) We may ask for the curve passing through a given point in the plane *with a given slope* at that point, i.e. not only is y_0 given, but also y_0' (as the slope of y at y_0 is often written).

(2) We may ask for the curve passing through *two* given points in the plane, or satisfying some other pair of conditions involving values and slopes at two points in the plane.

The first type, where all the conditions are relative to one point in the plane, is called an *initial-value* problem, or a problem with *initial conditions*. Theoretically, all such problems have a solution under very general conditions. The second type, where the constraints on the problem relate to two different points, is called a *two-point boundary problem*, and need not necessarily have a solution.

These ideas and definitions can be generalized to the case of higher-order equations if required.

12.9 Solution of differential equations: standard forms

Although there are many techniques for finding closed form solutions, in the last analysis the solution of a differential equation in this way always boils down at some stage to recognizing that the particular function in front of us at this point is the derivative or integral of some other function. The mixture of experience and low cunning which is of so much use in other scientific activities finds its place here as well. Useful relationships to keep in mind are (x and y being variables and all other quantities being constants):

(1) $\dfrac{d(x^n+C)}{dx}=nx^{n-1}$ $(n\neq 0)$ $\displaystyle\int x^n\,dx=\dfrac{x^{n+1}}{n+1}+C$ $(n\neq -1)$

(2) $\dfrac{d\ln(Cx)}{dx}=\dfrac{1}{x}$ $\displaystyle\int \dfrac{dx}{x}=\ln(x)+c$
$$=\ln(Cx)\,(\text{writing }\ln(C)\text{ for }c)$$

(3) $\dfrac{d}{dx}\{\ln(ax+b)\}=\dfrac{a}{ax+b}$ $\displaystyle\int\dfrac{dx}{ax+b}=\dfrac{1}{a}*\ln(ax+b)+c$
$$=\dfrac{1}{a}\ln[C(ax+b)]$$
$$(\text{writing }1/a\ln C\text{ for }c)$$
$$=\ln[\{C(ax+b)\}^{1/a}]$$

(4) $\dfrac{d}{dx}(\exp(ax)+c)=a\exp(ax)$ $\displaystyle\int\exp(ax)\,dx=\dfrac{\exp(ax)}{a}+c$

(5) $\dfrac{d}{dx}\sin(\omega x+\phi)=\omega\cos(\omega x+\phi)$
$$\int\sin(\omega x+\phi)\,dx=-\dfrac{1}{\omega}\cos(\omega x+\phi)+c$$

(6) $\dfrac{d}{dx}\cos(\omega x+\phi)=-\sin(\omega x+\phi)$
$$\int\cos(\omega x+\phi)\,dx=\dfrac{1}{\omega}\sin(\omega x+\phi)+c$$

So, for example, if we find that our unknown function y satisfies

$$\dfrac{dy}{dx}=\dfrac{a}{x}$$

then from (2) above, it follows that the general solution for y is

$$y=a*\ln(Cx)$$

where the value of C has to be determined by an initial condition on y in any given case. Alternatively, we can write

$$\int dy = \int \frac{dy}{dx} * dx = \int a \frac{dx}{x}$$

Performing the integrations we have

$$y + c = a * \ln (Cx)$$

i.e. $y = a * \ln (C'x)$

where C' is defined by $a * \ln (C') = a * \ln (C) - c$.

12.10

In the limited space available to us, it is out of the question to go into as vast a subject as differential equations to any extent. We will therefore confine our discussion to (a) certain types of equation which have found considerable application in medicine and biology, namely, *linear* differential equations, and (b) some aspects of the *numerical* solution of differential equations. In order to show that our theory is quite general, we will as a rule use x as the symbol for the independent variable rather than t, which usually has the special connotation of a time variable.

12.11   Linear differential equations

In Section 12.6, we defined a linear differential equation as one in which the dependent variable and its derivatives occur to at most the first degree and in which no products or quotients of the dependent variable and/or its derivatives occur. The most general form of such an equation is

$$a_n(x) \frac{d^n y}{dx^n} + a_{n-1}(x) \frac{d^{n-1} y}{dx^{n-1}} + \ldots + a_0(x) \, y = f(x) \tag{12.18}$$

the general nth order linear differential equation. The left-hand side of (12.18) is a *weighted sum* of derivatives (defining y as the zero derivative of y) in which the 'weights' or coefficients are functions of x. The coefficients $a_n(x)$, $a_{n-1}(x)$, ..., $a_0(x)$ may be also constants or zero, of course—in the latter case the corresponding term will not be present.

The function $f(x)$ on the right hand side of the equation is sometimes called the *forcing* function. The general solution of (12.18) will contain n arbitrary constants, whose values in any particular case will depend upon the boundary conditions.

To simplify the discussion, we will deal solely with first- or second-order equations from now on; the results can be generalized fairly readily to equations of higher order if necessary. We will make use of the notation

$$y' = \frac{dy}{dx}, \qquad y'' = \frac{d^2y}{dx^2}$$

and
$$\dot{p} = \frac{dp}{dt}, \qquad \ddot{p} = \frac{d^2p}{dt^2}$$

where t denotes time.

12.11.1 The reduced equation, and the complementary function

Consider the general second-order linear equation

$$a_2(x)\, y'' + a_1(x)\, y' + a_0(x)\, y = f(x) \tag{12.19}$$

Associated with this, we can define the equation

$$a_2(x)\, y'' + a_1(x)\, y' + a_0(x)\, y = 0 \tag{12.20}$$

called the *reduced* equation; it is the equation with the same left-hand side as (12.19), but with the forcing function identically zero.

The reason for introducing the reduced equation is that a knowledge of the general solution of the *reduced* equation enables us in theory to obtain the general solution of the *complete* equation—as the original equation (12.19) with non-zero forcing function is called—and the reduced equation is often quite easy to solve, certainly easier than the complete equation.

The general solution of the reduced equation is known as the *complementary function*. (Remember that these definitions and the ensuing results apply only to **linear** differential equations; they do **not** apply to non-linear equations.)

Example:

The reduced equation of

$$y'' + 6xy' - 2y = \sin 3x$$

is $$y'' + 6xy' - 2y = 0$$

The latter is also the reduced equation of, e.g.

$$y'' + 6xy' - 2y = \exp(-x^2)\ln(2x-7)$$

12.11.2   Relation between the complementary function and the complete solution

Suppose $y_r(x, c_1, c_2)$ is the general solution of the *reduced* equation (12.20). The quantities c_1, c_2 are the two arbitrary constants, and writing the solution as shown indicates that it depends on c_1 and c_2 as well as on x. In addition, let $y_p(x)$ be a particular solution of the *complete* equation (12.19).

Now consider the function

$$y_r(x, c_1, c_2) + y_p(x)$$

or $y_r + y_p$,   for short.

We have

$$a_2(x)\frac{d^2}{dx^2}[y_r+y_p] + a_1(x)\frac{d}{dx}[y_r+y_p] + a_0(x)[y_r+y_p]$$

$$= \left[a_2(x)\frac{d^2y_r}{dx^2} + a_1\frac{dy_r}{dx} + a_0(x)y_r\right] + \left[a_2(x)\frac{d^2y_p}{dx} + a_1(x)\frac{dy_p}{dx} + a_0(x)y_p\right]$$

$$(12.21)$$

But by the definition of y_r, the first bracketed expression on the right-hand side of (12.21) is zero, and the second one $=f(x)$, by the definition of y_p. Thus

$$a_2(x)\frac{d^2}{dx^2}[y_r+y_p] + a_1(x)\frac{d}{dx}[y_r+y_p] + a_0(x)[y_r+y_p] = f(x)$$

and therefore *the function* (y_r+y_p) *is a solution of the* complete *equation* (12.19). Since, however, it contains the two arbitrary constants c_1 and c_2, contributed by y_r, *it must be the* general *solution of the complete equation.*

12.11.3   The general solution of the complete equation

We see that the general solution of the complete equation can be represented as the sum of two components: (i) the general solution of the reduced equation, added to (ii) any particular solution of the complete equation. This result is true for linear differential equations of any order.

Example:

The equation

$$y'' + 5y' + 6y = 2 \exp(-x) \tag{12.22}$$

has as its reduced equation

$$y'' + 5y' + 6y = 0$$

The general solution of this latter equation—i.e. the complementary function —is

$$y_r = A \exp(-2x) + B \exp(-3x) \tag{12.23}$$

as can be proved by substitution (we will see how to obtain this solution later on). A and B are the arbitrary constants. Also, a particular solution of (12.22), obtained by intuition, guesswork, or whatever, is

$$y_p = \exp(-x)$$

Hence the general solution of (12.22) is

$$y = y_r + y_p = A \exp(-2x) + B \exp(-3x) + \exp(-x) \tag{12.24}$$

(check by substitution).

Note that if we are trying to solve the equation (12.22) subject to known boundary conditions, these must be applied to the complete solution, and not to the complementary function. In other words, solving for A and B must be based on (12.24), not (12.23). For example, suppose we wish to solve

$$y'' + 5y' + 6y = 2 \exp(-x)$$

but now subject to:

$$y = 1 \quad \text{when} \quad x = 0 \qquad \text{(i.e. } y(0) = 1)$$
$$y' = 0 \quad \text{when} \quad x = 0 \qquad \text{(i.e. } y'(0) = 0)$$

This is an initial-value problem. We proceed as follows: The general solution is:

$$y = A \exp(-2x) + B \exp(-3x) + \exp(-x)$$

Since $y(0) = 1$, we have

$$A \exp(-2 * 0) + B \exp(-3 * 0) + \exp(-0) = 1$$

i.e. $A \qquad\qquad\qquad + B \qquad\qquad\qquad + 1 \qquad\qquad = 1 \tag{12.25}$

Differentiating our general solution (12.24) with respect to x, we have
$$y' = -2A \exp(-2x) - 3B \exp(-3x) - \exp(-x)$$
and since $y'(0) = 0$, we have
$$-2A - 3B - 1 = 0 \tag{12.26}$$

Solving (12.25) and (12.26) for A and B, we have $A = 1$, $B = -1$, and therefore our solution is
$$y = \exp(-2x) - \exp(-3x) + \exp(-x)$$

On the face of it, the use of the reduced equation as a means of solving the complete equation would appear to be more trouble than it is worth, since we have to find the complementary function and also a particular solution. However, in the case of certain commonly-occurring classes of linear differential equations, there are formal quasi-algebraic techniques for obtaining both the complementary function and a particular solution (see, e.g. Ince (1956), Ross (1964)) and occasionally it is possible to solve the reduced equation fairly easily and then guess a particular solution of the complete equation. But the result is of more use in the theory than in the application of differential equations, especially since, as we will show, there is a technique available which leads us directly from the general solution of the reduced equation to that of the complete equation without our having to obtain a particular solution of the latter. Before developing this, however, we need some further theory.

12.11.4 The general form of the complementary function

Let us return to our equation
$$a_2(x)\, y'' + a_1(x)\, y' + a_0(x)\, y = 0 \tag{12.20}$$

If $y_1(x)$ is a particular solution of this, then so is $A_1 y_1(x)$, where A_1 is an arbitrary constant. For
$$a_2(x) \frac{d^2[A_1 y_1]}{dx^2} + a_1(x) \frac{d[A_1 y_1]}{dx} + a_0(x)\, [A_1 y_1(x)]$$
$$= A_1 \left[a_2(x) \frac{d^2 y_1}{dx^2} + a_1(x) \frac{dy_1}{dx} + a_0(x)\, y_1 \right] = 0$$

since from (12.20), the contents of the expression inside the brackets are equal to zero. Similarly, if $y_2(x)$ is another particular solution, then so is $A_2 y_2(x)$, where A_2 is another arbitrary constant. *And therefore so is $A_1 y_1(x) + A_2 y_2(x)$* (proved by substitution).

Now it can be shown that if the *particular* solutions $y_1(x)$ and $y_2(x)$ are inter-related in a certain way then $A_1y_1(x)+A_2y_2(x)$ will be in fact the *general* solution of (12.20)—i.e. A_1 and A_2 will become *essential* arbitrary constants (Section 12.7). The relationship between $y_1(x)$ and $y_2(x)$ is that they should be what is called *linearly independent*. This condition is defined as follows:

If $y_1(x)$ and $y_2(x)$ are such that

$$A_1y_1(x)+A_2y_2(x) \tag{12.27}$$

(A_1 and A_2 being constants) can be *identically* zero—i.e. zero for all values of x—only if *both* A_1 and A_2 are zero, then the functions $y_1(x)$ and $y_2(x)$ are said to be *linearly independent*.

Example:

The equation

$$y'' + \omega^2 y = 0 \tag{12.28}$$

has particular solutions

$$\sin \omega x, \quad \cos \omega x$$

Now $\sin \omega x$ and $\cos \omega x$ are linearly independent; it is impossible to find A_1 and A_2 such that $A_1 \sin \omega x + A_2 \cos \omega x$ is identically zero. (To see this, suppose it *was* possible to find A_1 and A_2 such that $A_1 \sin \omega x + A_2 \cos \omega x = 0$ for all values of x. Let $x=0$; whence $A_2=0$. Let $x=\pi/2$; whence $A_1=0$. Hence both A_1 and A_2 must be zero; and only if they are both zero can

$$A_1 \sin \omega x + A_2 \cos \omega x = 0$$

for all and any value of x.)

Since the two functions are linearly independent, our result (12.27) tells us that the general solution of (12.28) is

$$y = A \sin \omega x + B \cos \omega x$$

(cf. Section 12.4).

12.11.5 The linear equation with constant coefficients

A class of differential equations which are very important in biological work are linear equations with constant coefficients. These are of the general form

$$a_n \frac{d^n y}{dx^n} + a_{n-1} \frac{d^{n-1} y}{dx^{n-1}} + a_{n-2} \frac{d^{n-2} y}{dx^{n-2}} + \ldots + a_0 y = f(x)$$

where the coefficients $a_n, a_{n-1}, a_{n-2}, \ldots, a_0$ *are constants.*

Examples:

$$3y''' - 4y'' + 2y' - y = \sin x$$

$$\frac{d^2y}{dt^2} + \omega^2 y = 0 \qquad (\omega \text{ a constant})$$

Equations such as these occur in the mathematical modelling of, e.g. cell and enzyme kinetics, circulatory function, compartmental analysis, population growth and decay, etc. Their solution can be reduced to simple algebra, which makes them the easiest to handle of all differential equations. We consider first the case when $f(x) = 0$, i.e. the reduced equation.

12.11.6   First-order linear equations with constant coefficients

We have already seen that the first-order linear differential equation with constant coefficients

$$\frac{dp}{dt} + kp = 0$$

has as its general solution

$$p = \alpha \exp(-kt)$$

where α is an (essential) arbitrary constant.

This was in the context of a particular time-dependent variable $p(t)$. However, in the completely general situation of independent variable x and dependent variable y, we have similarly that

$$y' + ky = 0 \tag{12.29}$$

has the general solution

$$y = \alpha \exp(-kx)$$

Furthermore, given any equation of the form

$$a_1 y' + a_0 y = 0 \tag{12.30}$$

(a_1 and a_0 being constants)
we can reduce it to the form (12.29) by dividing across by a_1, giving

$$y' + (a_0/a_1)\, y = 0$$

and writing $k = -(a_0/a_1)$. Thus *the general solution of the first-order linear differential equation with constant coefficients*

$$a_1 y' + a_0 y = 0$$

is

$$y = \alpha \exp\left(-\frac{a_0}{a_1} x\right) \tag{12.31}$$

Examples:

(i) The general solution of

$$3\frac{dy}{dx}+4y=0$$

is

$$y=\alpha\exp\left(-\frac{4}{3}x\right)$$

(ii) The general solution of

$$\frac{dp}{dt}-3p=0$$

is

$$p=\beta\exp(3t)$$

If we require that $p(t)=70$, say, at $t=1$, this gives

$$70=\beta\exp(3*1)=\beta\exp(3)$$

whence $\beta=70\exp(-3)$, and the solution subject to the given boundary condition is

$$p=70\exp(-3)*\exp(3t)=70\exp\{3*(t-1)\}$$

Example (ii) above generalizes to the following result:
The solution of

$$a_1\frac{dy}{dx}+a_0y=0$$

subject to $y=Y$ at $x=X$ and where a_1 and a_0 are constants, is

$$y=Y\exp\left(-\frac{a_0}{a_1}*(x-X)\right)\qquad(12.32)$$

12.11.7 Second-order linear equations with constant coefficients

We have seen that the general solution of the first-order equation $a_1y'+a_0y=0$ is of the form $\alpha\exp\{-(a_0/a_1)x\}$. Let us see if the second-order equation of this type also has an exponential solution.

We have

$$a_2y''+a_1y'+a_0y=0\qquad(12.33)$$

as our general equation.

Let $y=\exp(rx)$. Then $y'=r\exp(rx)$, and $y''=r^2\exp(rx)$. Substituting in

(12.33), we have

$$a_2r^2 \exp(rx) + a_1r \exp(rx) + a_0 \exp(rx) = 0,$$

i.e. $(a_2r^2 + a_1r + a_0) \exp(rx) = 0$ (12.34)

for all x. Since $\exp(rx)$ is not zero for any finite x, (12.34) must mean that

$$a_2r^2 + a_1r + a_0 = 0 \qquad (12.35)$$

The equation (12.35) is called the *auxiliary equation* or the *characteristic equation*. It is a quadratic equation, which, if it admits of a solution at all, will have two roots, and hence give *two* values for r. Let these be r_1, r_2. Then the functions

$$y = \exp(r_1x), \quad y = \exp(r_2x)$$

are both possible solutions of (12.33). Except in the case $r_1 = r_2$, they are linearly independent, and hence the general solution of (12.33) in this case is

$$y = A \exp(r_1x) + B \exp(r_2x) \qquad (12.36)$$

Examples:

(i) $\dfrac{d^2y}{dx^2} - 7\dfrac{dy}{dx} + 12y = 0$

Here $a_2 = 1$, $a_1 = -7$, $a_0 = 12$. The auxiliary equation is

$r^2 - 7r + 12 = 0$

with roots

$r = 4, \quad r = 3$

Hence the general solution is

$y = A \exp(4x) + B \exp(3x)$

(ii) $3\dfrac{d^2p}{dt^2} - \dfrac{p}{3} = 0$ subject to $p(0) = 0$
                                                $\dot{p}(0) = 1$

The auxiliary equation is

$3r^2 - \tfrac{1}{3} = 0,$

solution

$r = \tfrac{1}{3}, \quad r = -\tfrac{1}{3}$

The differential equation solution is therefore

$p = A \exp(\tfrac{1}{3}t) + B \exp(-\tfrac{1}{3}t)$

Since $p(0) = 0$, we have

$0 = A + B$

Since $p'(0)=1$, we have also

$$1=\frac{A}{3}-\frac{B}{3}$$

The solution of this pair of simultaneous equations is

$$A=\tfrac{3}{2}, \quad B=-\tfrac{3}{2}$$

and the particular solution of the differential equation in this case is therefore

$$p=\tfrac{3}{2}\exp\left(\tfrac{1}{3}t\right)-\tfrac{3}{2}\exp\left(-\tfrac{1}{3}t\right)$$

We have seen that the solution (12.36) depends on $r_1\neq r_2$. If $r_1=r_2$ and we write $y=A\exp(r_1x)+B\exp(r_2x)$, this $=(A+B)\exp(r_1x)$. Since we may write $C=A+B$, giving $y=C\exp(r_1x)$, this is a solution with only one essential arbitrary constant. Clearly this is not the full solution. An even more unsettling situation confronts us if the auxiliary equation has no real roots at all—what can we do then?

It can be shown that these situations can be handled by extensions of the above approach; we will content ourselves here with listing the results in the various cases; for the theory, see e.g. the texts referred to in Section 12.11.3.

12.11.7.1

We define three distinct possibilities for the auxiliary equation

$$a_2r^2+a_1r+a_0=0.$$

(1) $a_1^2>4a_0a_2$

In this case, there are *two unequal distinct roots* to the auxiliary equation, given by

$$r_1=\frac{-a_1+\sqrt{(a_1^2-4a_0a_2)}}{2a_2}, \qquad r_2=\frac{-a_1-\sqrt{(a_1^2-4a_0a_2)}}{2a_2}$$

and the general solution of the differential equation (12.33) is

$$y=A\exp(r_1x)+B\exp(r_2x) \tag{12.37}$$

Example:

$$y''+5y'-6y=0$$

$$a_2=1, \quad a_1=5, \quad a_0=-6, \quad a_1^2=25, \quad a_0a_2=-6$$

$$r_1=\frac{-5+\sqrt{49}}{2}=1, \qquad r_2=\frac{-5-\sqrt{49}}{2}=-6$$

and therefore

$$y = A \exp(x) + B \exp(-6x)$$

The exact values to be given to A and B in any particular case have to be determined from the boundary conditions.

(2) $a_1^2 = 4a_0a_2$

In this case there are *two equal roots*, $r = -a_1/2a_2$. The general solution of the differential equation (12.33) can be shown to be

$$y = (A + Bx) \exp(rx) \qquad\qquad (12.38)$$

Example:

$$9y'' + 24y' + 16y = 0$$

$$a_1^2 = 576, \quad 4a_0a_2 = 576, \quad r = -\frac{24}{18} = -\frac{4}{3}$$

and therefore

$$y = (A + Bx) \exp(-\tfrac{4}{3}x)$$

Again, the values of A and B in any specific case are determined by the boundary conditions of the situation.

(3) $a_1^2 < 4a_0a_2$

In this case there are *no real roots*. We proceed as follows: write

$$\alpha = -\frac{a_1}{2a_2}$$

$$\beta = \frac{1}{2a_2} \sqrt{(4a_0a_2 - a_1^2)}$$

The general solution of the differential equation (12.33) can be shown to be

$$y = \exp(\alpha x) \{A \cos(\beta x) + B \sin(\beta x)\} \qquad\qquad (12.39)$$

Example:

$$\ddot{p} + \dot{p} + 2p = 0 \qquad p(0) = 0, \quad \dot{p}(0) = 0 \cdot 5$$

The auxiliary equation is $r^2 + r + 2 = 0$, which has no real roots. We have:

$$\alpha = -\tfrac{1}{2}$$

$$\beta = \tfrac{1}{2}\sqrt{(8-1)} = \frac{\sqrt{7}}{2}$$

and therefore

$$p = \exp\left(-\frac{t}{2}\right)\left[A \cos\frac{(\sqrt{7}t)}{2} + B \sin\frac{(\sqrt{7}t)}{2}\right]$$

Since $p(0) = 0$,   we have

$$0 = 1 * [A * 1 + B * 0], \quad \text{i.e.} \quad A = 0$$

Since $\dot{p}(0) = 0 \cdot 5$,   we have

$$0 \cdot 5 = B \frac{\sqrt{7}}{2}, \quad \text{i.e.} \quad B = \frac{1}{\sqrt{7}}$$

Whence:

$$p = \frac{\exp(-t/2)}{\sqrt{7}} \sin\left(\frac{\sqrt{7}t}{2}\right)$$

$$= \frac{\exp(-t/2)}{2 \cdot 646} \sin(1 \cdot 323t)$$

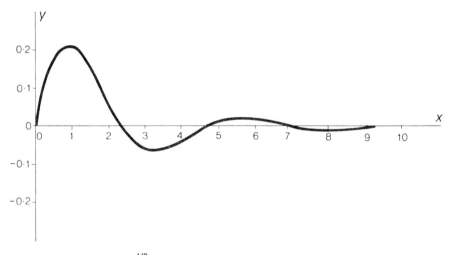

Fig 12·2 $y = \dfrac{e^{-t/2}}{2.646} \sin(1.323t)$

It is noteworthy in particular that the case $a_1^2 < 4a_0a_2$ gives an oscillatory solution.

A special case of this third type is of interest. If $a_1 = 0$, i.e. the term in y' is missing, the equation (12.33) becomes

$$a_2 y'' + a_0 y = 0$$

with $4a_0a_2 > 0$; this has the solution

$$y = A \cos \left\{ \sqrt{\left(\frac{a_0}{a_2}\right)} x \right\} + B \sin \left\{ \sqrt{\left(\frac{a_0}{a_2}\right)} x \right\} \tag{12.40}$$

This is a pure oscillation, with no exponential term as in (12.39). It is not perhaps obvious that the sum of sine and cosine terms as above is a single pure oscillation, but it can be shown that (12.40) is equivalent to

$$y = \sqrt{\{(A^2 + B^2)\}} * \sin(\omega x + \theta) \tag{12.41}$$

where $\omega = \sqrt{\dfrac{a_0}{a_2}}$

and $\sin\theta = \dfrac{A}{\sqrt{(A^2 + B^2)}}$

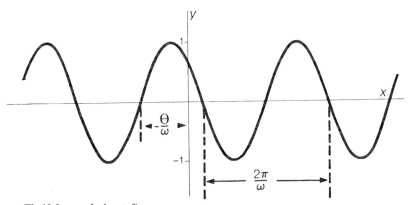

Fig 12.3 $y = \sin(\omega x + \theta)$

12.11.8   Solution of the complete equation: the method of variation of parameters

We now describe a general method for obtaining the solution of the complete equation directly from that of the reduced equation; the technique is known as *Variation of Parameters*.

The idea behind this is perhaps best illustrated by an example. We will use the equation

$$\frac{dS_b}{dt} = k_2 S_{a\max} * \{1 - \exp(-k_1 t)\} - (k_2 + k_3) S_b \tag{12.42}$$

with $S_b = 0$ at $t = 0$

considered by Waterlow and Stephen (1967) in a paper on lysine turnover. S_b is the specific activity of serum protein, $S_{a\text{max}} * \{1 - \exp(-k_1 t)\}$ is taken to be the specific activity of intracellular free lysine at time t. The quantities k_1, k_2 and k_3 are constants.†

Rearranging the terms, we can write (12.42) as

$$\frac{dS_b}{dt} + (k_2 + k_3) S_b = k_2 S_{a\text{max}} * \{1 - \exp(-k_1 t)\} \tag{12.43}$$

The reduced equation is

$$\frac{dS_b}{dt} + (k_2 + k_3) S_b = 0 \tag{12.44}$$

with solution

$$S_b = A \exp\{-(k_2 + k_3)t\} \tag{12.45}$$

Now the reduced equation is the same for all forcing functions. It is not unreasonable to speculate that if we could imagine the forcing function gradually settling down to being *identically* zero through a succession of functional forms, then the solution of the complete equation would gradually assume the form of the complementary function. This idea lies behind our next step.

We *assume* that the solution of the complete equation is of the form

$$S_b = A(t) \exp\{-(k_2 + k_3) t\} \tag{12.46}$$

which is of the same form as (12.45), our complementary function, except that the *constant* A has been replaced by a *function* $A(t)$. We now see if we can find an $A(t)$ which would make this assumption correct.

Now if $A(t) \exp\{-(k_2 + k_3)t\}$ *is* the solution of (12.42), then substituting it for S_b in the equation gives us

$$\frac{d}{dt}[A(t) \exp\{-(k_2 + k_3) t\}] + (k_2 + k_3) A(t) \exp\{-(k_2 + k_3) t\}$$

$$= k_2 S_{a\text{max}} * \{1 - \exp(-k_1 t)\}$$

Using the rule for differentiation of a product, we have:

$$\frac{dA(t)}{dt} \exp\{-(k_2 + k_3) t\} - A(t) (k_2 + k_3) \exp\{-(k_2 + k_3) t\}$$

$$+ (k_2 + k_3) A(t) \exp\{-(k_2 + k_3) t\} = k_2 S_{a\text{max}} * \{1 - \exp(-k_1 t)\} \tag{12.47}$$

i.e. $$\frac{dA(t)}{dt} = k_2 S_{a\text{max}} * [\exp\{(k_2 + k_3) t\} - \{\exp(k_2 + k_3 - k_1) t\}] \tag{12.48}$$

[multiplying (12.47) across by $\exp\{(k_2 + k_3)t\}$].

---

†It would be better to write $(k_2 + k_3)$ as a single constant—k, say—but we will use $(k_2 + k_3)$ throughout in order to make it easier to refer back to the original paper.

Integration of (12.48) with respect to t gives

$$\int \frac{dA(t)}{dt} \, dt = \int k_2 S_{a\max} * [\exp \{(k_2+k_3) \, t\} - \exp \{(k_2+k_3-k_1) \, t\}] dt$$

i.e. $$A(t) = k_2 S_{a\max} * \left[\frac{\exp \{(k_2+k_3) \, t\}}{k_2+k_3} - \frac{\exp \{(k_2+k_3-k_1) \, t\}}{k_2+k_3-k_1}\right] + C \quad (12.49)$$

where C is an arbitrary constant (cf. Section 12.9, ex. 4).

Our solution of the complete equation is therefore (from (12.46))

$$S_b = A(t) \{\exp -(k_2+k_3) \, t\}$$

$$= \left[k_2 S_{a\max} * \left[\frac{\exp \{(k_2+k_3) \, t\}}{k_2+k_3} - \frac{\exp \{(k_2+k_3-k_1) \, t\}}{k_2+k_3-k_1}\right] + C\right]$$

$$* \exp \{-(k_2-k_3) \, t\}$$

$$= k_2 S_{a\max} * \left[\frac{1}{k_2+k_3} - \frac{\exp (-k_1 t)}{k_2+k_3-k_1}\right] + C \exp \{-(k_2+k_3) \, t\} \quad (12.50)$$

The boundary condition $S_b = 0$ at $t = 0$ gives us

$$C = k_2 S_{a\max} * \left[\frac{1}{k_2+k_3-k_1} - \frac{1}{k_2+k_3}\right]$$

$$= k_2 S_{a\max} * \frac{k_1}{(k_2+k_3)(k_2+k_3-k_1)} \qquad \text{(cf. Section 1.8.3)}$$

Hence from (12.50)

$$S_b = k_2 S_{a\max} * \left[\frac{1}{k_2+k_3} - \frac{\exp (-k_1 t)}{k_2+k_3-k_1} + \frac{k_1 \exp \{-k_2+k_3) \, t\}}{(k_2+k_3)(k_2+k_3-k_1)}\right]$$

$$(12.51)$$

Note that (12.50) is the sum of two expressions: $C \exp \{-(k_2+k_3) \, t\}$, the general solution of the reduced equation, and

$$k_2 S_{a\max} * \left[\frac{1}{k_2+k_3} - \frac{\exp (-k_1 t)}{k_2+k_3-k_1}\right],$$

which it will be found is a particular solution of the complete equation. This is as predicted by the theorem in Section 12.11.2.

This example has involved an equation with constant coefficients, but the method can be extended to any ordinary linear differential equation. In broad terms, the technique is to solve the reduced equation with its arbitrary constants, replace these constants by functions of the independent variable, and then attempt to find the form of these functions by substituting the resulting expression in the original complete equation.

We give now without proofs the general formulae for first- and second-order equations; proofs are to be found in, e.g. Ince (1956) or Ross (1964). It is always most important to remember to include the constants of integration, as shown in the examples.

12.11.9   First-order equations

The general solution of the equation

$$a_1(x) \frac{dy}{dx} + a_0(x) y = f(x)$$

is $y = v(x) * u(x)$

where $u(x)$ is the complementary function without its arbitrary constant and

$$v(x) = \int \frac{f(x)}{a_1(x) * u(x)} \, dx$$

Example:

To find the general integral of the equation

$$y' + y = \sin x$$

The complementary function of this equation is $C e^{-x}$ where C is the arbitrary constant, and thus $u(x) = e^{-x}$. Also

$$v(x) = \int e^x \sin x \, dx$$

$$= \frac{e^x (\sin x - \cos x)}{2} + A$$

and so $y = A e^{-x} + \tfrac{1}{2}(\sin x - \cos x)$

12.11.10 Second-order equations

The general integral of the equation

$$a_2(x) \frac{d^2y}{dx^2} + a_1(x) \frac{dy}{dx} + a_0(x) y = f(x)$$

is $y = v_1(x) * u_1(x) + v_2(x) * u_2(x)$

N

where

$$C_1 u_1(x) + C_2 u_2(x)$$

is the complementary function, and

$$v_1(x) = -\int \frac{f(x)\, u_2(x)\, \mathrm{d}x}{a_2(x) * \{u_1(x)\, u_2'(x) - u_1'(x)\, u_2(x)\}}$$

$$v_2(x) = \int \frac{f(x)\, u_1(x)\, \mathrm{d}x}{a_2(x) * \{u_1(x)\, u_2'(x) - u_1'(x)\, u_2(x)\}}$$

Example:

The general integral of

$$y'' + y = e^{-x}$$

is $$v_1(x) * \sin x + v_2(x) * \cos x$$

where $$v_1(x) = -\int \frac{e^{-x} \cos x}{-\sin^2 x - \cos^2 x}\, \mathrm{d}x = \int e^{-x} \cos x\, \mathrm{d}x\dagger$$

$$= \frac{e^{-x}}{2} [\sin x - \cos x] + A_1$$

$$v_2(x) = -\int e^{-x} \sin x\, \mathrm{d}x = \frac{e^{-x}}{2} [\sin x + \cos x] + A_2$$

i.e. $$y = A_1 \sin x + A_2 \cos x + \tfrac{1}{2} e^{-x}$$

12.11.11 Systems of simultaneous linear differential equations with constant coefficients

Of frequent occurrence in quantitative biology and medicine are *systems* of simultaneous linear differential equations with constant coefficients. For example Samuel *et al* (1968) make use of a pair of equations

$$\frac{\mathrm{d}y_a}{\mathrm{d}t} = -Ay_a + By_b$$

$$\frac{\mathrm{d}y_b}{\mathrm{d}t} = Cy_a - Dy_b$$

(whose solutions y_a and y_b must satisfy *both* equations simultaneously) in their discussion on the effect of neomycin on exchangeable pools of cholesterol, and Matthews *et al* (1968–69) use a system of 12 simultaneous linear differential

† Section 6.11

equations in their construction of a model of CO_2 transport in the body.

The solution of such systems is a straightforward extension of the methods already developed for single equations, and usually matrix algebra (Chapter 7) is used as a simple and convenient way of handling them. However, an adequate treatment of this topic would take up more space than we have available; the reader is therefore referred to the standard texts for details, and we will merely quote the results for a simple two-equation constant coefficient system, as an indication of the way in which the generalization from single to multiple equation systems takes place:

The solution of the equations

$$\frac{dx}{dt} = Ax + By \tag{12.52a}$$

$$\frac{dy}{dt} = Cx + Dy \tag{12.52b}$$

(A, B, C, D being known constants) depends on the roots of the determinantal equation

$$\begin{vmatrix} A-r & B \\ C & D-r \end{vmatrix} = 0$$

i.e. $$r^2 - (A+D)r + (AD - BC) = 0 \tag{12.53}$$

(This links the solution of the equations with the problem of finding eigenvalues and eigenvectors of a matrix—see Section 7.11 and especially equation (7.32)).

As with the single linear equation, there are three cases:

(1) Two unequal roots

Let the roots of (12.53) be r_1 and r_2. Then the general solution of the system (12.52) is

$$x = K \exp(r_1 t) + L \exp(r_2 t) \tag{12.54a}$$

$$y = \frac{(r_1 - A)}{B} * K \exp(r_1 t) + \frac{(r_2 - A)}{B} * L \exp(r_2 t) \tag{12.54b}$$

There are thus two arbitrary constants (K and L) to be determined by the boundary conditions, one for each equation of the system (12.52).

The fact that each solution contains two arbitrary constants would seem to imply that x and y each satisfy a second-order differential equation. This is in fact the case; for example, if we differentiate the equation (12.52a) with respect to t, we obtain

$$\frac{d^2 x}{dt^2} = A \frac{dx}{dt} + B \frac{dy}{dt}$$

and if we substitute for dy/dt from (12.52b), the result is

$$\frac{d^2x}{dt^2} = A\frac{dx}{dt} + BCx + BDy$$

i.e. $$\frac{d^2x}{dt^2} = A\frac{dx}{dt} + BCx + D\left(\frac{dx}{dt} - Ax\right)$$

from (12.52a), i.e.

$$\frac{d^2x}{dt^2} - (A+D)\frac{dx}{dt} + (AD-BC)x = 0$$

whose auxiliary equation is (12.53). Similarly for y, we have

$$\frac{d^2y}{dt^2} - (A+D)\frac{dy}{dt} + (AD-BC)y = 0$$

with the same auxiliary equation. The existence of two second-order equations would seem to imply *four* arbitrary constants but the requirement that the solutions satisfy the simultaneous system (12.52) reduces the number of *essential* arbitrary constants to two.

(2) Two equal roots

The solutions are

$$x = (Kt+L) * \exp(rt)$$

$$y = \left[\frac{(r-A)K}{B} * t + \frac{(r-A)L+K}{B}\right]\exp(rt) \tag{12.55}$$

where r is the double root. Again there are only two arbitrary constants (K and L). (Compare the corresponding result in Section 12.11.7.)

(3) No (real) roots

Write: $$\alpha = \frac{A+D}{2}$$

$$\beta = \tfrac{1}{2}\sqrt{\{4(AD-BC)-(A+D)^2\}}$$

Then $$x = \{K * \cos(\beta t) + L * \sin(\beta t)\}\exp(\alpha t)$$

$$y = \left\{\frac{(\alpha-A)K+\beta L}{B} * \cos(\beta t) + \frac{(\alpha-A)L-\beta K}{B} * \sin(\beta t)\right\}\exp(\alpha t) \tag{12.56}$$

There is a special situation with the system (12.52) when $AD - BC = 0$: the two solutions x and y are linearly related, and the system can be reduced to a first order equation in one unknown. There are still, however, two arbitrary constants involved—one in the linear relationship between y and x, and the other in the solution of either y or x as a function of t.

12.12   Numerical solution of differential equations

In spite of the considerable body of theory which exists for the solution of differential equations, it quite frequently happens in practice that a theoretical solution is either not feasible or not really the best way to deal with a problem. Quite simple-looking differential equations can present formidable difficulties, and there is no real classification system for telling which equations will yield to mathematical ingenuity and which will not, although the solutions for various classes of equations are known. These, however, are mainly of linear type; very little general theory exists for non-linear equations. It is possible to develop the solution of certain types of differential equation as an infinite series. The most well-known examples of this are the *Bessel functions* (see e.g. Ince (1956)), which are series solutions of *Bessel's equation*

$$x^2 y'' + xy' + (x^2 - n^2) y = 0$$

However, series solutions are sometimes not very rapidly convergent, and in general are applicable only to linear equations.

When an equation cannot be solved exactly, one has to approximate the solution. This can sometimes be done purely by algebraic manipulations which take advantage of the particular physical situation which led to the equation. More often, however, such cases are treated by *numerical* methods.

Only specific applications, in which all constants and parameters have definite values, can be attacked this way, since the solution is actually *calculated*. Thus the equation

$$y' + \alpha y^{3/2} = \sin x^2, \quad y(0) = 1$$

cannot be solved numerically if the coefficient α is unknown; but the equations

$$y' + 0 \cdot 1 y^{3/2} = \sin x^2, \quad y(0) = 1$$

or $$y' + 0 \cdot 2 y^{3/2} = \sin x^2, \quad y(0) = 1$$

or $$y' + 0 \cdot 3 y^{3/2} = \sin x^2, \quad y(0) = 1$$

etc.

can each be solved this way. There are also techniques for determining which value of a parameter—such as α above—will give a solution which best fits experimental data, but these are very much outside the scope of this book.

To illustrate the approach, let us consider the simplest of all numerical methods for solving differential equations: *Euler's Method.*

12.12.1 *Euler's method*

Suppose y is a function of x such that

$$y'(x)=f(x, y), \quad \text{and} \quad y(x_0)=y_0 \quad \text{(a known value)} \tag{12.57}$$

(We will deal only with first-order equations from now on. This is not a great handicap, since an equation of order r can very frequently be reduced to a system of r first-order equations of the form (12.57), and numerical methods work as well for systems of equations as for single equations, as a rule.)

We already know the value of y at $x=x_0$—it is y_0. Let us consider the value of y at a nearby point x_0+h, at a distance h from x_0. Now if we know $y(x_0)$ and its derivatives, then from Taylor's theorem (Section 10.4) the value of y at x_0+h is given by

$$y(x_0+h)=y(x_0)+hy_0'(x)+\frac{h^2}{2!}y_0''(x)+\frac{h^3}{6!}y_0'''(x)+\ldots \tag{12.58}$$

From (12.57), however, we have $y'(x_0)=f(x_0, y_0)$, and therefore from (12.58),

$$y_0(x+h)=y_0(x)+hf(x_0, y_0)+\frac{h^2}{2!}f'(x_0, y_0)+\frac{h^3}{6!}f''(x_0, y_0)+\ldots \tag{12.59}$$

Euler's method consists of assuming that h is small enough to enable us to approximate (12.59) by

$$y(x_0+h)=y(x_0)+hf(x_0, y_0) \tag{12.60}$$

—in other words, we drop all terms after $hf(x_0, y_0)$ in (12.59) on the grounds that they are negligible.

Our initial conditions in (12.57) give us $y(x_0)=y_0$, and since $f(x, y)$ is a defined function, we can therefore compute $y_0(x+h)$ from (12.60). By repeating the process with (x_0+h) in place of x_0, we can compute $y(x_0+2h)$:

$$y(x_0+2h)=y(x_0+h)+hf(x_0+h, y_0+h)$$

where $y(x_0+h)$ has of course been computed from $y(x_0)$ as in (12.60). By repeated application of this process, we can compute $y(x_0+3h)$, $y(x_0+4h)$, etc. In other words, a series of discrete values of the solution of the differential equation (12.57) can be calculated.

The increment, h, is usually known as the *step-size* or *step-length*.

Let us now see how this method works out in practice.

Consider the equation

$$y'=4y \qquad y(0)=1 \tag{12.61}$$

integrated numerically with a step-size of $h=0\cdot1$ from $x_0=0$.

We have $y(0)=1$; and since the function $4y$ plays the part of $f(x, y)$, we have also

$$hf(x_0, y_0)=0\cdot1 * 4 * 1=0\cdot4$$

Hence $\quad y(0+0\cdot1)=y(0)+hf(x_0, y_0)$

i.e. $\quad y(0\cdot1)=1+0\cdot4=1\cdot4$

Similarly

$$y(0\cdot2)=y(0\cdot1)+0\cdot1 * 4 * y(0\cdot1)=1\cdot96$$

and $\quad y(0\cdot3)=y(0\cdot2)+0\cdot1 * 4 * y(0\cdot2)=2\cdot744$

etc., etc.

The tabulation of the values is as follows:

Table 12.1. Numerical solution of $y' = 4y$, $y(0) = 1$

	x	y	$f(x, y) = 4y$	$4yh$
Initial Values	$0\cdot0$	1	4	$0\cdot4$
	$0\cdot1$	$1\cdot4$	$5\cdot6$	$0\cdot56$
	$0\cdot2$	$1\cdot96$	$7\cdot84$	$0\cdot784$
	$0\cdot3$	$2\cdot744$	$10\cdot976$	$1\cdot0976$
	$0\cdot4$	$3\cdot8416$	.	.
	.	.	.	.
	.	.	.	.

Now as it happens, equation (12.61) is a linear equation, and with the given initial condition, its solution is $y=\exp(4x)$. Comparing the solution for y given in Table 12.1 with the corresponding values for $\exp(4x)$, we have

Table 12.2. Comparison of computed and theoretical
solutions of $y' = 4y$, $y(0) = 1$

x	y_{computed}	$y = \exp(4x)$
0·0	1·0	1·0
0·1	1·4	1·492
0·2	1·96	2·226
0·3	2·744	3·320
0·4	3·8416	4·953
.		
.		
.		

It is immediately obvious that there is increasing divergence between the computed and theoretical results. On the face of it, we could explain this away by deciding that our value of h is too large for us to be able to assume that the terms in h^2, h^3, ... etc. can be neglected in the Taylor expansion for $y(x_0+h)$. While it is true that reducing the step-size produces more accurate results over our interval $0 \leqslant x \leqslant 0·4$—e.g. $h=0·01$ gives for $x=0·4$ a computed y of 4·80 as against the true value of 4·95—reduction of the step-size increases the amount of calculation, and in addition, it can also be shown that *in this particular example no matter how much we reduce h, eventually the calculated solution will differ to an unacceptable extent from the true value*. The long-term divergence between computed and true solution is what is sometimes known as *instability*, though there are other definitions of this term. Not all equation solutions will suffer from instability if Euler's method is used, and there are criteria for determining whether instability will be likely or not.† And even if instability can occur, it is not necessarily a serious matter, as the point at which it becomes a nuisance may lie outside the range of interest of the problem under consideration; but it must be kept in mind as a possible hazard in *all* numerical methods.

Euler's method as applied in this case shows some aspects of all numerical methods. The first is this difference between true and computed values, which is due to what is known as *local truncation error*; it arises in this method through deriving Euler's formula by *truncating* the Taylor series expansion for $y(x+h)$ after the term $hy'(x)$, i.e. neglecting the terms of the expansion after $hy'(x)$. In other words, truncation error is that error due to an inexact or foreshortened formula.

Independently of truncation error, there is another type of error known as *round-off error*. If we examine the values of y in Table 12.1, we see that an

---

† See e.g. Fox & Mayers (1968), or Noble (1966).

increasing number of figures is needed to give the precise value of y. Sooner or later, the exact representation will become unwieldy, and we will have to round-off our values to some number of decimal places, or, more accurately, to some number of significant figures. Our values will thus become inexact, even if our formula is perfectly correct, and the occurrence of this at any point will affect subsequent values (even if these were to be computed exactly), though the effect may be unimportant. In a digital computer, all calculated values are correct at best only to the number of significant figures held in the computer's registers, and round-off error is always with us when we use computers.

(The cumulative build-up of error from truncation, round-off or any other cause is known as *cumulative* or *propagated* error.)

For this and other reasons, Euler's method is not used in practice, but it serves as a useful introduction. In the context of biological applications, it has one feature for which other, more sophisticated methods also have to be watched: it can give completely misleading answers to equations which should have negative exponential solutions (i.e. of the form $A \exp(-\lambda x)$, where λ is > 0). What is more, with any linear equation, it is the exponential term which tends to zero most rapidly—and is therefore the most readily neglected—which is the greatest source of instability in the solution. When we consider the importance of negative exponential solutions in biological problems, these are sobering facts. (See Fox & Mayers (1968) and Noble (1966) for further discussion of this.)

A large number of other methods, better than Euler's, have been developed, although care must be taken when using any numerical method. The methods fall into three categories: (a) 'Direct' methods, (b) 'Iterative' methods, also known as 'Predictor–Corrector' methods, and (c) 'Indirect' or 'Deferred-correction' methods. To give some idea of what is involved, we will discuss briefly an example of each of (a) and (b); for further information the reader must consult standard references (e.g. Redish (1961), Ralston & Wilf (1965), Noble (1966), Fox & Mayers (1968), and the publications 'Modern Computing Methods' (H.M.S.O. 1961) and 'Interpolation and Allied Tables' (H.M.S.O. 1956)).

12.12.2 Direct methods

Euler's is a direct method. In such methods, the variable being solved for, and its derivatives as required, are computed at each tabular point directly from their values at the previous point. Graphically speaking, we use the value of the function, its slope, rate of change of slope, etc., at the current point on the solution curve as a means of determining the next point on it. These methods usually involve considerable calculation, but offer advantages in other ways which have made them very popular as digital computer techniques.

The best-known of the direct methods is the *Runge-Kutta fourth-order* method, which runs as follows:

Given $y'=f(x, y)$,

let us write

$$x_r = x_0 + r * h$$

$$y_r = y(x_0 + r * h) \qquad r = 0, 1, 2, 3, \ldots$$

(this is a standard notation in numerical analysis).

Now suppose we know y_r. Then compute:

$$k_1 = h * f(x_r, y_r)$$

$$k_2 = h * f(x_r + \tfrac{1}{2}h, y_r + \tfrac{1}{2}k_1)$$

$$k_3 = h * f(x_r + \tfrac{1}{2}h, y_r + \tfrac{1}{2}k_2)$$

$$k_4 = h * f(x_r + h, y_r + k_3)$$

and finally

$$y_{r+1} = y_r + \tfrac{1}{6} * (k_1 + 2k_2 + 2k_3 + k_4)$$

The computation is then repeated to give y_{r+2}, y_{r+3}, etc.

Example:

$$y' + xy = 0, \quad y(0) = 1 \qquad\qquad (12.62)$$

For the purpose of applying the method, we write this as

$$y' = -xy$$

Let us take $h = 0 \cdot 1$. We have $y_0 = 1$, $x_0 = 0$, $x_0 + \tfrac{1}{2}h = 0 + 0 \cdot 05 = 0 \cdot 05$, $x_0 + h = 0 \cdot 1$.

Then $k_1 = -0 \cdot 1 * 0 * 1 = 0$

$$k_2 = -0 \cdot 1 * 0 \cdot 05 * \left(1 + \frac{0}{2}\right) = -0 \cdot 005$$

$$k_3 = -0 \cdot 1 * 0 \cdot 05 * \left(1 - \frac{0 \cdot 005}{2}\right) = -0 \cdot 0049875$$

$$k_4 = -0 \cdot 1 * 0 \cdot 1 * (1 - 0 \cdot 0049875) = -0 \cdot 009950125$$

and $y(0 \cdot 1) = y_1 = 1 + \tfrac{1}{6} [0 - 2 * 0 \cdot 005 - 2 * 0 \cdot 0049875 - 0 \cdot 009950125]$

$$= 0 \cdot 99501248$$

Already we see that we are going to be forced to round-off. Let us do so to four significant figures throughout. We have then $y_1 = 0.9950$, $x_1 = 0.1$. Repeating the process we have

$$k_1 = -0.1 * 0.1 * 0.9950 = -0.009950 \text{ to 4 significant figures}$$

$$k_2 = -0.1 * 0.15 * 0.9900 = -0.01485 \text{ to 4 significant figures}$$

$$k_3 = -0.1 * 0.15 * 0.9876 = -0.01481 \text{ to 4 significant figures}$$

$$k_4 = -0.1 * 0.2 * 0.9802 = -0.01960 \text{ to 4 significant figures}$$

and hence

$$y(0.2) = y_2 = 0.9950 + \tfrac{1}{6} * [-0.009950 - 2 * 0.01485$$
$$- 2 * 0.01481 - 0.01960]$$
$$= 0.9803$$

Similarly for $y(0.3)$, $y(0.4)$ etc.

As with the previous example, the equation (12.62) can be integrated exactly—the solution is $y = \exp(-x^2/2)$. We have deliberately chosen it as an example so that we can compare computed and true results. From tables,[†] $\exp(-x^2/2)$ has the value 0.99501248 at $x = 0.1$, and 0.98019867 at $x = 0.2$. We see that agreement is very good, although—as we might expect with round-off to the fourth significant figure—there is an error in the fourth significant figure of the computed answer for $x = 0.2$.

The Runge-Kutta method is generally reliable, although it too can give rise to instability in, among others, the case of negative exponential solutions. However, this may not be important within the range of integration, and it is possible to determine the step-size so that error build-up is kept under control. One method advocated for automatically dealing with this difficulty is to repeat the integration over a step as two steps of half the step-size and compare the results, i.e. we integrate first from (x_r, y_r) to (x_{r+1}, y_{r+1}), and then from (x_r, y_r) to $(x_{r+1/2}, y_{r+1/2})$ and thence to a second estimate of (x_{r+1}, y_{r+1}). If the two results for (x_{r+1}, y_{r+1}) are acceptably close, continue to use the same step-size, otherwise try again, comparing the results for half the step-size and quarter step-size for estimates of $(x_{r+1/2}, y_{r+1/2})$. This is an extremely time-consuming process, however, even on a computer. There is a refinement of Runge-Kutta, due to Merson (1957) which subject to certain assumptions, automatically computes the step-size to use by an estimate of the error at each step. As always, care is needed in using it, as its assumptions cannot be checked in actual cases (Fox & Mayers, 1968).

---

† Abramowitz and Stegun (1965).

12.12.3 *Predictor–corrector methods*

Unlike direct methods, these use the computed values of the solution at earlier points, and their derivatives, as well as those of the current tabular point, to make a first estimate of the value at the next tabular point. There are always at least two formulae involved: the *predictor*, used to make the first estimate, and the *corrector*, used to refine this estimate, often *iteratively*. One disadvantage of such formulae is that they cannot be used to start an integration, since for this they need values previous to the starting point and which are therefore not known. The usual practice is to use a direct method to start the integration off, and switch to a predictor–corrector method as soon as sufficient starting values have become available. They have the advantage of considerably easier arithmetic, and error checking is also easier than with, e.g. Runge-Kutta. They can be rather more sensitive to round-off error than are direct methods, however, as well as involving the usual risks of truncation errors and instability. But then no method is 100% safe.

One of the simplest predictor–corrector methods is the following: the 'predictor' formula (using our previous notation) is the *modified Euler formula*

$$y_{r+1}^* = y_{r-1} + 2hy_r' \tag{12.63}$$

where y_{r+1}^* is our first estimate of y_{r+1}. Assuming our equation to be in the standard form $y' = f(x, y)$, (12.63) gives an estimate $(y_{r+1}')^* = f(x_{r+1}, y_{r+1}^*)$. The 'corrector' formula is the so-called *trapezoidal rule*

$$y_{r+1} = y_r + \frac{h}{2}(y_r' + y_{r+1}') \tag{12.64}$$

which is then used to refine our estimate of y_{r+1}, using the estimate $(y_{r+1}')^*$ for y_{r+1}' in (12.64). From this new estimate of y_{r+1}, we can obtain a new estimate of y_{r+1}' from the differential equation, which is substituted in (12.64) again to give yet another estimate of y_{r+1}. The process is continued until successive estimates of y_{r+1} coincide. It often happens that no more than two applications of the corrector formula are needed.

Example:

Let us continue the integration of $y' = -xy$ from where we left off in the Runge-Kutta example (equation (12.62)) but now using the above method.
We already have:

$$y_0 = 1$$
$$y_1 = 0.9950$$
$$y_2 = 0.9803$$
and $\quad h = 0.1, r = 2$

Predictor:

$$y_3^* = y_1 + 2hy_2'$$
$$= y_1 - 2hx_2y_2 \quad (\text{since } y' = -xy)$$
$$= 0 \cdot 9950 - 0 \cdot 2 * 0 \cdot 2 * 0 \cdot 9803$$
$$= 0 \cdot 9558$$

Corrector:

$$y_3 = y_2 + \frac{h}{2}(y_2' + y_3')$$

$$= y_2 + \frac{h}{2}(-x_2y_2 - x_3y_3^*)$$

$$= 0 \cdot 9803 + 0 \cdot 05(-0 \cdot 1961 - 0 \cdot 2867)$$

$$= 0 \cdot 9562 \quad \text{—quite close, in fact, to } y_3^*$$

Repeat of corrector:

$$y_3 = 0 \cdot 9803 + 0 \cdot 05(-0 \cdot 1961 - 0 \cdot 3 * 0 \cdot 9562)$$

$$\uparrow \qquad \uparrow$$
$$x_3 * \text{latest } y_3 \text{ estimate}$$

$$= 0 \cdot 9561$$

We cannot refine our estimate further. The true value for y_3 is $0 \cdot 9560$, to four significant figures, but our working is not precise enough to hope to obtain four significant figures correctly.

This method, which does not seem to have a formal name, is easy to carry out, as we saw above. It also has the advantage in the medical and biological context that it is stable for equations with exponentially decreasing solutions. Indeed, *it can be shown to give stable solutions for any equation $y' = f(x, y)$ for which $\partial f / \partial y$ is < 0.*

Apart from stability, however, there is the question as to the size of step, h, which can be used. In our example, two repetitions or *iterations*, as they are called, of the corrector formula were enough to produce a result which could not be further refined. If a finite number of iterations produces such a result, the process is said to *converge* to a solution. However, if the step-size is too big convergence will not take place, successive estimates of y_{r+1} oscillating either steadily or else more and more wildly. It can be shown with this particular predictor–corrector method that if the equation is *$y' = f(x, y)$ where $f(x, y)$ is such that*

$$\left| \frac{\partial f}{\partial y} \right| \quad \text{remains} < \text{some constant } K$$

throughout a sequence of corrector iterations, then the process will converge for any step-size h satisfying $h < 2/K$. So, taking our equation $y' = -xy$, we have

$$f(x, y) = -xy$$

and therefore

$$\frac{\partial f}{\partial y} = -x$$

Our previous discussion then shows us that for positive x, (i) our numerical solution will be stable, since $\partial f/\partial y = -x < 0$, and (ii) if $0 \leqslant x < K$ then since $|\partial f/\partial y|$ will be $< K$ for any value of y, the corrector will converge at all points inside $0 \leqslant x < K$ if $h < 2/K$, or to put it another way, a given step-size h will give convergence for the corrector for points in the range $0 \leqslant x < 2/k$, $k > h$. Thus our step-size $h = 0 \cdot 1$ could be used over, e.g., the range $0 \leqslant x < 2/0 \cdot 2$, i.e. $0 \leqslant x < 10$ (though in fact the solution would have become sensibly zero long before this).

Note that convergence of the iteration is not the only criterion determining h in this method. If h is taken close to its upper limit $2/K$ convergence can become very slow, and also the larger h is, the more the truncation error will be increased, leading to inaccuracy in the answer. On the other hand, if h is made very small, the risk of round-off error increases and so does the amount of computation. As with all numerical work, a proper balance has to be struck.

A very thorough discussion of the predictor–corrector system (12.63)–(12.64) is given in McCracken & Dorn (1968) and the reader is referred to this source for further information. Details of other predictor–corrector methods are given in the texts referred to in Section 12.12.1.

12.13   Some general remarks

The numerical methods mentioned in this chapter are only a small sample of the large number of available techniques. Thanks to the development of the desk calculator and the digital computer, numerical analysis—i.e. the theory and application of numerical solutions and techniques to mathematical problems in general and differential equations in particular—has grown from a relatively small-scale, specialized subject to become *the* dominating influence in modern applied mathematics, and new methods of numerical analysis are continually being developed.

The program library of any computer centre involved with scientific work normally contains programs for the more widely used methods of solving differential equations numerically, and this makes it feasible to employ quite sophisticated techniques. Their very availability however, can have its drawbacks; there is a natural tendency to believe that anything as high-powered as an electronic digital computer *must* be producing the right answers, but the previous sections have shown us that these methods have their weak points which can be possible sources of error. It is true of course, that mathematicians and numerical analysts are now well aware of the difficulties, and a great deal of work has been and is being carried out to devise methods of coping with them. But the numerical solution of differential equations is really a specialist subject with wide ramifications, and perhaps the best way for the novice to avoid repeating the mistakes which others have learned to watch for by long (and frequently bitter) experience is to seek the guidance of an experienced numerical analyst before starting on one of these exercises. An unexpected numerical solution *may* be a new physiological or biochemical phenomenon, but could also be an old mathematical phenomenon such as round-off, truncation or some other painfully-documented instability!

Appendix

The appendix is arranged in approximately the same order as the text: figures in the margin are references to chapters or sections in the text.

The Greek alphabet

A	α	Alpha	I	ι	Iota	P	ρ	Rho
B	β	Beta	K	κ	Kappa	Σ	σ	Sigma
Γ	γ	Gamma	Λ	λ	Lambda	T	τ	Tau
Δ	δ	Delta	M	μ	Mu	Y	υ	Upsilon
E	ϵ	Epsilon	N	ν	Nu	Φ	ϕ	Phi
Z	ζ	Zeta	Ξ	ξ	Xi	X	χ	Chi
H	η	Eta	O	o	Omicron	Ψ	ψ	Psi
Θ	θ	Theta	Π	π	Pi	Ω	ω	Omega

Useful constants (12 places of decimals)

$$\pi = 3 \cdot 141\ 592\ 653\ 590 \qquad 1/\pi = 0 \cdot 318\ 309\ 886\ 184$$

$$\log_{10} e = 0 \cdot 434\ 294\ 481\ 903 \qquad \log_e 10 = 2 \cdot 302\ 585\ 092\ 994$$

$$\log_{10} 2 = 0 \cdot 301\ 029\ 995\ 664 \qquad e = 2 \cdot 718\ 281\ 828\ 459$$

$$\log_{10} \tfrac{1}{2} = -0 \cdot 301\ 029\ 995\ 664 \qquad \log_e \tfrac{1}{2} = -0 \cdot 693\ 147\ 180\ 560$$

$$\sqrt{2} = 1 \cdot 414\ 213\ 562\ 373 \qquad \sqrt{3} = 1 \cdot 732\ 050\ 807\ 569$$

$$1\ \text{radian} = 57 \cdot 295\ 779\ 513\ 082° \qquad 1° = 0 \cdot 017\ 453\ 292\ 520 \text{ radian}$$

1.2 ### Powers of 2 in decimal

2^n	n	2^{-n}	2^n	n	2^{-n}
2	1	·5	64	6	·015 625
4	2	·25	128	7	·007 812 5
8	3	·125	256	8	·003 906 25
16	4	·062 5	512	9	·001 953 125
32	5	·031 25	1024	10	·000 976 562 5

1.8.2   Factors

$$(a \pm b)^2 = a^2 \pm 2ab + b^2$$
$$(a+b+c)^2 = a^2 + b^2 + c^2 + 2ab + 2ac + 2bc$$
$$(a \pm b)^3 = a^3 \pm 3a^2b + 3ab^2 \pm b^3$$

$$a^2 - b^2 = (a+b)(a-b) \quad [N.B. \ a^2 + b^2 \text{ has no factors}]$$
$$a^3 + b^3 = (a+b)(a^2 - ab + b^2)$$
$$a^3 - b^3 = (a-b)(a^2 + ab + b^2)$$
$$a^3 + b^3 + c^3 - 3abc = (a+b+c)(a^2 + b^2 + c^2 - ab - ac - bc)$$
$$a^4 + a^2b^2 + b^4 = (a^2 + ab + b^2)(a^2 - ab + b^2)$$

$$a(b^2 - c^2) + b(c^2 - a^2) + c(a^2 - b^2) = (b-c)(c-a)(a-b)$$
$$a^2(b-c) + b^2(c-a) + c^2(a-b) = -(b-c)(c-a)(a-b)$$
$$bc(b-c) + ca(c-a) + ab(a-b) = -(b-c)(c-a)(a-b)$$

1.8.3   Ratios

If $\dfrac{a}{b} = \dfrac{c}{d}$, then

$$\frac{a}{c} = \frac{b}{d}; \quad \frac{d}{b} = \frac{c}{a}; \quad \frac{a+b}{b} = \frac{c+d}{d}; \quad \frac{a-b}{b} = \frac{c-d}{d}; \quad \frac{a}{a+b} = \frac{c}{c+d};$$

$$\frac{a}{a-b} = \frac{c}{c-d}; \quad \frac{3a+2c}{3b+2d} = \frac{a}{b}; \quad \text{etc.}$$

1.3.2 & Powers and indices
4.1

$$a^m * a^n = a^{m+n}; \quad a^{1/n} = \sqrt[n]{a}; \quad (a^m)^n = a^{mn};$$
$$a^m / a^n = a^{m-n}; \quad a^{-n} = 1/a^n;$$
$$a^0 = 1; \quad a^{-1} = 1/a$$

1.10   Equations

Quadratic: $ax^2 + bx + c = 0$

$$x = \{-b + \sqrt{(b^2 - 4ac)}\}/(2a) \quad \text{or} \quad x = \{-b - \sqrt{(b^2 - 4ac)}\}/(2a)$$

Cubic: $x^3+px^2+qx+r=0$

This can be solved by the following scheme:
Let

$A=(p/3)^2-q/3, \quad B=-(p/3)^3+(q/2)(p/3)-r/2$ and $D=B^2-A^3$

If $D>0$ there is one real root viz:

$x=(B+\sqrt{D})^{1/3}+(B-\sqrt{D})^{1/3}-p/3$

If $D=0$ there are three real roots viz:

$x=2B^{1/3}-p/3$ and a repeated root $x=-B^{1/3}-p/3$

If $D<0$ there are three distinct real roots which may be obtained as follows:

Let $\theta=\arctan\{(A^3/B^2-1)^{1/2}\}$, then

$x=2A^{1/2}\cos(\theta/3)-p/3$

or

$x=2A^{1/2}\cos(\theta/3+2\pi/3)-p/3$

or

$x=2A^{1/2}\cos(\theta/3+4\pi/3)-p/3$

Quartic: See Abramowitz and Stegun (1965) section 3.8.3.

1.10 & 11.3.1 Upper and lower bounds for the real roots of a polynomial

Arrange the polynomial equation in the form:

$a_nx^n+a_{n-1}x^{n-1}+\ldots+a_1x+a_0=0$ where $a_n>0$.

Upper bound: if none of the coefficients $a_{n-1}, a_{n-2}\ldots a_0$ are negative then any real root of this equation must be less than or equal to zero. If there are negative coefficients select the coefficient with largest absolute value, i.e. the most negative. We will denote its absolute value by $|a_i|$. Then any real root of the equation must be less *than*

$1+|a_i|/a_n$

To find the lower bound for the roots, put

$b_n=a_n, b_{n-1}=-a_{n-1}, b_{n-2}=a_{n-2}, b_{n-3}=-a_{n-3}$ etc.

If none of the b's are negative then any real roots must be greater than or equal to zero. Otherwise, define $|b_i|$ in a similar fashion to $|a_i|$ above, then any real root must be greater than

$-1-|b_i|/b_n$

Having found the upper and lower bounds, this gives a range within which to search for roots (see 11.3.1). This inequality and others due to Lagrange and Tillot may be found in Rektorys (1969) p. 1169.

4.2.   Binomial theorem

$$(a+x)^n = a^n + na^{n-1}x + \frac{n(n-1)}{2!}a^{n-2}x^2 + \frac{n(n-1)(n-2)}{3!}a^{n-3}x^3 + \dots$$

when n is fractional or negative, condition for validity $|x| < |a|$.

$(1 \pm x)^{-1} = 1 \mp x + x^2 \mp x^3 + x^4 \mp x^5 + \dots$ $(x^2 < 1)$

$(1 \pm x)^{-2} = 1 \mp 2x + 3x^2 \mp 4x^3 + 5x^4 \mp 6x^5 + \dots$ $(x^2 < 1)$

Use the upper or lower sign throughout each formula.

4.2.3   Factorial function

$r!$ also written $\lfloor r$ and $\Gamma(r-1)$ for r integer.

$r! = 1 * 2 * 3 * 4 * \dots * r$

$r!$ is the number of arrangements of r different objects.

r	$r!$	$\log(r!)$	r	$r!$	$\log_{10} r!$
1	1	0·00000	6	720	2·85733
2	2	0·30103	7	5040	3·70243
3	6	0·77815	8	40320	4·60552
4	24	1·38021	9	362880	5·55976
5	120	2·07918	10	3628800	6·55976

Stirling's Formula and similar approximations for large values of r:

$$r! \doteqdot (r/e)^r \sqrt{(2r\pi)}$$

$$\ln(r!) \doteqdot \tfrac{1}{2}\ln(2\pi) + (r+\tfrac{1}{2})\ln(r) - r + 1/(12r)$$

$r!$ lies between $(r/e)^r \sqrt{(2r\pi)}$ and $(r/e)^r \exp{(1/12r)} \sqrt{(2r\pi)}$

4.2.3 Binomial coefficients

$$^nC_r \text{ also written } \binom{n}{r} = \frac{n(n-1)\ldots(n-r+1)}{r(r-1)\ldots 1} = \frac{n!}{(n-r)!\,r!}$$

The number of different combinations of r objects from n different objects is ^nC_r.

n	$\binom{n}{0}$	$\binom{n}{1}$	$\binom{n}{2}$	$\binom{n}{3}$	$\binom{n}{4}$	$\binom{n}{5}$	$\binom{n}{6}$	$\binom{n}{7}$	$\binom{n}{8}$	$\binom{n}{9}$	$\binom{n}{10}$
0	1										
1	1	1									
2	1	2	1								
3	1	3	3	1							
4	1	4	6	4	1						
5	1	5	10	10	5	1					
6	1	6	15	20	15	6	1				
7	1	7	21	35	35	21	7	1			
8	1	8	28	56	70	56	28	8	1		
9	1	9	36	84	126	126	84	36	9	1	
10	1	10	45	120	210	252	210	120	45	10	1

4.3.2 Logarithms

$\log(xy) = \log x + \log y$ (same base on both sides)

$\log\left(\dfrac{x}{y}\right) = \log x - \log y$ (same base on both sides), $\log(1/y) = -\log y$

$\log x^n = n \log x$ (same base on both sides)

$\log_b x = \log_a x * \log_b a = \log_a x / \log_a b, \quad \log_b a = 1/\log_a b$

$x^s = a^{s \log_a x}$

$\log_e x = 2 \cdot 30259 \log_{10} x, \quad \log_{10} x = 0 \cdot 43429 \log_e x$

4.3.12 $y = Ax^m$ can be investigated for $x, y > 0$ by plotting $\log y$ against $\log x$ (log/log paper). It will appear as a straight line with slope m.

4.3.12   Decay constant and half life

$y = Ar^t$ or $y = A \exp(-\lambda t)$ can be investigated for $y > 0$ by plotting $\log y$ against t (log/linear paper). It will appear as a straight line. λ is called the *decay constant* or *time constant*.

In simple exponential decay $A \exp(-\lambda t)$, the time to half value is called the *half life*, $t_{1/2}$.

$\lambda = 0 \cdot 69315/t_{1/2}, \quad t_{1/2} = 0 \cdot 69315/\lambda.$

This relationship is not affected by the starting value A.

5.8   Limits

If $\quad n \to \infty \quad$ then

$$x^n \to \infty \quad x > 1$$
$$\qquad\quad 1 \quad x = 1$$
$$\qquad\quad 0 \quad -1 < x < 1$$
$$x^{-n} \to 0 \quad x > 1, \quad x < -1$$
$$\qquad\quad 1 \quad x = 1$$
$$\qquad\quad \infty \quad 0 < x < 1$$
$$n^{1/n} \to 1$$
$$\frac{x^n}{n!} \to 0$$
$$n^r x^n \to \infty \quad x \geqslant 1$$
$$\qquad\quad 0 \quad -1 < x < 1 \Big\} r > 1$$
$$\log x \to \infty \quad \text{as} \quad x \to \infty$$
$$\log x \to -\infty \quad \text{as} \quad x \to 0$$
$$x^r/e^x \to 0 \quad \text{as} \quad x \to \infty, \quad r > 0$$
$$x^r \log x \to 0 \quad \text{as} \quad x \to 0, \quad r > 0$$
$$x^{-r} \log x \to 0 \quad \text{as} \quad x \to \infty, \quad r > 0$$

5.14

$$\left(1 + \frac{y}{x}\right)^x \to e^y \quad \text{as} \quad x \to \infty$$
$$(1 + yx)^{1/x} \to e^y \quad \text{as} \quad x \to 0$$

L'Hospital's rule

If as $x \to a$, $f(x) \to 0$ and $g(x) \to 0$ then

$$\lim_{x \to a} f(x)/g(x) = \lim_{x \to a} (df/dx)/(dg/dx)$$

6.12   Limits of trigonometric functions

x in radians, $a \neq 0,$

$\quad \sin (ax)/x \to a \qquad$ as $\quad x \to 0$

$\quad \tan (ax)/x \to a \qquad$ as $\quad x \to 0$

$\quad x \sin (a/x) \to a \qquad$ as $\quad x \to \infty$

$\quad x \tan (a/x) \to a \qquad$ as $\quad x \to \infty$

$\quad x \operatorname{cosec} (ax) \to 1/a \quad$ as $\quad x \to 0$

$\quad x \cot (ax) \to 1/a \quad$ as $\quad x \to 0$

6.3.2   **Conventions of trigonometry**

Direction of rotation:

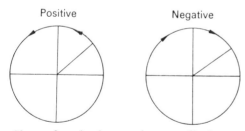

Signs of projections and perpendiculars:

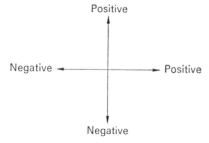

Basic trigonometric relationships

$\sin^2 x$ is the notation for $(\sin x)^2$, i.e. $(\sin x) * (\sin x)$; similar notations apply to the other functions and powers. However $\sin^{-1} x$ is a notation for 'the angle whose sine is x' it is also written arcsin x, and similarly for the other trigonometric functions.

6.4 $\tan x = \dfrac{\sin x}{\cos x}$; $\operatorname{cosec} x = \dfrac{1}{\sin x}$; $\sec x = \dfrac{1}{\cos x}$; $\cot x = \dfrac{1}{\tan x}$

If $-\dfrac{\pi}{2} \leqslant x \leqslant \dfrac{\pi}{2}$ then

$\sin x = (\tan x)/(1 + \tan^2 x)^{1/2}$; $\cos x = 1/(1 + \tan^2 x)^{1/2}$

6.11 $\cos^2 A + \sin^2 A = 1$; $1 + \tan^2 A = \sec^2 A$; $1 + \cot^2 A = \operatorname{cosec}^2 A$

6.4

Second Quadrant		First Quadrant	
SIN	+	SIN	+
COS	−	COS	+
TAN	−	TAN	+
Third Quadrant		Fourth Quadrant	
SIN	−	SIN	−
COS	−	COS	+
TAN	+	TAN	−

Equivalences between an angle X and an angle A
where $0 \leqslant A \leqslant 90°(0 \leqslant A \leqslant \pi/2)$

	Angle $X=$		
	$90°-A°$ $(\pi/2-A)$	$90°+A°$ $(\pi/2+A)$	$180°-A°$ $(\pi-A)$
$\sin X=\ldots$	$\cos A$	$\cos A$	$\sin A$
$\cos X=\ldots$	$\sin A$	$-\sin A$	$-\cos A$
$\tan X=\ldots$	$\cot A$	$-\cot A$	$-\tan A$
$\cot X=\ldots$	$\tan A$	$-\tan A$	$-\cot A$
$\sec X=\ldots$	$\operatorname{cosec} A$	$-\operatorname{cosec} A$	$-\sec A$
$\operatorname{cosec} X=\ldots$	$\sec A$	$\sec A$	$\operatorname{cosec} A$

	Angle $X=$		
	$180°+A°$ $(\pi+A)$	$270°-A°$ $(3\pi/2-A)$	$270°+A°$ $(3\pi/2+A)$
$\sin X=\ldots$	$-\sin A$	$-\cos A$	$-\cos A$
$\cos X=\ldots$	$-\cos A$	$-\sin A$	$\sin A$
$\tan X=\ldots$	$\tan A$	$\cot A$	$-\cot A$
$\cot X=\ldots$	$\cot A$	$\tan A$	$-\tan A$
$\sec X=\ldots$	$-\sec A$	$-\operatorname{cosec} A$	$\operatorname{cosec} A$
$\operatorname{cosec} X=\ldots$	$-\operatorname{cosec} A$	$-\sec A$	$-\sec A$

	Angle $X=$		
	$360°-A°$ $(2\pi-A)$	$360°+A°$ $(2\pi+A)$	$-A$
$\sin X=\ldots$	$-\sin A$	$\sin A$	$-\sin A$
$\cos X=\ldots$	$\cos A$	$\cos A$	$\cos A$
$\tan X=\ldots$	$-\tan A$	$\tan A$	$-\tan A$
$\cot X=\ldots$	$-\cot A$	$\cot A$	$-\cot A$
$\sec X=\ldots$	$\sec A$	$\sec A$	$\sec A$
$\operatorname{cosec} X=\ldots$	$-\operatorname{cosec} A$	$\operatorname{cosec} A$	$-\operatorname{cosec} A$

6.10   **Functions of special angles**

$x°$	x radians	$\sin x$	$\cos x$	$\tan x$	$\cot x$	$\sec x$	$\operatorname{cosec} x$
0°	0	0	1	0	∞	1	∞
30°	$\dfrac{\pi}{6}$	$\dfrac{1}{2}$	$\dfrac{\sqrt{3}}{2}$	$\dfrac{1}{\sqrt{3}}$	$\sqrt{3}$	$\dfrac{2}{\sqrt{3}}$	2
45°	$\dfrac{\pi}{4}$	$\dfrac{1}{\sqrt{2}}$	$\dfrac{1}{\sqrt{2}}$	1	1	$\sqrt{2}$	$\sqrt{2}$
60°	$\dfrac{\pi}{3}$	$\dfrac{\sqrt{3}}{2}$	$\dfrac{1}{2}$	$\sqrt{3}$	$\dfrac{1}{\sqrt{3}}$	2	$\dfrac{2}{\sqrt{3}}$
90°	$\dfrac{\pi}{2}$	1	0	∞	0	∞	1
120°	$\dfrac{2\pi}{3}$	$\dfrac{\sqrt{3}}{2}$	$-\dfrac{1}{2}$	$-\sqrt{3}$	$-\dfrac{1}{\sqrt{3}}$	-2	$\dfrac{2}{\sqrt{3}}$
135°	$\dfrac{3\pi}{4}$	$\dfrac{1}{\sqrt{2}}$	$-\dfrac{1}{\sqrt{2}}$	-1	-1	$-\sqrt{2}$	$\sqrt{2}$
150°	$\dfrac{5\pi}{6}$	$\dfrac{1}{2}$	$-\dfrac{\sqrt{3}}{2}$	$-\dfrac{1}{\sqrt{3}}$	$-\sqrt{3}$	$-\dfrac{2}{\sqrt{3}}$	2
180°	π	0	-1	0	∞	-1	∞
210°	$\dfrac{7\pi}{6}$	$-\dfrac{1}{2}$	$-\dfrac{\sqrt{3}}{2}$	$\dfrac{1}{\sqrt{3}}$	$\sqrt{3}$	$-\dfrac{2}{\sqrt{3}}$	-2
225°	$\dfrac{5\pi}{4}$	$-\dfrac{1}{\sqrt{2}}$	$-\dfrac{1}{\sqrt{2}}$	1	1	$-\sqrt{2}$	$-\sqrt{2}$
240°	$\dfrac{4\pi}{3}$	$-\dfrac{\sqrt{3}}{2}$	$-\dfrac{1}{2}$	$\sqrt{3}$	$\dfrac{1}{\sqrt{3}}$	-2	$-\dfrac{2}{\sqrt{3}}$
270°	$\dfrac{3\pi}{2}$	-1	0	∞	0	∞	-1
300°	$\dfrac{4\pi}{3}$	$-\dfrac{\sqrt{3}}{2}$	$\dfrac{1}{2}$	$-\sqrt{3}$	$-\dfrac{1}{\sqrt{3}}$	2	$-\dfrac{2}{\sqrt{3}}$
315°	$\dfrac{7\pi}{4}$	$-\dfrac{1}{\sqrt{2}}$	$\dfrac{1}{\sqrt{2}}$	-1	-1	$\sqrt{2}$	$-\sqrt{2}$
330°	$\dfrac{11\pi}{6}$	$-\dfrac{1}{2}$	$\dfrac{\sqrt{3}}{2}$	$-\dfrac{1}{\sqrt{3}}$	$-\sqrt{3}$	$\dfrac{2}{\sqrt{3}}$	-2
360°	2π	0	1	0	∞	1	∞

Compound and multiple angle formulae

$\sin (A \pm B) = \sin A \cos B \pm \cos A \sin B$

$\cos (A \pm B) = \cos A \cos B \mp \sin A \sin B$

$\tan (A \pm B) = \dfrac{\tan A \pm \tan B}{1 \mp \tan A \tan B}$

Use upper or lower sign throughout each formula.

$\sin 2x = 2 \sin x \cos x$

$\cos 2x = \cos^2 x - \sin^2 x = 2 \cos^2 x - 1 = 1 - 2 \sin^2 x$

$\sin 3x = 3 \sin x - 4 \sin^3 x$

$\cos 3x = 4 \cos^3 x - 3 \cos x$

$\tan 2x = \dfrac{2 \tan x}{1 - \tan^2 x}$

6.13 $\qquad \tan 3x = \dfrac{3 \tan x - \tan^3 x}{1 - 3 \tan^2 x}$

$\dagger \sin \tfrac{1}{2}x = \pm \sqrt{\left(\dfrac{1 - \cos x}{2}\right)}$

$\cos \tfrac{1}{2}x = \pm \left(\sqrt{\dfrac{1 + \cos x}{2}}\right)$

$\tan \tfrac{1}{2}x = \pm \sqrt{\left(\dfrac{1 - \cos x}{1 + \cos x}\right)} = \dfrac{1 - \cos x}{\sin x} = \dfrac{\sin x}{1 + \cos x}$

If $\qquad t = \tan \tfrac{1}{2}x$

$\cos x = \dfrac{1 - t^2}{1 + t^2}; \quad \sin x = \dfrac{2t}{1 + t^2}$

6.15 **Inverse circular functions**

For $0 \leqslant x \leqslant 1$ $\arcsin (x) = \arctan (x/(1 - x^2)^{1/2})$;

$\arccos (x) = \arctan \{(1 - x^2)^{1/2}/x\}$

$= \dfrac{\pi}{2} - \arcsin (x)$

$\dagger$ The sign in front of root depends on quadrant in which $\tfrac{1}{2}x$ falls.

Function	Interval containing the principal value	
	$x \geqslant 0$	$x < 0$
$y = \arcsin x$ and $\arctan x$	$0 \leqslant y \leqslant \pi/2$	$-\pi/2 \leqslant y < 0$
6.14.2 $y = \arccos x$ and $\operatorname{arcsec} x$	$0 \leqslant y \leqslant \pi/2$	$\pi/2 < y \leqslant \pi$
& 6.15 $y = \operatorname{arccot} x$ and $\operatorname{arccosec} x$	$0 \leqslant y \leqslant \pi/2$	$-\pi/2 \leqslant y < 0$

6.16   Hyperbolic functions

$$\sinh x = \tfrac{1}{2}(e^x - e^{-x}); \quad \cosh x = \tfrac{1}{2}(e^x + e^{-x})$$

$$\tanh x = \frac{\sinh x}{\cosh x}; \quad \operatorname{sech} x = \frac{1}{\cosh x}$$

$$\coth x = \frac{1}{\tanh x}; \quad \operatorname{csch} x = \frac{1}{\sinh x}$$

$$\tanh x = (e^x - e^{-x})/(e^x + e^{-x})$$

$$\sinh x = -\sinh(-x); \quad \operatorname{sech} x = \operatorname{sech}(-x)$$

$$\cosh x = \cosh(-x); \quad \operatorname{csch} x = -\operatorname{csch}(-x)$$

$$\tanh x = -\tanh(-x); \quad \coth x = -\coth(-x)$$

$$\sinh x = \frac{2 \tanh \tfrac{1}{2}x}{1 - \tanh^2 \tfrac{1}{2}x} = \frac{\tanh x}{\sqrt{(1 - \tanh^2 x)}}$$

$$\cosh x = \frac{1 + \tanh^2 \tfrac{1}{2}x}{1 - \tanh^2 \tfrac{1}{2}x} = \frac{1}{\sqrt{(1 - \tanh^2 x)}}$$

$$\cosh^2 x - \sinh^2 x = 1$$

$$\tanh x = \sqrt{(1 - \operatorname{sech}^2 x)}; \quad \operatorname{sech} x = \sqrt{(1 - \tanh^2 x)}$$

$$\coth x = \sqrt{(\operatorname{csch}^2 x + 1)}; \quad \operatorname{csch} x = \sqrt{(\coth^2 x - 1)}$$

	$x = 0$	$x = 0 \cdot 5$	$x = 1$	$x = 2$	$x = 4$
$\sinh x$	0	$0 \cdot 521$	$1 \cdot 175$	$3 \cdot 627$	$27 \cdot 29$
$\cosh x$	1	$1 \cdot 128$	$1 \cdot 543$	$3 \cdot 762$	$27 \cdot 31$
$\tanh x$	0	$0 \cdot 462$	$0 \cdot 762$	$0 \cdot 964$	$0 \cdot 999$

Matrix arithmetic

If $\mathbf{C} = \mathbf{A} + \mathbf{B}$ then $c_{i,j} = a_{i,j} + b_{i,j}$

7.5.2 $\mathbf{C} = \mathbf{A} - \mathbf{B}$ $c_{i,j} = a_{i,j} - b_{i,j}$

7.6 $\mathbf{C} = \mathbf{A} * \mathbf{B}$ $c_{i,j} = \sum a_{i,k} * b_{k,j}$ $(k = 1, 2, 3, \ldots)$

7.5.1 $\mathbf{C} = \mathbf{A}^{\mathrm{T}}$ $c_{i,j} = a_{j,i}$ (transpose also written $\mathbf{A}'$)

7.6.1   If $\mathbf{x}$ and $\mathbf{y}$ are column vectors $\begin{pmatrix} x_1 \\ x_2 \\ \cdot \\ \cdot \\ \cdot \\ x_n \end{pmatrix}$ and $\begin{pmatrix} y_1 \\ \cdot \\ \cdot \\ \cdot \\ \cdot \\ y_n \end{pmatrix}$

$\mathbf{x}^{\mathrm{T}}\mathbf{x} = \sum x_1^2$ $(i = 1, 2 \ldots n)$

$\mathbf{x}^{\mathrm{T}}\mathbf{y} = \sum x_i y_i$ $(i = 1, 2 \ldots n)$

7.9   Determinants

Determinant of a square matrix $\mathbf{A}$ is denoted by

$\det | \mathbf{A} |$, $| \mathbf{A} |$,   or Δ.

Two dimensions:

$$\begin{vmatrix} a_{1,1} & a_{1,2} \\ a_{2,1} & a_{2,2} \end{vmatrix} = a_{1,1}a_{2,2} - a_{1,2}a_{2,1}$$

Three dimensions:

$$\begin{vmatrix} a_{1,1} & a_{1,2} & a_{1,3} \\ a_{2,1} & a_{2,2} & a_{2,3} \\ a_{3,1} & a_{3,2} & a_{3,3} \end{vmatrix} = a_{1,1} * \begin{vmatrix} a_{2,2} & a_{2,3} \\ a_{3,2} & a_{3,3} \end{vmatrix} - a_{1,2} * \begin{vmatrix} a_{2,1} & a_{2,3} \\ a_{3,1} & a_{3,3} \end{vmatrix}$$

$$+ a_{1,3} * \begin{vmatrix} a_{2,1} & a_{2,2} \\ a_{3,1} & a_{3,2} \end{vmatrix}$$

$$= a_{1,1}\, a_{2,2}\, a_{3,3} - a_{1,1}\, a_{2,3}\, a_{3,2}$$
$$- a_{1,2}\, a_{2,1}\, a_{3,3} + a_{1,2}\, a_{2,3}\, a_{3,1}$$
$$+ a_{1,3}\, a_{2,1}\, a_{3,2} - a_{1,3}\, a_{2,2}\, a_{3,1}$$

Rules for the simplification of determinants:

If the rows are made into columns and columns into rows, the determinant (Δ) is unaltered.

If two rows or two columns are interchanged, Δ is altered in sign but unaltered in absolute value. Δ becomes $-\Delta$.

If two rows or two columns are identical then $\Delta = 0$.

If a row (or a column) is multiplied by a factor, k say, then the new determinant $= k\Delta$.

If the elements of any row (or column) are increased or diminished by equimultiples of corresponding elements in any other row or column, Δ is unaltered.

7.7.2   Inverse matrix

A has an inverse, denoted by $\mathbf{A}^{-1}$, if $\mathbf{A}^{-1}\mathbf{A} = \mathbf{A}\mathbf{A}^{-1} = \mathbf{I}$ where **I** is the *identity* or *unit* matrix.

Two dimensions:

$$\mathbf{A} = \begin{pmatrix} a & b \\ c & d \end{pmatrix}, \quad \text{let determinant of } \mathbf{A} \text{ be } \Delta$$

$$\Delta = ad - bc$$

then

$$\mathbf{A}^{-1} = \begin{pmatrix} d/\Delta & -b/\Delta \\ -c/\Delta & a/\Delta \end{pmatrix}$$

$$\mathbf{A}\mathbf{A}^{-1} = \begin{pmatrix} 1 & 0 \\ 0 & 1 \end{pmatrix} \quad \text{i.e. } \mathbf{I}$$

Three dimensions:

$$\mathbf{A} = \begin{pmatrix} a & b & e \\ c & d & f \\ g & h & i \end{pmatrix}, \quad \text{let determinant of } \mathbf{A} \text{ be } \Delta$$

$$\Delta = a(di - fh) - b(ci - fg) + e(ch - dg)$$

then

$$\mathbf{A}^{-1} = \begin{pmatrix} (di - fh)/\Delta & -(bi - eh)/\Delta & (bf - ed)/\Delta \\ -(ci - fg)/\Delta & (ai - eg)/\Delta & -(af - ec)/\Delta \\ (ch - dg)/\Delta & -(ah - gb)/\Delta & (ad - bc)/\Delta \end{pmatrix}$$

$$AA^{-1}=\begin{pmatrix}1&0&0\\0&1&0\\0&0&1\end{pmatrix} \quad \text{i.e. } \mathbf{I}$$

Inverse of a diagonal matrix:

$$A=\begin{pmatrix}a&0&0&0\\0&b&0&0\\0&0&c&0\\0&0&0&d\end{pmatrix} \quad \text{then} \quad A^{-1}=\begin{pmatrix}a^{-1}&0&0&0\\0&b^{-1}&0&0\\0&0&c^{-1}&0\\0&0&0&d^{-1}\end{pmatrix}$$

7.4.1   Partitioned matrices

Multiplication (the rule is similar to that for unpartitioned matrices).

$$\left(\begin{array}{c:c}\mathbf{A}&\mathbf{B}\\\hline\mathbf{C}&\mathbf{D}\end{array}\right)\left(\begin{array}{c:c}\mathbf{E}&\mathbf{F}\\\hline\mathbf{G}&\mathbf{H}\end{array}\right)=\left(\begin{array}{c:c}\mathbf{AE+BG}&\mathbf{AF+BH}\\\hline\mathbf{CE+DG}&\mathbf{CF+DH}\end{array}\right)$$

AE is the matrix product of **A** with **E**, similarly for **BG** etc.

Inversion

It is possible to invert large matrices by partitioning the matrix and then inverting smaller matrices. If the matrix is partitioned as

$$\left(\begin{array}{c:c}\mathbf{A}&\mathbf{B}\\\hline\mathbf{C}&\mathbf{D}\end{array}\right) \quad \text{with inverse} \quad \left(\begin{array}{c:c}\mathbf{P}&\mathbf{Q}\\\hline\mathbf{R}&\mathbf{S}\end{array}\right)$$

(**A, D, P, S** are square, the others can be rectangular), the submatrices of the inverse are given by

$$\mathbf{P}=(\mathbf{A}-\mathbf{BD}^{-1}\mathbf{C})^{-1}$$

$$\mathbf{S}=(\mathbf{D}-\mathbf{CA}^{-1}\mathbf{B})^{-1}$$

$$\mathbf{Q}=-\mathbf{A}^{-1}\mathbf{BS}$$

$$\mathbf{R}=-\mathbf{D}^{-1}\mathbf{CP}$$

Special definitions for square matrices

The sum of the terms on the principal diagonal is called the *trace* and is denoted by tr (**A**).

The expansion of the determinant $|x\mathbf{I}-\mathbf{A}|$ in powers of x is called the *characteristic polynomial* of **A**.

7.11   The roots of $|xI - A| = 0$ are the *eigenvalues* of A, usually denoted by λ_1, λ_2 etc.

7.10   If A is *singular* then $|A| = 0$ and A^{-1} does not exist.

If A is *non singular* then $|A| \neq 0$.

7.4   If A is *symmetric* then $A = A^T$.

7.7.4   If A is *orthogonal* then $A^T A = I$, i.e. $A^{-1} = A^T$

If A is *normal* then $A^T A = A A^T$

7.11   If A is *positive semidefinite* then the eigenvalues of A are all real and greater than or equal to zero.

If A is *positive definite* then the eigenvalues of A are all real and greater than zero.

If A is *hermitian* and its elements are real numbers then this is the same as saying A is symmetric.

If A is *unitary* and its elements are real numbers then this is the same as saying A is orthogonal.

Correlation and covariance matrices are symmetric and positive semi-definite.

7.7   Matrix operations

$$A^2 = A*A, \ A^3 = A*A*A, \ A^{-1}*A = I$$

$$(A+C)*B = A*B + C*B$$

$$(A*B)*C = A*(B*C)$$

$$(A*B)^T = B^T*A$$

$$(A*B)^{-1} = B^{-1}*A^{-1}$$

$$|A^{-1}| = (|A|)^{-1}$$

$$|A*B| = |A|*|B|$$

$$|A^T| = |A|$$

$$|S^{-1}AS| = |A| \text{ for any non-singular S.}$$

Determinant of an orthogonal matrix $= 1$.

$|\mathbf{A}| = $ product of the eigenvalues of $\mathbf{A}$

tr $(\mathbf{A}) = $ sum of the eigenvalues of $\mathbf{A}$

tr $(\mathbf{S}^{-1}\mathbf{A}\mathbf{S}) = $ tr $(\mathbf{S})$

7.11   For every real symmetric matrix $\mathbf{V}$ there is an orthogonal matrix $\mathbf{L}$ such that the matrix $\mathbf{L}^T\mathbf{V}\mathbf{L}$ or $\mathbf{L}^{-1}\mathbf{V}\mathbf{L}$ is diagonal with the diagonal elements equal to the eigenvalues.

7.8.3   **Complex numbers** (many texts use i instead of j).

The number $(x+jy)$ is called a *complex* number. The *real* part is x; the *imaginary* part is jy.

The sum of $(a+jb)$ and $(c+jd)$ is $(a+c)+j(b+d)$.

$(a+jb)-(c+jd)=(a-c)+j(b-d)$.

The product of $(a+jb)$ and $(c+jd)$ is $(ac-bd)+j(bc+ad)$.

This product may be determined by replacing j^2 by -1 in the algebraic product of $(a+jb)(c+jd)$.

$j^3=-j; \quad j^4=1$.

If $z=x+jy$, then $\bar{z}=x-jy$ is called the *conjugate* of z.

$z\bar{z}=x^2+y^2$.

$(x+jy)$ may always be put in the form $r * (\cos\theta+j\sin\theta)$ where r is positive and θ lies between $\pm180°$.

r is called the *modulus* and θ the *amplitude* or *argument*.

The modulus of $(x+jy)$ is written $|x+jy|$ and equals $\sqrt{(x^2+y^2)}$.

The amplitude of $(x+jy)$ is written amp $(x+jy)$ and equals arctan (y/x).

de Moivre's theorem states that

$(\cos\theta+j\sin\theta)^n=\cos n\theta+j\sin n\theta$.

$(\cos\alpha+j\sin\alpha)(\cos\beta+j\sin\beta)=\cos(\alpha+\beta)+j\sin(\alpha+\beta)$.

The product of $r_1(\cos\theta_1+j\sin\theta_1)$ and $r_2(\cos\theta_2+j\sin\theta_2)$ is

$r_1 r_2\{\cos(\theta_1+\theta_2)+j\sin(\theta_1+\theta_2)\}$.

The modulus of a product is the product of the moduli; the amplitude of a product is the sum of the separate amplitudes.

$$\frac{r_1(\cos\theta_1+j\sin\theta_1)}{r_2(\cos\theta_2+j\sin\theta_2)}=\frac{r_1}{r_2}\{\cos(\theta_1-\theta_2)+j\sin(\theta_1-\theta_2)\}.$$

$r(\cos\theta+j\sin\theta)$ can be put in the form $re^{j\theta}$ and is usually easier to handle algebraically in this form.

O

Co-ordinate geometry: straight line

8.4.2   Length of line joining (x_1, y_1) and $(y_2, y_2) = \sqrt{((x_2 - x_1)^2 + (y_2 - y_1)^2)}$.

8.4.1   Co-ordinates of point dividing above line internally in ratio $k_1 : k_2$ are

$$\left(\frac{k_2 x_1 + k_1 x_2}{k_1 + k_2}, \frac{k_2 y_1 + k_1 y_2}{k_1 + k_2} \right)$$

Co-ordinates of the mid point of above line are

$$\left(\frac{x_1 + x_2}{2}, \frac{y_1 + y_2}{2} \right)$$

8.5   *Equations of a straight line*

General format $ax + by + c = 0$

Slope m, and thro' points (x_1, y_1):	$y - y_1 = m(x - x_1)$
Thro' points (x_1, y_1) and (x_2, y_2):	$\dfrac{y - y_1}{y_2 - y_1} = \dfrac{x - x_1}{x_2 - x_1}$
Intercept a on the X axis and intercept b on the Y axis:	$\dfrac{x}{a} + \dfrac{y}{b} = 1$
Slope m, intercept on Y axis c:	$y = mx + c$
Line parallel to X axis:	$y = k$
	(k = distance from x axis)
Line parallel to Y axis:	$x = k$
	(k = distance from y axis)

Angle between two lines whose slopes are m_1 and m_2:

8.5.4 $\tan \theta = \dfrac{m_1 - m_2}{1 + m_1 m_2}$

8.5.7   *Length of perpendicular* from (x_1, y_1) to the line $ax + by + c = 0$ is

$$\frac{ax_1 + by_1 + c}{\sqrt{(a^2 + b^2)}}$$

8.6   **Transformation of co-ordinates**

Translation only of axes parallel to themselves.

The co-ordinates of new origin with respect to the old axes are:
$x = h$, $y = k$. Primed letters designate new co-ordinates.

$x' = x - h \qquad x = x' + h$
$y' = y - k \qquad y = y' + k$

Rotation of axes with fixed origin.

Angle of rotation $= \theta$

$$x' = x \cos \theta + y \sin \theta \qquad x = x' \cos \theta - y' \sin \theta$$

$$y' = y \cos \theta - x \sin \theta \qquad y = y' \cos \theta + x' \sin \theta$$

Origin translated and axes rotated.

Symbols same as above

$$x' = (x - h) \cos \theta + (y - k) \sin \theta$$

$$y' = (y - k) \cos \theta - (x - h) \sin \theta$$

$$x = x' \cos \theta - y' \sin \theta + h$$

$$y = y' \cos \theta + x' \sin \theta + k$$

7.6.2 & **Transformation of points**
8.6.3

If $\mathbf{A}$ is a $(2 \times n)$ matrix and the columns represent n points on a *Cartesian* x, y system of co-ordinates, then

$\begin{pmatrix} 1 & 0 \\ 0 & -1 \end{pmatrix} * \mathbf{A}$ represents the reflection of the points in the x axis

$\begin{pmatrix} -1 & 0 \\ 0 & 1 \end{pmatrix} * \mathbf{A}$ represents the reflection of the points in the y axis

$\begin{pmatrix} 0 & 1 \\ 1 & 0 \end{pmatrix} * \mathbf{A}$ represents the reflection of the points in the line $x = y$

$\begin{pmatrix} \cos \alpha & -\sin \alpha \\ \sin \alpha & \cos \alpha \end{pmatrix} * \mathbf{A}$ rotates the points through angle α in an anti-clockwise direction.

8.8   **Relation between rectangular and polar co-ordinates**

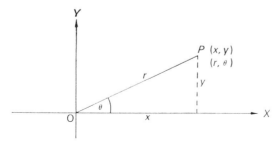

$P=(x, y)=(r, \theta)$ then $x=r \cos \theta$, $y=r \sin \theta$,

$r=\sqrt{(x^2+y^2)}$, $\theta=\arctan (y/x)$; not necessarily the principal value, if $x<0$ then $\theta=$ principal value $+\pi$.

Polar co-ordinate forms

8.7   *The equation of a straight line*, to which the perpendicular from the origin makes an *angle* α with the x axis and is of length p, is

$r \cos (\theta-\alpha)=p$

The equation of a straight line through (r_1, θ_1) and (r_2, θ_2) is

$r_1 r \sin (\theta-\theta_1)-r r_2 \sin (\theta-\theta_2)+r_1r_2 \sin (\theta_1-\theta_2)=0$

The equation of a circle with centre at (r_1, θ_1) and radius a is

$r^2-2r r_1 \cos (\theta-\theta_1)+r_1^2-a^2=0$

The equation of a conic, with the focus as origin, is

8.10 $r=\dfrac{l}{1+e \cos \theta}$

where e is the eccentricity and $2l$ the width of the conic measured on a line through the focus perpendicular to its axis. l is called the *semi-latus rectum*.

The equation of the tangent to a conic at the point (r_1, θ_1) on it is

$\dfrac{l}{r}=\cos (\theta-\theta_1)+e \cos \theta$

8.10.1   **Classification of second degree curves (conics)**

General form: $ax^2+2hxy+by^2+2gx+2fy+c=0$

Let $I=a+b$, $J=ab-h^2$, $K=\{c(a+b)-f^2-g^2\}/I^2$ and

$\Delta = \begin{vmatrix} a & h & g \\ h & b & f \\ g & f & c \end{vmatrix}$

Type of conic	Conditions
Ellipse	$\Delta \neq 0,\ J > 0,\ \Delta/I < 0$
Circle	$\Delta \neq 0,\ \Delta/I < 0,\ h=0,\ a=b$
Hyperbola	$\Delta \neq 0,\ J < 0$
Rectangular hyperbola	$\Delta \neq 0,\ J < 0,\ I=0$
Parabola	$\Delta \neq 0,\ J=0,\ \Delta/I < 0$
Straight lines (intersecting)	$\Delta = 0,\ J < 0$
Perpendicular lines	$\Delta = 0,\ J < 0,\ I=0$
Parallel lines	$\Delta = 0,\ J=0,\ K < 0$
Coincident lines	$\Delta = 0,\ J=0,\ K=0$

The centres of the conics are at the point:

$$((hf-bg)/J,\ (gh-af)/J)$$

Examples of the variety of shapes which may be defined by simple equations.

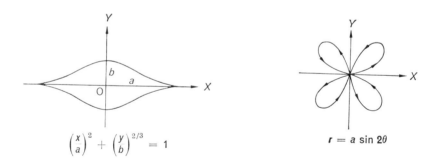

$$\left(\frac{x}{a}\right)^2 + \left(\frac{y}{b}\right)^{2/3} = 1 \qquad\qquad r = a\sin 2\theta$$

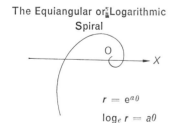

The Equiangular or Logarithmic Spiral

$$r = e^{a\theta}$$
$$\log_e r = a\theta$$

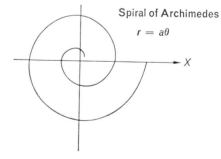

Spiral of Archimedes

$$r = a\theta$$

8.12   **Co-ordinate geometry in three dimensions**

Space co-ordinate systems

1. Rectangular system x, y, z.
2. Cylindrical system r, θ, z.
3. Spherical system ρ, θ, ϕ. In certain situations it is desirable to interchange the symbol ϕ for θ and vice versa.
4. Polar space system ρ, α, β, γ.

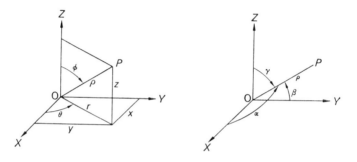

Relations of co-ordinates of systems in terms of x, y, z

Cylindrical	Spherical	Polar space
$r=\sqrt{(x^2+y^2)}$	$\rho=\sqrt{(x^2+y^2+z^2)}$	$\rho=\sqrt{(x^2+y^2+z^2)}$
$\theta=\arctan\dfrac{y}{x}$	$\theta=\arctan\dfrac{y}{x}$	$\alpha=\arccos\left(\dfrac{x}{\sqrt{(x^2+y^2+z^2)}}\right)$
$z=z$	$\phi=\arccos\left(\dfrac{z}{\sqrt{(x^2+y^2+z^2)}}\right)$	$\beta=\arccos\left(\dfrac{y}{\sqrt{(x^2+y^2+z^2)}}\right)$
		$\gamma=\arccos\left(\dfrac{z}{\sqrt{(x^2+y^2+z^2)}}\right)$

Relations of rectangular co-ordinates (x, y, z) in terms of cylindrical, spherical and polar space co-ordinates

Cylindrical	Spherical	Polar space
$x=r\cos\theta$	$x=\rho\sin\phi\cos\theta$	$x=\rho\cos\alpha$
$y=r\sin\theta$	$y=\rho\sin\phi\sin\theta$	$y=\rho\cos\beta$
$z=z$	$z=\rho\cos\phi$	$z=\rho\cos\gamma$

Distance from (x_1, y_1, z_1) to (x_2, y_2, z_2):

$d=\sqrt{\{(x_1-x_2)^2+(y_1-y_2)^2+(z_1-z_2)^2\}}$

'Direction cosines' l, m, and n of the line joining
$(x_1\ y_1\ z_1)$ to $(x_2\ y_2\ z_2)$:

$l=(x_2-x_1)/d,\quad m=(y_2-y_1)/d,\quad \text{and}\quad n=(z_2-z_1)/d$

$l^2+m^2+n^2=1$ (l, m, and n are the cosines of the angles between the line and the axes).

Equation of line through (x_1, y_1, z_1) and (x_2, y_2, z_2):

$$\frac{x-x_1}{l}=\frac{y-y_1}{m}=\frac{z-z_1}{n}$$

(N.B.: Two simultaneous equations for a line.)

Equation of a plane at right angles to a line from the origin with direction cosines l, m, and n intersecting it at distance p from the origin:

$lx+my+nz=p$

Sphere centre $(0, 0, 0)$: $x^2+y^2+z^2=r^2$ (radius $=r$)

Ellipsoid, centre $(0, 0, 0)$: $x^2/a^2+y^2/b^2+z^2/c^2=1$
(Length of axes $=2a$, $2b$, and $2c$).

9.5 & 9.8   Standard derivatives and integrals

For extensive tables of derivatives and integrals see James and James (1968), Rektorys (1969) or the Handbooks published by the Chemical Rubber Co. These present the integrals for about 500 different functions. The Table gives the differential of $f(t)$ with respect to t in the column headed $f'(t)$. The integral of a function can be found by finding the function in the column headed $f'(t)$, when its integral will be found in the column headed $f(t)=\int f'(t)\,dt$. a, k and n are constants, all trigonometric functions are in radians.

$f(t)=\int f'(t)\,\mathrm{d}t$	$f'(t)=\mathrm{d}f/\mathrm{d}t$
k	0
$(kt+a)^n$	$nk(kt+a)^{n-1}$
$t^{n+1}/(n+1)$	t^n
$k\ln(t)$	k/t
ka^{nt}	$kn\ln(a)\,a^{nt}$
$a^t/\ln(a)$	a^t
e^t	e^t
$\sin(kt)$	$k\cos(kt)$
$\cos(kt)$	$-k\sin(kt)$
$\tan(kt)$	$k\sec^2(kt)$
$\sec(kt)$	$k\sec(kt)\tan(kt)$
$\operatorname{cosec}(kt)$	$-k\operatorname{cosec}(kt)\cot(kt)$
$\cot(kt)$	$-k\operatorname{cosec}^2(kt)$
$\ln(\sec(kt))$	$k\tan(kt)$
$\ln(\sin(kt))$	$k\cot(kt)$
$\arcsin(kt)$	$k(1-k^2t^2)^{-1/2}$
$\arctan(kt)$	$k(1+k^2t^2)^{-1}$

9.8.4   Definite integrals

Gamma function:

$$\int_0^\infty x^{n-1}\exp(-x)\,\mathrm{d}x=\int_0^1\left(\log\frac{1}{x}\right)^{n-1}\mathrm{d}x=\Gamma(n)$$

$\Gamma(n)$ is finite if $n>0$, $\Gamma(n+1)=n\Gamma(n)$

$$\Gamma(n)\cdot\Gamma(1-n)=\frac{\pi}{\sin n\pi}$$

$\Gamma(n)=(n-1)!$ if $n=\text{integer}>0$

$\Gamma(\tfrac12)-\sqrt{n}.$

Beta function:

$$\int_0^1 x^{m-1}(1-x)^{n-1}\,\mathrm{d}x=B(m,\,n)$$

$$B(m, n) = B(n, m) = \frac{\Gamma(m)\,\Gamma(n)}{\Gamma(m+n)}, \quad \text{where } m \text{ and } n \text{ are any positive real}$$

numbers.

$$\int_0^\infty \frac{x^{m-1}\,\mathrm{d}x}{(1+x)^{m+n}} = \frac{\Gamma(m)\,\Gamma(n)}{\Gamma(m+n)} = B(m, n)$$

$$\int_0^{\pi/2} \sin^{n-1} x \, \cos^{m-1} x \, \mathrm{d}x = \tfrac{1}{2} B\left(\frac{n}{2}, \frac{m}{2}\right) \qquad m \text{ and } n \text{ positive integers}$$

Error function erf:

$$\mathrm{erf}\,(x) = \frac{2}{\sqrt{\pi}} \int_0^x \exp(-t^2)\,\mathrm{d}t$$

Normal or Gaussian distribution function:

$$N(x \mid \mu, \sigma) = \frac{1}{\sigma\sqrt{(2\pi)}} \int_{-\infty}^x \exp\{-(t-\mu)^2/(2\sigma^2)\}\,\mathrm{d}t$$

$$= \tfrac{1}{2}\left(1 + \mathrm{erf}\left(\frac{x-\mu}{\sigma\sqrt{2}}\right)\right)$$

Chi square, χ^2 *(cf. Gamma function):*

$$P(\chi^2 \mid v) = 2^{-v/2}\left(\Gamma\left(\frac{v}{2}\right)\right)^{-1} \int_0^{\chi^2} t^{v/2-1} \exp(-t/2)\,\mathrm{d}t$$

Other integrals:

$$\int_0^\infty \exp(-ax)\,\mathrm{d}x = \frac{1}{a} \qquad\qquad\qquad\qquad [a>0]$$

$$\int_0^\infty x^n \exp(-ax)\,\mathrm{d}x = \frac{\Gamma(n+1)}{a^{n+1}}, \qquad\qquad [n>-1, a>0]$$

$$= \frac{n!}{a^{n+1}} \qquad\qquad [n \text{ pos. integ., } a>0]$$

$$\int_0^\infty \exp(-a^2 x^2)\,\mathrm{d}x = \frac{1}{2a}\sqrt{\pi} = \frac{1}{2a}\Gamma(\tfrac{1}{2}) \qquad\qquad [a>0]$$

$$\int_0^\infty x \exp(-x^2)\,\mathrm{d}x = \tfrac{1}{2}$$

$$\int_0^\infty x^2 \exp(-x^2)\,\mathrm{d}x = \frac{\sqrt{\pi}}{4}$$

$$\int_0^1 \frac{\log x}{1+x}\,dx = -\frac{\pi^2}{12}$$

$$\int_0^\pi \sin^2 mx\,dx = \int_0^\pi \cos^2 mx\,dx = \frac{\pi}{2}$$

11.7.2 $$\int_0^\pi \sin kx \sin mx\,dx = \int_0^\pi \cos kx \cos mx\,dx = 0$$

$$[k \neq m;\ m,\ k = \text{integers}]$$

$$\int_0^{\pi/2} \frac{dx}{a^2 \sin^2 x + b^2 \cos^2 x} = \frac{\pi}{2ab}$$

Integral transforms

Transforms are rules which convert a function of a variable t, say $f(t)$, into another function of another variable p, say $F(p)$. The inverse transform will recover $f(t)$ from $F(p)$. The transformed function usually has useful properties which simplify the handling of the original function. Tables of such transforms are available, e.g. Abramowitz and Stegun (1965) for a list of Laplace transforms.

Laplace transform $$L(p) = \int_0^\infty \exp(-pt) f(t)\,dt$$

Inverse Laplace transform $$f(t) = \frac{1}{2\pi j} \int_{c-j\infty}^{c+j\infty} L(p) \exp(pt)\,dp$$

$$(j^2 = -1)$$

Fourier transform $$F(p) = \int_{-\infty}^\infty f(t) \exp(-j\omega t)\,dt$$

$$(j^2 = -1)$$

Inverse Fourier transform $$f(t) = \frac{1}{2\pi} \int_{-\infty}^\infty F(p) \exp(j\omega t)\,dp$$

9.7.2   **Maxima and minima, turning points**

Turning points of a function of several variables, say $f(x, y, z)$—for functions of one variable $f(t)$ replace the partial differential coefficients by d/dt:

Turning points $\partial f/\partial x=0$, $\partial f/\partial y=0$, $\partial f/\partial z=0$

One variable functions

Maxima	$d^2f/dx^2<0$
Minima	$d^2f/dx^2>0$
Inflection	$d^2f/dx^2=0$

Constrained maxima and minima (Lagrange's method)

To find turning points subject to constraints on $f(x, y, z)$:

(i) Express the constraints in the form of functions equal to zero, i.e.

$g(x, y, z)=0$, $h(x, y, z)=0$, etc.

(ii) Form a new function

$\phi(x, y, z)=f(x, y, z)+t_1g(x, y, z)+t_2h(x, y, z)+$etc.

where the values of t_1, t_2, etc. are at this point unknown.

(iii) Solve the equations:

$g(x, y, z)=0$, $h(x, y, z)=0$, etc.; $\partial\phi/\partial x=0$, $\partial\phi/\partial y=0$, $\partial\phi/\partial z=0$

for the values of x, y, z and t_1 and t_2 etc. The quantities t_1 and t_2 etc. are called *undetermined multipliers*; the x, y and z found from the equations represent turning points of the function subject to the constraints.

Integration formulae for $\int_a^b f(t)\,dt$

Each formula is followed by the difference between the integral and the formula. This is called the *error term* and is a function of the second or fourth differential of $f(t)$ evaluated somewhere in the interval $[a, b]$, the exact place in the interval is not specified.

1st order Newton Cotes (trapezoidal rule)

Evaluate $f(t)$ at $n+1$ equally spaced points distance $h=(b-a)/n$ apart

$t_0=a$, $t_1=a+h$, $t_2=a+2h$, $t_3=a+3h$ ... $t_n=b$

$$\int_a^b f(t)\,dt = \frac{h}{2}\,(f(t_0)+2f(t_1)+2f(t_2)+\ldots+2f(t_{n-1})+f(t_n)) + \text{error term}$$

$$\text{error term} = -\frac{nh^3}{12}\,f^{(2)}(t)$$

1st order Gaussian (midpoint method)

Evaluate $f(t)$ at n equally spaced points distance $h=(b-a)/n$

$$t_0 = a+h/2, \quad t_1 = a+3h/2, \quad t_2 = a+5h/2. \ldots t_{n-1} = b-h/2$$

Then

$$\int_a^b f(t)\,dt = h(f(t_0)+f(t_1)+f(t_2)+\ldots+f(t_{n-2})+f(t_{n-1})) + \text{error term}$$

$$\text{error term} = \frac{nh^3}{24}\,f^{(2)}(t)$$

2nd order Newton Cotes (Simpson's rule)

Evaluate $f(t)$ at same points as 1st order Newton Cotes formula. *n must be even.* Then

$$\int_a^b f(t)\,dt = \frac{h}{3}\,(f(t_0)+4f(t_1)+2f(t_2)+4f(t_3)+\ldots+2f(t_{n-2})$$

$$+4f(t_{n-1})+f(t_n)) + \text{error term}$$

$$\text{error term} = -\frac{nh^5}{180}\,f^{(4)}(t)$$

2nd order Gaussian

Evaluate $f(t)$ at n points (n even) as follows

$$h=(b-a)/n$$

$$t_0 = a+0\cdot42265h \quad t_2 = a+2\cdot42265h \quad t_4 = a+3\cdot42265h$$

$$t_1 = a+1\cdot57735h \quad t_3 = a+3\cdot57735h \quad \ldots\ldots\ldots \quad t_{n-1} = b-0\cdot42265h$$

The rather odd fractions $0\cdot57735$ and $0\cdot42265$ are $1/\sqrt{3}$ and $1-1/\sqrt{3}$ respectively. Then

$$\int_a^b f(t)\,\mathrm{d}t = h(f(t_0)+f(t_1)+f(t_2)+\ldots+f(t_{n-1}))+\text{error term}$$

$$\text{error term} = \frac{nh^5}{270}f^{(4)}(t)$$

Series

10.3.1   *Geometric series:* Equal ratio between successive terms

e.g. $2+4+8+16+32\ldots$

$a=$first term, $l=$last term, $n=$number of terms

$r=$ratio between successive terms, $s=$sum of terms,

$l=ar^{n-1}$; $n=\{(\log l-\log a)/\log r\}+1$

$s=a(1-r^n)/(1-r)$; $s=a(r^n-1)/(r-1)$

If $-1<r<1$ then $s\to a/(1-r)$ as $n\to\infty$

10.3.2   *Arithmetic series:* Equal differences between successive terms.

e.g. $2+4+6+8+10$

$a=$first term, $l=$last term, $n=$number of terms

$d=$difference between successive terms, $s=$sum of terms

$l=a+(n-1)\,d$; $n=\{(l-a)/d\}+1$; $d=(l-a)/(n-1)$

$s=\frac{1}{2}n(2a+(n-1)\,d)$; $s=\frac{1}{2}n(a+l)$

10.2   *Miscellaneous series*

$1+2+3+4+\ldots+n=\frac{1}{2}n(n+1)$

$1^2+2^2+3^2+4^2+\ldots+n^2=\frac{1}{6}n(n+1)\,(2n+1)$

$1^3+2^3+3^3+4^3+\ldots+n^3=\frac{1}{4}n^2(n+1)^2$

$1+\dfrac{1}{2^2}+\dfrac{1}{3^2}+\dfrac{1}{4^2}+\ldots\dfrac{1}{n^2}\to\dfrac{\pi^2}{6}$ as $n\to\infty$

$1+\dfrac{1}{2^4}+\dfrac{1}{3^4}+\dfrac{1}{4^4}+\ldots+\dfrac{1}{n^4}\to\dfrac{\pi^4}{90}$ as $n\to\infty$

$1+\dfrac{1}{2^6}+\dfrac{1}{3^6}+\dfrac{1}{4^6}+\ldots+\dfrac{1}{n^6}\to\dfrac{\pi^6}{945}$ as $n\to\infty$

10.4   *Taylor's formula* for expansion of a function $f(x)$ near the point $x=R$.

$f(R+x)=a_0+a_1x+a_2x^2+a_3x^3+\ldots+a_nx^n+$ 'remainder'

where

$a_0=f(R),\ a_1=f^{(1)}(R),\ a_2=\dfrac{f^{(2)}(R)}{2!},\ a_3=\dfrac{f^{(3)}(R)}{3!}\ \ldots\ a_n=\dfrac{f^{(n)}(R)}{n!}$

'remainder' (sometimes called '*error*') $=\dfrac{x^{n+1}}{(n+1)!}f^{(n+1)}\ (R+\theta x)$

$$0\leqslant\theta\leqslant1$$

The value of θ is unspecified.

Maclaurin's formula for the expansion of a function f near the point $x=0$: as Taylor's formula with $R=0$.

10.4   **Series expansions of common functions**

Alternative series and more accurate computing formulae may be found in Chapter 4 of Abramowitz and Stegun (1965); the relevant paragraphs are indicated thus [A & S 4.1.24–29]. See also Hastings (1955). The error bounds quoted below have been found by computation at steps of at most 1/30th of the stated range.

Log (x)

Taylor's series [A & S 4.1.24–29]

$\ln(1+x)=x-x^2/2+x^3/3-x^4/4+\ldots$

valid for $-1<x\leqslant1$

$|\text{error in taking terms to } x^n|\leqslant\left|\dfrac{x^{n+1}}{n+1}\right|\quad\text{if}\quad x\geqslant0$

$\text{or}\leqslant\left|\dfrac{1}{n+1}\left(\dfrac{x}{1+x}\right)^{n+1}\right|\quad\text{if}\quad x<0$

Approximation [A & S 4.1.41–45]

$\log_{10}(x)=0\cdot86304t+0\cdot36415t^3\quad\text{where}\quad t=(x-1)/(x+1)$

applicable for $\dfrac{1}{\sqrt{10}}\leqslant x\leqslant\sqrt{10}\qquad|\text{ error }|<7\times10^{-4}$

e^x

Taylor's series

$$e^x = 1 + x + \frac{x^2}{2!} + \frac{x^3}{3!} + \frac{x^4}{4!} + \cdots$$

$$e^{-\lambda t} = 1 - \lambda t + \frac{\lambda^2 t^2}{2!} - \frac{\lambda^3 t^3}{3!} + \frac{\lambda^4 t^4}{4!} - \cdots$$

applicable for any x (or λt)

$$|\text{ error in taking terms to } x^n| \leqslant \left| \frac{x^{n+1}}{(n+1)!} \right| e^x, \quad x \geqslant 0$$

$$\text{or} \leqslant \left| \frac{x^{n+1}}{(n+1)!} \right|, \quad x < 0$$

Approximation [A & S 4.2.43–48]

$e^{-x} = 1 - 0 \cdot 9664x + 0 \cdot 3536x^2$

applicable for $0 \leqslant x \leqslant \ln(2)$ | error $| < 3 \times 10^{-3}$

Binomial expansion $(1+x)^r$

4.2   Taylor's series

$$(1+x)^r = 1 + rx + \frac{r(r-1)}{1.2} x^2 + \frac{r(r-1)(r-2)}{1.2.3} x^3 + \cdots$$

valid for r any positive integer or $-1 < x < 1$

| error in taking terms to x^n | is the greatest of

$$\left| \frac{r(r-1)\dots(r-n)}{(n+1)!} x^{n+1} \right| \quad \text{and} \quad \left| \frac{r(r-1)\dots(r-n)}{(n+1)!} x^{n+1}(1+x)^{r-n-1} \right|$$

Trigonometric functions $\sin(x)$ etc. (x in radians)

Taylor's series [A & S 4.3.65–73]

6.7 & $\sin(x) = x - \frac{x^3}{3!} + \frac{x^5}{5!} - \frac{x^7}{7!} + \cdots$
10.4

$$\cos(x) = 1 - \frac{x^2}{2!} + \frac{x^4}{4!} - \frac{x^6}{6!} + \cdots$$

valid for all x. | error in taking terms to x^n $| \leqslant \left| \frac{x^{n+1}}{(n+1)!} \right|$

$$\tan (x) = x + \frac{x^3}{3} + \frac{2x^5}{15} + \frac{17x^7}{315} + \ldots$$

Valid for $-\frac{\pi}{2} < x < \frac{\pi}{2}$

Approximations [A & S 4.3.96–4.3.104]

$\sin (x) = x - 0 \cdot 16605x^3 + 0 \cdot 00761x^5$

applicable for $0 \leqslant x < \pi/2$ | error | $< 2 \times 10^{-4}$

$\cos (x) = 1 - 0 \cdot 49670x^2 + 0 \cdot 03705x^4$

applicable for $0 \leqslant x \leqslant \pi/2$ | error | $< 2 \times 10^{-3}$

$\tan (x) = x + 0 \cdot 31755x^3 + 0 \cdot 20330x^5$

applicable for $0 \leqslant x \leqslant \pi/4$ | error | $< 9 \times 10^{-4}$

$$\cot (x) = \frac{1}{x} - 0 \cdot 332867x - 0 \cdot 024369x^3$$

applicable for $0 \leqslant x \leqslant \pi/4$ | error | $< 9 \times 10^{-5}$

Note if: $\pi/4 < x < \pi/2$ one can use the relation $\tan (x) = \cot (\pi/2 - x)$

Inverse circular functions (in radians)

Taylor's series [A & S 4.4.40–42]

$$\arctan (x) = x - \frac{x^3}{3} + \frac{x^5}{5} - \frac{x^7}{7} \ldots$$

valid for $-1 \leqslant x \leqslant 1$

$$\arctan (x) = \pi/2 - \frac{1}{x} + \frac{1}{3x^3} - \frac{1}{5x^5} \ldots$$

valid for $x < -1$ and $x > 1$

Approximation [A & S 4.4.45–51]

$$\arctan (x) = \frac{x}{1 + 0 \cdot 28x^3}$$

valid for $-1 \leqslant x \leqslant 1$

For $| x | > 1$ use $\arctan (x) = \pi/2 - \arctan (1/x)$

| error | $< 5 \times 10^{-3}$

10.6   **Fourier series**. Period of $f(t) = 2\pi$

$f(t) = a_0 + a_1 \sin (p_1 + t) + a_2 \sin (p_2 + 2t) + \ldots + \text{remainder}$

or

$f(t) = a_0 + b_1 \sin (t) + b_2 \sin (2t) + b_3 \sin (3t) + \ldots$

$\qquad\qquad c_1 \cos (t) + c_2 \cos (2t) + c_3 \cos (3t) + \ldots + \text{remainder}$

$$a_0 = \frac{1}{2\pi} \int_0^{2\pi} f(t) \, dt \quad b_n = \frac{1}{\pi} \int_0^{2\pi} f(t) \sin (nt) \, dt \quad c_n = \frac{1}{\pi} \int_0^{2\pi} f(t) \cos (nt) \, dt$$

$$a_n = (b_n^2 + c_n^2)^{1/2} \qquad\qquad p_n = \arctan (c_n / b_n)$$

for $n = 1, 2$, etc.

Remainder: for continuous functions with continuous derivatives, the remainder after considering terms up to $\sin (nt)$ and $\cos (nt)$ satisfies

$$\text{remainder}^2 \leqslant \left(\frac{1}{\pi} \int_0^{2\pi} (f'(t))^2 \, dt \right) \left(\frac{\pi^2}{6} - 1 - \frac{1}{2^2} - \frac{1}{3^2} \cdots - \frac{1}{n^2} \right)$$

Least squares:

If $\quad f_N(t) = a_0 + \displaystyle\sum_{n=1}^{N} \{b_n \sin (nt) + c_n \cos (nt)\}$

then

$\displaystyle\int_0^{2\pi} (f(t) - f_N(t))^2 \, dt$, i.e. mean square error is

$\displaystyle\int_0^{2\pi} (f(t))^2 \, dt - 2\pi a_0^2 - \pi \sum_{n=1}^{N} (b_n^2 + c_n^2)$

The Fourier Series gives the least mean square error when fitting $f(t)$ by functions of the form

$a_0 + \displaystyle\sum_{n=1}^{N} \{b_n \sin (nt) + c_n \cos (nt)\}$

Discrete observations:

$f(t_r) = \alpha_0 + \displaystyle\sum_{p=1}^{N} \{\alpha_p \sin (pt_r) + \beta_p \cos (pt_r)\}$

$t_r = 2\pi r / (2N + 1)$

Then

$$\alpha_0 = \frac{1}{2N+1} \sum_{r=0}^{2N} f(t_r)$$

$$\alpha_p = \frac{2}{2N+1} \sum_{r=0}^{2N} f(t_r) \cos (pt_r) \quad \beta_p = \frac{2}{2N+1} \sum_{r=0}^{2N} f(t_r) \sin (pt_r)$$

(Ralston and Wilf (1960), ch. 24). Many texts use $\frac{1}{2}a_0$ or $\frac{1}{2}\alpha_0$ as the first term.

Differential equations

In this section a_0, a_1 and a_2 are constants

12.11.6 *First order:*

$$a_1 y'(x) + a_0 y(x) = 0 \quad \text{subject to} \quad y = Y \quad \text{at} \quad x = X$$

has solution

$$y = Y \exp (-(x-X) a_0/a_1)$$

12.11.7 *Second order:*

$$a_2 y''(x) + a_1 y'(x) + a_0 y(x) = 0$$

has as general solution:

(i) $a_1^2 > 4a_0 a_2$

$$y = A \exp (r_1 x) + B \exp (r_2 x)$$

where r_1 and r_2 are the roots of $a_2 r^2 + a_1 r + a_0 = 0$

(ii) $a_1^2 = 4a_0 a_2$

$$y = (A + Bx) \exp (rx)$$

where $r = \dfrac{-a_1}{2a_2}$

(iii) $a_1^2 < 4a_0 a_2$

$$y = \exp (\alpha x) \{A \cos (\beta x) + B \sin (\beta x)\}$$

where $\alpha = \dfrac{-a_1}{2a_2}$

$$\beta = \frac{1}{2a_2} \sqrt{(4a_0 a_2 - a_1^2)}$$

In all cases A and B are determined by the boundary conditions.

Named polynomials

A number of named polynomials, of degree n, have three important features:

1. They are solutions of a similarly named differential equation of the form

$$g_2 y_n'' + g_1 y_n' + g_0 y_n = 0$$

where g_2 and g_1 are functions of x, y_n is the polynomial of degree n in x and g_0 is a constant depending on n.

11.7.2   2. They are orthogonal with respect to a weighting function $w(x)$,

i.e. $\int_A^B w(x)\, y_n y_m\, dx = 0$ if $n \neq m$

3. They may be generated by assuming $y_0 = 1$ and $y_1 = x$, then repeatedly applying a formula of the form

$$y_{n+1} = c_1 x y_n - c_2 y_{n-1}$$

The table below gives the values of c_1, c_2, g_2, g_1, g_0, $w(x)$, A and B for the commonest named polynomials. Others may be found in Abramowitz and Stegun (1965) chapter 22.

Name	Symbol	c_1	c_2	g_2	g_1	g_0	$w(x)$	A	B
Chebychev	$T_n(x)$	2	1	$1-x^2$	$-x$	n^2	$(1-x^2)^{-1/2}$	-1	1
Hermite	$H_n(x)$	2	$2n$	1	$-2x$	$2n$	$\exp(-x^2/2)$	$-\infty$	∞
Legendre	$P_n(x)$	$\frac{2n+1}{n+1}$	$\frac{n}{n+1}$	$1-x^2$	$-2x$	$n(n+1)$	1	-1	1

Bessel's functions and equations

Bessel's equation is   modified equation is

$$x^2 y'' + xy' + (x^2 - p^2)\, y = 0 \qquad\qquad x^2 y'' + xy' - (x^2 + p^2)\, y = 0$$

Solutions of this equation are called Bessel Functions of order p. Different kinds of solution are referred to as 1st, 2nd or 3rd kind of Bessel Function and are denoted by various symbols such as $J_p(x)$, $J_{-p}(x)$, $Y_p(x)$, $H_p(x)$, $K_p(x)$. They are infinite series and are extensively tabled and documented (e.g. Abramowitz & Stegun (1965)).

Notes for the Preparation of Mathematical Papers

The notes below are reproduced from the *Journal of the Royal Statistical Society*, Series B, by kind permission of the Royal Statistical Society. It is our hope that these notes will ease the troubles of authors and editors when mathematical work is submitted to medical journals. We have not always kept to these conventions in this book.

1 General

A lot of time and patience are necessary to prepare adequately the manuscript of a mathematical paper. Not only must the precise nature and position of each symbol be plain, but the lay-out of the formulae should be such as to lead to a clear and pleasing printed page.

Best results are usually obtained when an experienced typist works from a well-arranged manuscript. The following notes are intended to cover some of the points that commonly cause difficulty.

2 Clarity

It is particularly important to distinguish between the following:

(a) capitals and small letters;
(b) ordinary and bold-faced letters; the latter must be underlined in pencil with a wavy line.
(c) certain Greek letters and similar roman letters;
(d) subscripts, superscripts and 'ordinary' symbols.

The following are particularly liable to confusion:

$$a, d, \alpha, \propto; \quad c, C, n, r, \eta; \quad s, S; \quad v, V, \nu, \gamma; \quad u, U, \mu; \quad \xi, \zeta; \quad l, i, I, 1;$$

$$e, \in, \epsilon, l, \rho; \quad w, W, \omega, \varpi; \quad o, O, 0, \sigma; \quad x, X, \chi, \times; \quad t, \tau; \quad k, K, \kappa; \quad p, P, \rho.$$

Symbols should not be used at the start of a sentence. For special symbols make a pencil marginal note, enclosed in a circle. Exotic characters, however, are to be avoided.

3 Arrangement of formulae

Equations and long formulae should be displayed (i.e. shown on a separate line), where necessary being numbered at the right of the page. Short isolated formulae should usually be left in the text and then must be arranged so as not to be more than one line high.

Example. $\sum\limits_{i=1}^{n} x_i$ must *not* be left in the text. It should be written $\sum x_i$ (if the limits of summation are obvious), or $x_1 + \ldots + x_n$; otherwise displayed.

The solidus sign (/) will be needed frequently in formulae in the text (see paragraph 4(d)).

Equations involving lengthy expressions should, where possible, be avoided by introducing suitable notation.

Equations must be punctuated in the usual way.

4   Some special points

The following remarks concern more detailed matters.

(a) *Brackets.* Where several sets of brackets occur inside one another in the same formula, the order should be [{()}].

(b) *Square roots.* These should be denoted by the sign $\sqrt{\ }$ or by a superscript $\frac{1}{2}$. The former should be used in simple expressions, the latter in complicated ones; in intermediate cases, the usage should be consistent. Where the sign refers to a group of symbols, the group must be in brackets. Where the sign $\sqrt{\ }$ refers to one symbol or number in a group, the sign and the symbol or number to which it refers, should be at the right of the group. Note that the sign $\sqrt{\quad}$ is never used.

Examples. $\sqrt{(2\pi)}$, $\pi\sqrt{2}$ are correct, but not $\sqrt{2\pi}$, which is ambiguous without a special convention.

(c) *Exponential function.* The expression 'exp' should be used for the exponential function when the argument is longer than a single compact group of symbols.

Examples. The following are correct:

$$\exp(a + bt + ct^2), \exp\{(a + bt)/(c + dt)\}.$$

(d) *The solidus.* This should always be used for fractions in the text and where possible in displayed formulae. It is essential to bracket a group of symbols to the right of the solidus if they are to be included in the denominator. This point is a very common source of error.

Examples. $(a + b)(c + d)/(h + k)l$ is wrong, being ambiguous without a special convention. $(a + b)(c + d)/\{(h + k)l\}$ is correct.

(e) *Simple numerical fractions.* Except in certain displayed formulae, the simple fractions $\frac{1}{2}, \frac{1}{3}, \frac{2}{3}, \frac{1}{4}, \frac{3}{4}, \frac{1}{5}, \frac{3}{5}, \frac{1}{6}, \frac{1}{8}, \frac{3}{8}, \frac{5}{8}, \frac{7}{8}, \frac{1}{16}, \frac{3}{16}, \frac{5}{16}, \ldots$ should be written as one-line fractions.

Example. In the text $\frac{1}{2}t$ is better than $t/2$; $\dfrac{t}{2}$ is bad (see Section 3).

(f) *Range of running variables.* This is given as in the following examples:

$$p_{i+1} = ap_i + bp_{i-1} \qquad (i = 1, 2, \ldots, n),$$

$$p_{i+1} = ap_i + bp_{i-1} \qquad (1 \leqslant i \leqslant n).$$

(g) *Roman characters.* Certain standard abbreviations that occur in mathematical work are set in roman fount, not in the italic fount used for mathematical symbols. Examples are: exp, log, lim, max, min, sup, inf, var, cov, sin, cos, and so on.

Example. $\exp(t + \frac{1}{2}t^2)$, but $e^{\frac{1}{2}}$.

If there is a danger of confusion, letters to be set in roman fount should be underlined lightly in red pencil.

References

Whosoever reports a thing in the name of him that said it brings deliverance into the world. . . . R. Meir

ABRAMOWITZ M. & STEGUN I.A. (Eds) (1965) *Handbook of Mathematical Functions.* New York: Dover.

AITKEN A.C. (1948) *Determinants and Matrices.* Edinburgh: Oliver & Boyd.

BARTON D., BOURNE S.R. & FITCH J.P. (1970) An algebra system. *Computer Journal,* **13**, 32.

BELL M. & PIKE M.C. (1966) Algorithm 178: Direct search. *Communications of the ACM,* **9**, 684. See also *ibid* **11**, 498.

BERENBAUM M.C. (1969) Dose response curves for agents that impair cell reproductive integrity. *British Journal of Cancer,* **23**, 429.

BIRKHOFF G. & MACLANE S. (1953) *A Survey of Modern Algebra.* New York: Macmillan.

B.S. 1991 (1961–67) *Letter Symbols, Signs and Abbreviations.* London: British Standards Institution.

COOLEY J.W. & TUKEY J.W. (1965) An algorithm for the machine calculation of complex Fourier series. *Mathematics of Computation,* **19**, 297.

COOLIDGE J.L. (1931) *A Treatise on Algebraic Plane Curves.* Oxford: Clarendon Press. Also (1959) New York: Dover.

COURANT R. (1934) *Differential and Integral Calculus.* Glasgow: Blackie.

DAVIS H.F. (1963) *Fourier Series and Orthogonal Functions.* Boston: Allyn and Bacon.

DAY M.H. & WOOD B.A. (1968) Functional affinities of the Olduvai Hominid 8 talus. *Man,* **3**, 440.

Documenta Geigy, 6th Edition (ed. Diem) 'Synopsis of Blood—Erythrocytes'. 577.

DU BOIS D. & DU BOIS E.F. (1916) A formula to estimate the approximate surface area if height and weight be known. *Arch. Intern. Med.,* **17**, 863.

EKINS R.P., NEWMAN G.B. & O'RIORDAN J.L.H. (1968) Theoretical aspects of 'saturation' and radioimmunoassay. In *Radioisotopes in Medicine: In Vitro Studies.* (Edited by Hayes R.L., Goswitz F.A. & Pearson-Murphy B.E.). Oak Ridge: U.S. Atomic Energy Commission.

EKINS R.P., WILLIAMS E.S. & ELLIS S. (1969) The sensitive and precise measurement of serum thyroxcine by saturation analysis (competitive protein binding assay). *Clinical Biochemistry,* **2**, 253.

ELLIS J.R. (1955) Note on Carpet graphs. *The Engineer,* June 24th, 869–870.

FERRAR W.L. (1938) *Convergence.* Oxford: Clarendon Press.

FERRAR W.L. (1957) *Algebra.* London: Oxford University Press.

FINNEY D.J. (1952) *Statistical Method in Biological Assay.* London: Griffin.

FISCHER J. & WOLF R. (1964) Resultats de l'application clinque de la scintigraphie de la rate dans 500 cas: possibilites et limites. In *Medical Radioisotopic Scanning,* Vol. 2, p. 337. Vienna: International Atomic Energy Commission.

FISHER R.F. (1969) Elastic constants of the human lens capsule. *Journal of Physiology* **201**, 1.

FORKER E.L. (1967) Two sites of bile formation as determined by mannitol and erythritol clearance in the guinea pig. *Journal of Clinical Investigation,* **46**, 1189.

FOX L. & MAYERS D.F. (1968) *Computing Methods for Scientists and Engineers.* London: Oxford University Press.

FROST P. (1960) *An Elementary Treatise on Curve Tracing.* New York: Chelsea Publ. Co.

429

HALL H.S. & KNIGHT S.R. (1946) *Elementary Trigonometry*. London: Macmillan.

HARDY G.H. (1967) *A Course of Pure Mathematics*. Cambridge: Cambridge University Press.

HASTINGS C. (1955) *Approximations for Digital Computers*. Princeton: Princeton University Press.

HEWITT H.B. & BLAKE E.R. (1968) Transplanted tumours in pre-irradiated mice. *British Journal of Cancer*, **22**, 808.

HILTON H. (1932) *Plane Algebraic Curves*. London: Oxford University Press.

HLAVOVÁ A., LINHART J., PŘEROVSKÝ I. & GANZ V. (1968) Lactate and pyruvate changes in the leg during and after exercise in normal subjects and in patients with femoral artery occlusion. *Clinical Science*, **34**, 397.

H.M.S.O. (1956) *Interpolation and Allied Tables*. London: Her Majesty's Stationery Office.

H.M.S.O. (1961) *Modern Computing Methods*. London: Her Majesty's Stationery Office.

HYSLOP J.M. (1950) *Infinite Series*. Edinburgh: Oliver & Boyd.

INCE E.L. (1956) *Integration of Ordinary Differential Equations*. Edinburgh: Oliver & Boyd.

JAMES G. & JAMES R.C. (Eds) (1968) *Mathematics Dictionary*. New York: Van Nostrand.

KENDALL M.G. (1951) *The Advanced Theory of Statistics*, Vol. II. London: Griffin.

KENDALL M.G. (1961) *A Course in Multivariate Analysis*. London: Griffin.

KINDLE J.H. (1950) *Theory and Problems of Plane and Solid Analytic Geometry*. New York: Schaum's Outline Series; McGraw-Hill.

KING V. (1969) A study of the mechanism of water transfer across frog skin by a comparison of the permeability of the skin to deuterated and tritiated water. *Journal of Physiology*, **200**, 529.

KORN G.A. & KORN T.M. (1961) *Mathematical Handbook for Scientists and Engineers*. New York: McGraw-Hill.

LEDERMANN W. (Ed.) *Library of Mathematics*. London: Routledge Kegan & Paul.

LEDLEY R.S. & WILSON J.B. (1965) *Computers in Biology and Medicine*. New York: McGraw-Hill.

MARCUS M. (1960) *Basic Theorems in Matrix Theory*. Applied Mathematics Series, 57. Washington: National Bureau of Standards.

MATTHEWS C.M.E., LASZLO G., CAMPBELL E.J.M. & READ D.J.C. (1968–69) A model for the distribution and transport of CO_2 in the body and the ventilatory response to CO_2. *Respiration Physiology*, **6**, 45.

MAYNARD SMITH J. (1968) *Mathematical Ideas in Biology*. Cambridge: Cambridge University Press.

McCRACKEN D.D. and DORN W.S. (1968) *Numerical Methods and Fortran Programming*. New York: Wiley.

MERSON R.H. (1957) An operational method for the study of integration processes. *Proceedings of a Conference on Data Processing and Automatic Computing Machines, Weapons Research Establishment, Salisbury, South Australia.*

MORI K.F. (1969) Antigenic structure of human gonadotrophins: contribution of carbohydrate moiety to the antigenic structure of pituitary follicle-stimulating hormone. *Endocrinology*, **85**, 330.

NOBLE B. (1964) *Numerical Methods* (2 Vols). Edinburgh: Oliver & Boyd.

OWEN D.B. (1962) *Handbook of Statistical Tables*. Reading, Mass.: Addison-Wesley.

PECKHAM G. (1970) A new method for minimising a sum of squares without calculating gradients. *Computer Journal*, **13**, 418.

PROTTER M.H. & MORREY C.B. (1966) *Analytic Geometry*. Reading, Mass.: Addison-Wesley.

RALSTON A. & WILF H.S. (Eds) (1960) *Mathematical Methods for Digital Computers*. New York: Wiley.

REDISH K.A. (1961) *An Introduction to Computational Methods*. London: English Universities Press.

REGISTRAR GENERAL (1941–67) *Statistical Review for England and Wales. Part I. Tables Medical*. London: Her Majestys' Stationery Office.

REKTORYS K. (1969) *Survey of Applicable Mathematics*. London: Iliffe.

ROSENFIELD A. (1969) *Picture Processing by Computer*. New York: Academic Press.

ROSS S.L. (1964) *Differential Equations*. New York: Blaisdell Publ. Co.

SAMUEL P., HOLTZMANN C.M., MEILMAN E. & PERL W. (1968) Effect of neomycin on exchangeable pools of cholesterol in the steady state. *Journal of Clinical Investigation*, **47**, 1806.

SCHAFF W.L. (1963) *The Calculus*. New York: Doubleday.

SCHMID-SCHONBEIN H., GAEHTGENS P. & HIRSCH H. (1968) On the shear rate dependence of red cell aggregation in vitro. *Journal of Clinical Investigation*, **47**, 1447.

SHAW D.F. (1962) *An Introduction to Electronics*. London: Longmans.

SIEGAL J.H. & WILLIAMS J.B. (1969) A computer based index for the prediction of operative survival in patients with cirrhosis and portal hypertension. *Annals of Surgery*, **169**, 191.

SINGLETON R.C. (1968) Algorithm 339. An algol procedure for the fast Fourier transform with arbitrary factors. *Communications of the ACM*, **11**, 776.

SOMMERVILLE D.M.Y. (1943) *Analytical Geometry of Three Dimensions*. Cambridge: Cambridge University Press.

SOMMERVILLE D.M.Y. (1949) *Analytical Conics*. London: G. Bell & Sons Ltd.

SPRENT P. (1969) *Models in Regression and Related Topics*. London: Methuen.

STEPHENSON G. (1967) *An Introduction to Matrices, Sets and Groups for Science Students*. London: Longmans.

TODD-POKROPEK A.E. (1969) Theoretical considerations when using various computer enhancing methods for the radioisotope scan. In *Proc. Symp. Utilisation des Ordinateurs en Radiologie*. Brussels September 1969. Basle: Karger (1970).

WATERLOW J.C. & STEPHEN JOAN M.C. (1967) The measurement of total lysine turnover in the rat by intravenous infusion of L-[U-^{14}C] lysine. *Clinical Science*, **33**, 489.

WAYNE D.J. & CHAMNEY ANNE R. (1969) Oxygen tent performance. *Physics in Medicine and Biology*, **14**, 9.

WEATHERBURN C.E. (1950) *Elementary Vector Analysis*. London: Bell.

WHITNEY R.J. (1953) The measurement of volume changes in human limbs. *Journal of Physiology*, **121**, 1.

WILKINSON I.M.S., BULL J.W.D., DU BOULAY G.H., MARSHALL J., ROSS RUSSELL R.W. & SYMON L. (1969) Regional blood flow in the normal cerebral hemisphere. *Journal of Neurology, Neurosurgery and Psychiatry*, **32**, 367.

WILKINSON J.H. (1963) *Rounding Errors in Algebraic Processes. Notes on Applied Science* No. 32. London: Her Majesty's Stationery Office.

WISE M.E. (1966) Tracer dilution curves in cardiology and random walk and log normal distributions. *Acta Physiologica Pharmacologica Neerlandica*, **14**, 175.

WORSLEY B.H. & LAX L.C. (1962) Selection of a numerical technique for analysing experimental data of the decay type with special reference to the use of tracers in biological systems. *Biochimica et Biophysica Acta*, **59**, 1.

Tables

LOGARITHMS

Mean Differences

	0	1	2	3	4	5	6	7	8	9	1 2 3	4 5 6	7 8 9
10	0000	0043	0086	0128	0170						5 9 13	17 21 26	30 34 38
						0212	0253	0294	0334	0374	4 8 12	16 20 24	28 32 36
11	0414	0453	0492	0531	0569						4 8 12	16 20 23	27 31 35
						0607	0645	0682	0719	0755	4 7 11	15 18 22	26 29 33
12	0792	0828	0864	0899	0934						3 7 11	14 18 21	25 28 32
						0969	1004	1038	1072	1106	3 7 10	14 17 20	24 27 31
13	1139	1173	1206	1239	1271						3 6 10	13 16 19	23 26 29
						1303	1335	1367	1399	1430	3 7 10	13 16 19	22 25 29
14	1461	1492	1523	1553	1584						3 6 9	12 15 19	22 25 28
						1614	1644	1673	1703	1732	3 6 9	12 14 17	20 23 26
15	1761	1790	1818	1847	1875						3 6 9	11 14 17	20 23 26
						1903	1931	1959	1987	2014	3 6 8	11 14 17	19 22 25
16	2041	2068	2095	2122	2148						3 6 8	11 14 16	19 22 24
						2175	2201	2227	2253	2279	3 5 8	10 13 16	18 21 23
17	2304	2330	2355	2380	2405						3 5 8	10 13 15	18 20 23
						2430	2455	2480	2504	2529	3 5 8	10 12 15	17 20 22
18	2553	2577	2601	2625	2648						2 5 7	9 12 14	17 19 21
						2672	2695	2718	2742	2765	2 4 7	9 11 14	16 18 21
19	2788	2810	2833	2856	2878						2 4 7	9 11 13	16 18 20
						2900	2923	2945	2967	2989	2 4 6	8 11 13	15 17 19
20	3010	3032	3054	3075	3096	3118	3139	3160	3181	3201	2 4 6	8 11 13	15 17 19
21	3222	3243	3263	3284	3304	3324	3345	3365	3385	3404	2 4 6	8 10 12	14 16 18
22	3424	3444	3464	3483	3502	3522	3541	3560	3579	3598	2 4 6	8 10 12	14 15 17
23	3617	3636	3655	3674	3692	3711	3729	3747	3766	3784	2 4 6	7 9 11	13 15 17
24	3802	3820	3838	3856	3874	3892	3909	3927	3945	3962	2 4 5	7 9 11	12 14 16
25	3979	3997	4014	4031	4048	4065	4082	4099	4116	4133	2 3 5	7 9 10	12 14 15
26	4150	4166	4183	4200	4216	4232	4249	4265	4281	4298	2 3 5	7 8 10	11 13 15
27	4314	4330	4346	4362	4378	4393	4409	4425	4440	4456	2 3 5	6 8 9	11 13 14
28	4472	4487	4502	4518	4533	4548	4564	4579	4594	4609	2 3 5	6 8 9	11 12 14
29	4624	4639	4654	4669	4683	4698	4713	4728	4742	4757	1 3 4	6 7 9	10 12 13
30	4771	4786	4800	4814	4829	4843	4857	4871	4886	4900	1 3 4	6 7 9	10 11 13
31	4914	4928	4942	4955	4969	4983	4997	5011	5024	5038	1 3 4	6 7 8	10 11 12
32	5051	5065	5079	5092	5105	5119	5132	5145	5159	5172	1 3 4	5 7 8	9 11 12
33	5185	5198	5211	5224	5237	5250	5263	5276	5289	5302	1 3 4	5 6 8	9 10 12
34	5315	5328	5340	5353	5366	5378	5391	5403	5416	5428	1 3 4	5 6 8	9 10 11
35	5441	5453	5465	5478	5490	5502	5514	5527	5539	5551	1 2 4	5 6 7	9 10 11
36	5563	5575	5587	5599	5611	5623	5635	5647	5658	5670	1 2 4	5 6 7	8 10 11
37	5682	5694	5705	5717	5729	5740	5752	5763	5775	5786	1 2 3	5 6 7	8 9 10
38	5798	5809	5821	5832	5843	5855	5866	5877	5888	5899	1 2 3	5 6 7	8 9 10
39	5911	5922	5933	5944	5955	5966	5977	5988	5999	6010	1 2 3	4 5 7	8 9 10
40	6021	6031	6042	6053	6064	6075	6085	6096	6107	6117	1 2 3	4 5 6	8 9 10
41	6128	6138	6149	6160	6170	6180	6191	6201	6212	6222	1 2 3	4 5 6	7 8 9
42	6232	6243	6253	6263	6274	6284	6294	6304	6314	6325	1 2 3	4 5 6	7 8 9
43	6335	6345	6355	6365	6375	6385	6395	6405	6415	6425	1 2 3	4 5 6	7 8 9
44	6435	6444	6454	6464	6474	6484	6493	6503	6513	6522	1 2 3	4 5 6	7 8 9
45	6532	6542	6551	6561	6571	6580	6590	6599	6609	6618	1 2 3	4 5 6	7 8 9
46	6628	6637	6646	6656	6665	6675	6684	6693	6702	6712	1 2 3	4 5 6	7 7 8
47	6721	6730	6739	6749	6758	6767	6776	6785	6794	6803	1 2 3	4 5 5	6 7 8
48	6812	6821	6830	6839	6848	6857	6866	6875	6884	6893	1 2 3	4 4 5	6 7 8
49	6902	6911	6920	6928	6937	6946	6955	6964	6972	6981	1 2 3	4 4 5	6 7 8

Example: Log $20 \cdot 24 = 1 \cdot 0 + 0 \cdot 3054 + 0 \cdot 0008 = 1 \cdot 3062$

LOGARITHMS

	0	1	2	3	4	5	6	7	8	9	1 2 3	4 5 6	7 8 9
50	6990	6998	7007	7016	7024	7033	7042	7050	7059	7067	1 2 3	3 4 5	6 7 8
51	7076	7084	7093	7101	7110	7118	7126	7135	7143	7152	1 2 3	3 4 5	6 7 8
52	7160	7168	7177	7185	7193	7202	7210	7218	7226	7235	1 2 2	3 4 5	6 7 7
53	7243	7251	7259	7267	7275	7284	7292	7300	7308	7316	1 2 2	3 4 5	6 6 7
54	7324	7332	7340	7348	7356	7364	7372	7380	7388	7396	1 2 2	3 4 5	6 6 7
55	7404	7412	7419	7427	7435	7443	7451	7459	7466	7474	1 2 2	3 4 5	5 6 7
56	7482	7490	7497	7505	7513	7520	7528	7536	7543	7551	1 2 2	3 4 5	5 6 7
57	7559	7566	7574	7582	7589	7597	7604	7612	7619	7627	1 2 2	3 4 5	5 6 7
58	7634	7642	7649	7657	7664	7672	7679	7686	7694	7701	1 1 2	3 4 4	5 6 7
59	7709	7716	7723	7731	7738	7745	7752	7760	7767	7774	1 1 2	3 4 4	5 6 7
60	7782	7789	7796	7803	7810	7818	7825	7832	7839	7846	1 1 2	3 4 4	5 6 6
61	7853	7860	7868	7875	7882	7889	7896	7903	7910	7917	1 1 2	3 4 4	5 6 6
62	7924	7931	7938	7945	7952	7959	7966	7973	7980	7987	1 1 2	3 3 4	5 6 6
63	7993	8000	8007	8014	8021	8028	8035	8041	8048	8055	1 1 2	3 3 4	5 5 6
64	8062	8069	8075	8082	8089	8096	8102	8109	8116	8122	1 1 2	3 3 4	5 5 6
65	8129	8136	8142	8149	8156	8162	8169	8176	8182	8189	1 1 2	3 3 4	5 5 6
66	8195	8202	8209	8215	8222	8228	8235	8241	8248	8254	1 1 2	3 3 4	5 5 6
67	8261	8267	8274	8280	8287	8293	8299	8306	8312	8319	1 1 2	3 3 4	5 5 6
68	8325	8331	8338	8344	8351	8357	8363	8370	8376	8382	1 1 2	3 3 4	4 5 6
69	8388	8395	8401	8407	8414	8420	8426	8432	8439	8445	1 1 2	2 3 4	4 5 6
70	8451	8457	8463	8470	8476	8482	8488	8494	8500	8506	1 1 2	2 3 4	4 5 6
71	8513	8519	8525	8531	8537	8543	8549	8555	8561	8567	1 1 2	2 3 4	4 5 5
72	8573	8579	8585	8591	8597	8603	8609	8615	8621	8627	1 1 2	2 3 4	4 5 5
73	8633	8639	8645	8651	8657	8663	8669	8675	8681	8686	1 1 2	2 3 4	4 5 5
74	8692	8698	8704	8710	8716	8722	8727	8733	8739	8745	1 1 2	2 3 4	4 5 5
75	8751	8756	8762	8768	8774	8779	8785	8791	8797	8802	1 1 2	2 3 3	4 5 5
76	8808	8814	8820	8825	8831	8837	8842	8848	8854	8859	1 1 2	2 3 3	4 5 5
77	8865	8871	8876	8882	8887	8893	8899	8904	8910	8915	1 1 2	2 3 3	4 5 5
78	8921	8927	8932	8938	8943	8949	8954	8960	8965	8971	1 1 2	2 3 3	4 4 5
79	8976	8982	8987	8993	8998	9004	9009	9015	9020	9025	1 1 2	2 3 3	4 4 5
80	9031	9036	9042	9047	9053	9058	9063	9069	9074	9079	1 1 2	2 3 3	4 4 5
81	9085	9090	9096	9101	9106	9112	9117	9122	9128	9133	1 1 2	2 3 3	4 4 5
82	9138	9143	9149	9154	9159	9165	9170	9175	9180	9186	1 1 2	2 3 3	4 4 5
83	9191	9196	9201	9206	9212	9217	9222	9227	9232	9238	1 1 2	2 3 3	4 4 5
84	9243	9248	9253	9258	9263	9269	9274	9279	9284	9289	1 1 2	2 3 3	4 4 5
85	9294	9299	9304	9309	9315	9320	9325	9330	9335	9340	1 1 2	2 3 3	4 4 5
86	9345	9350	9355	9360	9365	9370	9375	9380	9385	9390	1 1 2	2 3 3	4 4 5
87	9395	9400	9405	9410	9415	9420	9425	9430	9435	9440	0 1 1	2 2 3	3 4 4
88	9445	9450	9455	9460	9465	9469	9474	9479	9484	9489	0 1 1	2 2 3	3 4 4
89	9494	9499	9504	9509	9513	9518	9523	9528	9533	9538	0 1 1	2 2 3	3 4 4
90	9542	9547	9552	9557	9562	9566	9571	9576	9581	9586	0 1 1	2 2 3	3 4 4
91	9590	9595	9600	9605	9609	9614	9619	9624	9628	9633	0 1 1	2 2 3	3 4 4
92	9638	9643	9647	9652	9657	9661	9666	9671	9675	9680	0 1 1	2 2 3	3 4 4
93	9685	9689	9694	9699	9703	9708	9713	9717	9722	9727	0 1 1	2 2 3	3 4 4
94	9731	9736	9741	9745	9750	9754	9759	9763	9768	9773	0 1 1	2 2 3	3 4 4
95	9777	9782	9786	9791	9795	9800	9805	9809	9814	9818	0 1 1	2 2 3	3 4 4
96	9823	9827	9832	9836	9841	9845	9850	9854	9859	9863	0 1 1	2 2 3	3 4 4
97	9868	9872	9877	9881	9886	9890	9894	9899	9903	9908	0 1 1	2 2 3	3 4 4
98	9912	9917	9921	9926	9930	9934	9939	9943	9948	9952	0 1 1	2 2 3	3 4 4
99	9956	9961	9965	9969	9974	9978	9983	9987	9991	9996	0 1 1	2 2 3	3 3 4

ANTILOGARITHMS

Mean Differences

	0	1	2	3	4	5	6	7	8	9	1 2 3	4 5 6	7 8 9
·00	1000	1002	1005	1007	1009	1012	1014	1016	1019	1021	0 0 1	1 1 1	2 2 2
·01	1023	1026	1028	1030	1033	1035	1038	1040	1042	1045	0 0 1	1 1 1	2 2 2
·02	1047	1050	1052	1054	1057	1059	1062	1064	1067	1069	0 0 1	1 1 1	2 2 2
·03	1072	1074	1076	1079	1081	1084	1086	1089	1091	1094	0 0 1	1 1 1	2 2 2
·04	1096	1099	1102	1104	1107	1109	1112	1114	1117	1119	0 1 1	1 1 2	2 2 2
·05	1122	1125	1127	1130	1132	1135	1138	1140	1143	1146	0 1 1	1 1 2	2 2 2
·06	1148	1151	1153	1156	1159	1161	1164	1167	1169	1172	0 1 1	1 1 2	2 2 2
·07	1175	1178	1180	1183	1186	1189	1191	1194	1197	1199	0 1 1	1 1 2	2 2 2
·08	1202	1205	1208	1211	1213	1216	1219	1222	1225	1227	0 1 1	1 1 2	2 2 3
·09	1230	1233	1236	1239	1242	1245	1247	1250	1253	1256	0 1 1	1 1 2	2 2 3
·10	1259	1262	1265	1268	1271	1274	1276	1279	1282	1285	0 1 1	1 1 2	2 2 3
·11	1288	1291	1294	1297	1300	1303	1306	1309	1312	1315	0 1 1	1 2 2	2 2 3
·12	1318	1321	1324	1327	1330	1334	1337	1340	1343	1346	0 1 1	1 2 2	2 2 3
·13	1349	1352	1355	1358	1361	1365	1368	1371	1374	1377	0 1 1	1 2 2	2 3 3
·14	1380	1384	1387	1390	1393	1396	1400	1403	1406	1409	0 1 1	1 2 2	2 3 3
·15	1413	1416	1419	1422	1426	1429	1432	1435	1439	1442	0 1 1	1 2 2	2 3 3
·16	1445	1449	1452	1455	1459	1462	1466	1469	1472	1476	0 1 1	1 2 2	2 3 3
·17	1479	1483	1486	1489	1493	1496	1500	1503	1507	1510	0 1 1	1 2 2	2 3 3
·18	1514	1517	1521	1524	1528	1531	1535	1538	1542	1545	0 1 1	1 2 2	2 3 3
·19	1549	1552	1556	1560	1563	1567	1570	1574	1578	1581	0 1 1	1 2 2	3 3 3
·20	1585	1589	1592	1596	1600	1603	1607	1611	1614	1618	0 1 1	1 2 2	3 3 3
·21	1622	1626	1629	1633	1637	1641	1644	1648	1652	1656	0 1 1	2 2 2	3 3 3
·22	1660	1663	1667	1671	1675	1679	1683	1687	1690	1694	0 1 1	2 2 2	3 3 3
·23	1698	1702	1706	1710	1714	1718	1722	1726	1730	1734	0 1 1	2 2 2	3 3 4
·24	1738	1742	1746	1750	1754	1758	1762	1766	1770	1774	0 1 1	2 2 2	3 3 4
·25	1778	1782	1786	1791	1795	1799	1803	1807	1811	1816	0 1 1	2 2 2	3 3 4
·26	1820	1824	1828	1832	1837	1841	1845	1849	1854	1858	0 1 1	2 2 3	3 3 4
·27	1862	1866	1871	1875	1879	1884	1888	1892	1897	1901	0 1 1	2 2 3	3 3 4
·28	1905	1910	1914	1919	1923	1928	1932	1936	1941	1945	0 1 1	2 2 3	3 4 4
·29	1950	1954	1959	1963	1968	1972	1977	1982	1986	1991	0 1 1	2 2 3	3 4 4
·30	1995	2000	2004	2009	2014	2018	2023	2028	2032	2037	0 1 1	2 2 3	3 4 4
·31	2042	2046	2051	2056	2061	2065	2070	2075	2080	2084	0 1 1	2 2 3	3 4 4
·32	2089	2094	2099	2104	2109	2113	2118	2123	2128	2133	0 1 1	2 2 3	3 4 4
·33	2138	2143	2148	2153	2158	2163	2168	2173	2178	2183	0 1 1	2 2 3	3 4 4
·34	2188	2193	2198	2203	2208	2213	2218	2223	2228	2234	1 1 2	2 3 3	4 4 5
·35	2239	2244	2249	2254	2259	2265	2270	2275	2280	2286	1 1 2	2 3 3	4 4 5
·36	2291	2296	2301	2307	2312	2317	2323	2328	2333	2339	1 1 2	2 3 3	4 4 5
·37	2344	2350	2355	2360	2366	2371	2377	2382	2388	2393	1 1 2	2 3 3	4 4 5
·38	2399	2404	2410	2415	2421	2427	2432	2438	2443	2449	1 1 2	2 3 3	4 4 5
·39	2455	2460	2466	2472	2477	2483	2489	2495	2500	2506	1 1 2	2 3 3	4 5 5
·40	2512	2518	2523	2529	2535	2541	2547	2553	2559	2564	1 1 2	2 3 4	4 5 5
·41	2570	2576	2582	2588	2594	2600	2606	2612	2618	2624	1 1 2	2 3 4	4 5 5
·42	2630	2636	2642	2649	2655	2661	2667	2673	2679	2685	1 1 2	2 3 4	4 5 6
·43	2692	2698	2704	2710	2716	2723	2729	2735	2742	2748	1 1 2	3 3 4	4 5 6
·44	2754	2761	2767	2773	2780	2786	2793	2799	2805	2812	1 1 2	3 3 4	4 5 6
·45	2818	2825	2831	2838	2844	2851	2858	2864	2871	2877	1 1 2	3 3 4	5 5 6
·46	2884	2891	2897	2904	2911	2917	2924	2931	2938	2944	1 1 2	3 3 4	5 5 6
·47	2951	2958	2965	2972	2979	2985	2992	2999	3006	3013	1 1 2	3 3 4	5 5 6
·48	3020	3027	3034	3041	3048	3055	3062	3069	3076	3083	1 1 2	3 4 4	5 6 6
·49	3090	3097	3105	3112	3119	3126	3133	3141	3148	3155	1 1 2	3 4 4	5 6 6

Example: Antilog $0 \cdot 3062 = 2 \cdot 023 + 0 \cdot 001 = 2 \cdot 024$

ANTILOGARITHMS

Mean Differences

	0	1	2	3	4	5	6	7	8	9	1	2	3	4	5	6	7	8	9
·50	3162	3170	3177	3184	3192	3199	3206	3214	3221	3228	1	1	2	3	4	4	5	6	7
·51	3236	3243	3251	3258	3266	3273	3281	3289	3296	3304	1	2	2	3	4	5	5	6	7
·52	3311	3319	3327	3334	3342	3350	3357	3365	3373	3381	1	2	2	3	4	5	5	6	7
·53	3388	3396	3404	3412	3420	3428	3436	3443	3451	3459	1	2	2	3	4	5	6	6	7
·54	3467	3475	3483	3491	3499	3508	3516	3524	3532	3540	1	2	2	3	4	5	6	6	7
·55	3548	3556	3565	3573	3581	3589	3597	3606	3614	3622	1	2	2	3	4	5	6	7	7
·56	3631	3639	3648	3656	3664	3673	3681	3690	3698	3707	1	2	3	3	4	5	6	7	8
·57	3715	3724	3733	3741	3750	3758	3767	3776	3784	3793	1	2	3	3	4	5	6	7	8
·58	3802	3811	3819	3828	3837	3846	3855	3864	3873	3882	1	2	3	4	4	5	6	7	8
·59	3890	3899	3908	3917	3926	3936	3945	3954	3963	3972	1	2	3	4	5	5	6	7	8
·60	3981	3990	3999	4009	4018	4027	4036	4046	4055	4064	1	2	3	4	5	6	6	7	8
·61	4074	4083	4093	4102	4111	4121	4130	4140	4150	4159	1	2	3	4	5	6	7	8	9
·62	4169	4178	4188	4198	4207	4217	4227	4236	4246	4256	1	2	3	4	5	6	7	8	9
·63	4266	4276	4285	4295	4305	4315	4325	4335	4345	4355	1	2	3	4	5	6	7	8	9
·64	4365	4375	4385	4395	4406	4416	4426	4436	4446	4457	1	2	3	4	5	6	7	8	9
·65	4467	4477	4487	4498	4508	4519	4529	4539	4550	4560	1	2	3	4	5	6	7	8	9
·66	4571	4581	4592	4603	4613	4624	4634	4645	4656	4667	1	2	3	4	5	6	7	9	10
·67	4677	4688	4699	4710	4721	4732	4742	4753	4764	4775	1	2	3	4	5	7	8	9	10
·68	4786	4797	4808	4819	4831	4842	4853	4864	4875	4887	1	2	3	4	6	7	8	9	10
·69	4898	4909	4920	4932	4943	4955	4966	4977	4989	5000	1	2	3	5	6	7	8	9	10
·70	5012	5023	5035	5047	5058	5070	5082	5093	5105	5117	1	2	4	5	6	7	8	9	11
·71	5129	5140	5152	5164	5176	5188	5200	5212	5224	5236	1	2	4	5	6	7	8	10	11
·72	5248	5260	5272	5284	5297	5309	5321	5333	5346	5358	1	2	4	5	6	7	9	10	11
·73	5370	5383	5395	5408	5420	5433	5445	5458	5470	5483	1	3	4	5	6	8	9	10	11
·74	5495	5508	5521	5534	5546	5559	5572	5585	5598	5610	1	3	4	5	6	8	9	10	12
·75	5623	5636	5649	5662	5675	5689	5702	5715	5728	5741	1	3	4	5	7	8	9	10	12
·76	5754	5768	5781	5794	5808	5821	5834	5848	5861	5875	1	3	4	5	7	8	9	11	12
·77	5888	5902	5916	5929	5943	5957	5970	5984	5998	6012	1	3	4	5	7	8	10	11	12
·78	6026	6039	6053	6067	6081	6095	6109	6124	6138	6152	1	3	4	6	7	8	10	11	13
·79	6166	6180	6194	6209	6223	6237	6252	6266	6281	6295	1	3	4	6	7	9	10	11	13
·80	6310	6324	6339	6353	6368	6383	6397	6412	6427	6442	1	3	4	6	7	9	10	12	13
·81	6457	6471	6486	6501	6516	6531	6546	6561	6577	6592	2	3	5	6	8	9	11	12	14
·82	6607	6622	6637	6653	6668	6683	6699	6714	6730	6745	2	3	5	6	8	9	11	12	14
·83	6761	6776	6792	6808	6823	6839	6855	6871	6887	6902	2	3	5	6	8	9	11	13	14
·84	6918	6934	6950	6966	6982	6998	7015	7031	7047	7063	2	3	5	6	8	10	11	13	15
·85	7079	7096	7112	7129	7145	7161	7178	7194	7211	7228	2	3	5	7	8	10	12	13	15
·86	7244	7261	7278	7295	7311	7328	7345	7362	7379	7396	2	3	5	7	8	10	12	13	15
·87	7413	7430	7447	7464	7482	7499	7516	7534	7551	7568	2	3	5	7	9	10	12	14	16
·88	7586	7603	7621	7638	7656	7674	7691	7709	7727	7745	2	4	5	7	9	11	12	14	16
·89	7762	7780	7798	7816	7834	7852	7870	7889	7907	7925	2	4	5	7	9	11	13	14	16
·90	7943	7962	7980	7998	8017	8035	8054	8072	8091	8110	2	4	6	7	9	11	13	15	17
·91	8128	8147	8166	8185	8204	8222	8241	8260	8279	8299	2	4	6	8	9	11	13	15	17
·92	8318	8337	8356	8375	8395	8414	8433	8453	8472	8492	2	4	6	8	10	12	14	15	17
·93	8511	8531	8551	8570	8590	8610	8630	8650	8670	8690	2	4	6	8	10	12	14	16	18
·94	8710	8730	8750	8770	8790	8810	8831	8851	8872	8892	2	4	6	8	10	12	14	16	18
·95	8913	8933	8954	8974	8995	9016	9036	9057	9078	9099	2	4	6	8	10	12	15	17	19
·96	9120	9141	9162	9183	9204	9226	9247	9268	9290	9311	2	4	6	8	11	13	15	17	19
·97	9333	9354	9376	9397	9419	9441	9462	9484	9506	9528	2	4	7	9	11	13	15	17	20
·98	9550	9572	9594	9616	9638	9661	9683	9705	9727	9750	2	4	7	9	11	13	16	18	20
·99	9772	9795	9817	9840	9863	9886	9908	9931	9954	9977	2	5	7	9	11	14	16	18	20

P

HYPERBOLIC OR NATURAL LOGARITHMS

	0	1	2	3	4	5	6	7	8	9	Mean Differences 1 2 3	4 5 6	7 8 9
1·0	0·0000	0099	0198	0296	0392	0488	0583	0677	0770	0862	10 19 29	38 48 57	67 76 86
1·1	·0953	1044	1133	1222	1310	1398	1484	1570	1655	1740	9 17 26	35 44 52	61 70 78
1·2	·1823	1906	1989	2070	2151	2231	2311	2390	2469	2546	8 16 24	32 40 48	56 64 72
1·3	·2624	2700	2776	2852	2927	3001	3075	3148	3221	3293	7 15 22	30 37 44	52 59 67
1·4	·3365	3436	3507	3577	3646	3716	3784	3853	3920	3988	7 14 21	28 35 41	48 55 62
1·5	·4055	4121	4187	4253	4318	4383	4447	4511	4574	4637	6 13 19	26 32 39	45 52 58
1·6	·4700	4762	4824	4886	4947	5008	5068	5128	5188	5247	6 12 18	24 30 36	42 48 55
1·7	·5306	5365	5423	5481	5539	5596	5653	5710	5766	5822	6 11 17	24 29 34	40 46 51
1·8	·5878	5933	5988	6043	6098	6152	6206	6259	6313	6366	5 11 16	22 27 32	38 43 49
1·9	·6419	6471	6523	6575	6627	6678	6729	6780	6831	6881	5 10 15	20 26 31	36 41 46
2·0	·6931	6981	7031	7080	7129	7178	7227	7275	7324	7372	5 10 15	20 24 29	34 39 44
2·1	·7419	7467	7514	7561	7608	7655	7701	7747	7793	7839	5 9 14	19 23 28	33 37 42
2·2	·7885	7930	7975	8020	8065	8109	8154	8198	8242	8286	4 9 13	18 22 27	31 36 40
2·3	·8329	8372	8416	8459	8502	8544	8587	8629	8671	8713	4 9 13	17 21 26	30 34 38
2·4	·8755	8796	8838	8879	8920	8961	9002	9042	9083	9123	4 8 12	16 20 24	29 33 37
2·5	·9163	9203	9243	9282	9322	9361	9400	9439	9478	9517	4 8 12	16 20 24	27 31 35
2·6	·9555	9594	9632	9670	9708	9746	9783	9821	9858	9895	4 8 11	15 19 23	26 30 34
2·7	·9933	9969	1·0006	0043	0080	0116	0152	0188	0225	0260	4 7 11	15 18 22	25 29 33
2·8	1·0296	0332	0367	0403	0438	0473	0508	0543	0578	0613	4 7 11	14 18 21	25 28 32
2·9	1·0647	0682	0716	0750	0784	0818	0852	0886	0919	0953	3 7 10	14 17 20	24 27 31
3·0	1·0986	1019	1053	1086	1119	1151	1184	1217	1249	1282	3 7 10	13 16 20	23 26 30
3·1	1·1314	1346	1378	1410	1442	1474	1506	1537	1569	1600	3 6 10	13 16 19	22 25 29
3·2	1·1632	1663	1694	1725	1756	1787	1817	1848	1878	1909	3 6 9	12 15 18	22 25 28
3·3	1·1939	1969	1·2000	2030	2060	2090	2119	2149	2179	2208	3 6 9	12 15 18	21 24 27
3·4	1·2238	2267	2296	2326	2355	2384	2413	2442	2470	2499	3 6 9	12 15 17	20 23 26
3·5	1·2528	2556	2585	2613	2641	2669	2698	2726	2754	2782	3 6 8	11 14 17	20 23 25
3·6	1·2809	2837	2865	2892	2920	2947	2975	3002	3029	3056	3 5 8	11 14 16	19 22 25
3·7	1·3083	3110	3137	3164	3191	3218	3244	3271	3297	3324	3 5 8	11 13 16	19 21 24
3·8	1·3350	3376	3403	3429	3455	3481	3507	3533	3558	3584	3 5 8	10 13 16	18 21 23
3·9	1·3610	3635	3661	3686	3712	3737	3762	3788	3813	3838	3 5 8	10 13 15	18 20 23
4·0	1·3863	3888	3913	3938	3962	3987	4012	4036	4061	4085	2 5 7	10 12 15	17 20 22
4·1	1·4110	4134	4159	4183	4207	4231	4255	4279	4303	4327	2 5 7	10 12 14	17 19 22
4·2	1·4351	4375	4398	4422	4446	4469	4493	4516	4540	4563	2 5 7	9 12 14	16 19 21
4·3	1·4586	4609	4633	4656	4679	4702	4725	4748	4770	4793	2 5 7	9 12 14	16 18 21
4·4	1·4816	4839	4861	4884	4907	4929	4951	4974	4996	5019	2 5 7	9 11 14	16 18 20
4·5	1·5041	5063	5085	5107	5129	5151	5173	5195	5217	5239	2 4 7	9 11 13	15 18 20
4·6	1·5261	5282	5304	5326	5347	5369	5390	5412	5433	5454	2 4 6	9 11 13	15 17 19
4·7	1·5476	5497	5518	5539	5560	5581	5602	5623	5644	5665	2 4 6	8 11 13	15 17 19
4·8	1·5686	5707	5728	5748	5769	5790	5810	5831	5851	5872	2 4 6	8 10 12	14 16 19
4·9	1·5892	5913	5933	5953	5974	5994	6014	6034	6054	6074	2 4 6	8 10 12	14 16 18
5·0	1·6094	6114	6134	6154	6174	6194	6214	6233	6253	6273	2 4 6	8 10 12	14 16 18
5·1	1·6292	6312	6332	6351	6371	6390	6409	6429	6448	6467	2 4 6	8 10 12	14 16 18
5·2	1·6487	6506	6525	6544	6563	6582	6601	6620	6639	6658	2 4 6	8 10 11	13 15 17
5·3	1·6677	6696	6715	6734	6752	6771	6790	6808	6827	6845	2 4 6	7 9 11	13 15 17
5·4	1·6864	6882	6901	6919	6938	6956	6974	6993	7011	7029	2 4 5	7 9 11	13 15 17

Hyperbolic or natural logarithms of 10^{+n}

n	1	2	3	4	5	6	7	8	9
$\log_e 10^n$	2·3026	4·6052	6·9078	9·2103	11·5129	13·8155	16·1181	18·4207	20·7233

HYPERBOLIC OR NATURAL LOGARITHMS

	0	1	2	3	4	5	6	7	8	9	1 2 3	4 5 6	7 8 9
5·5	1·7047	7066	7084	7102	7120	7138	7156	7174	7192	7210	2 4 5	7 9 11	13 14 16
5·6	1·7228	7246	7263	7281	7299	7317	7334	7352	7370	7387	2 4 5	7 9 11	12 14 16
5·7	1·7405	7422	7440	7457	7475	7492	7509	7527	7544	7561	2 3 5	7 9 10	12 14 16
5·8	1·7579	7596	7613	7630	7647	7664	7681	7699	7716	7733	2 3 5	7 9 10	12 14 15
5·9	1·7750	7766	7783	7800	7817	7834	7851	7867	7884	7901	2 3 5	7 8 10	12 13 15
6·0	1·7918	7934	7951	7967	7984	8001	8017	8034	8050	8066	2 3 5	7 8 10	12 13 15
6·1	1·8083	8099	8116	8132	8148	8165	8181	8197	8213	8229	2 3 5	6 8 10	11 13 15
6·2	1·8245	8262	8278	8294	8310	8326	8342	8358	8374	8390	2 3 5	6 8 10	11 13 14
6·3	1·8405	8421	8437	8453	8469	8485	8500	8516	8532	8547	2 3 5	6 8 9	11 13 14
6·4	1·8563	8579	8594	8610	8625	8641	8656	8672	8687	8703	2 3 5	6 8 9	11 12 14
6·5	1·8718	8733	8749	8764	8779	8795	8810	8825	8840	8856	2 3 5	6 8 9	11 12 14
6·6	1·8871	8886	8901	8916	8931	8946	8961	8976	8991	9006	2 3 5	6 8 9	11 12 14
6·7	1·9021	9036	9051	9066	9081	9095	9110	9125	9140	9155	1 3 4	6 7 9	10 12 13
6·8	1·9169	9184	9199	9213	9228	9242	9257	9272	9286	9301	1 3 4	6 7 9	10 12 13
6·9	1·9315	9330	9344	9359	9373	9387	9402	9416	9430	9445	1 3 4	6 7 9	10 12 13
7·0	1·9459	9473	9488	9502	9516	9530	9544	9559	9573	9587	1 3 4	6 7 9	10 11 13
7·1	1·9601	9615	9629	9643	9657	9671	9685	9699	9713	9727	1 3 4	6 7 8	10 11 13
7·2	1·9741	9755	9769	9782	9796	9810	9824	9838	9851	9865	1 3 4	6 7 8	10 11 12
7·3	1·9879	9892	9906	9920	9933	9947	9961	9974	9988	2·0001	1 3 4	5 7 8	10 11 12
7·4	2·0015	0028	0042	0055	0069	0082	0096	0109	0122	0136	1 3 4	5 7 8	9 11 12
7·5	2·0149	0162	0176	0189	0202	0215	0229	0242	0255	0268	1 3 4	5 7 8	9 11 12
7·6	2·0281	0295	0308	0321	0334	0347	0360	0373	0386	0399	1 3 4	5 7 8	9 10 12
7·7	2·0412	0425	0438	0451	0464	0477	0490	0503	0516	0528	1 3 4	5 6 8	9 10 12
7·8	2·0541	0554	0567	0580	0592	0605	0618	0631	0643	0656	1 3 4	5 6 8	9 10 11
7·9	2·0669	0681	0694	0707	0719	0732	0744	0757	0769	0782	1 3 4	5 6 8	9 10 11
8·0	2·0794	0807	0819	0832	0844	0857	0869	0882	0894	0906	1 3 4	5 6 7	9 10 11
8·1	2·0919	0931	0943	0956	0968	0980	0992	1005	1017	1029	1 2 4	5 6 7	9 10 11
8·2	2·1041	1054	1066	1078	1090	1102	1114	1126	1138	1150	1 2 4	5 6 7	9 10 11
8·3	2·1163	1175	1187	1199	1211	1223	1235	1247	1258	1270	1 2 4	5 6 7	8 10 11
8·4	2·1282	1294	1306	1318	1330	1342	1353	1365	1377	1389	1 2 4	5 6 7	8 9 11
8·5	2·1401	1412	1424	1436	1448	1459	1471	1483	1494	1506	1 2 4	5 6 7	8 9 11
8·6	2·1518	1529	1541	1552	1564	1576	1587	1599	1610	1622	1 2 3	5 6 7	8 9 10
8·7	2·1633	1645	1656	1668	1679	1691	1702	1713	1725	1736	1 2 3	5 6 7	8 9 10
8·8	2·1748	1759	1770	1782	1793	1804	1815	1827	1838	1849	1 2 3	5 6 7	8 9 10
8·9	2·1861	1872	1883	1894	1905	1917	1928	1939	1950	1961	1 2 3	4 6 7	8 9 10
9·0	2·1972	1983	1994	2006	2017	2028	2039	2050	2061	2072	1 2 3	4 6 7	8 9 10
9·1	2·2083	2094	2105	2116	2127	2138	2148	2159	2170	2181	1 2 3	4 5 7	8 9 10
9·2	2·2192	2203	2214	2225	2235	2246	2257	2268	2279	2289	1 2 3	4 5 7	8 9 10
9·3	2·2300	2311	2322	2332	2343	2354	2364	2375	2386	2396	1 2 3	4 5 6	8 9 10
9·4	2·2407	2418	2428	2439	2450	2460	2471	2481	2492	2502	1 2 3	4 5 6	7 8 10
9·5	2·2513	2523	2534	2544	2555	2565	2576	2586	2597	2607	1 2 3	4 5 6	7 8 9
9·6	2·2618	2628	2638	2649	2659	2670	2680	2690	2701	2711	1 2 3	4 5 6	7 8 9
9·7	2·2721	2732	2742	2752	2762	2773	2783	2793	2803	2814	1 2 3	4 5 6	7 8 9
9·8	2·2824	2834	2844	2854	2865	2875	2885	2895	2905	2915	1 2 3	4 5 6	7 8 9
9·9	2·2925	2935	2946	2956	2966	2976	2986	2996	3006	3016	1 2 3	4 5 6	7 8 9
10·0	2·3026												

Examples:

$$\log_e 0·6 = \log_e 6·0 - \log_e 10 = -0·5108$$
$$\log_e 12·0 = \log_e 1·2 + \log_e 10 = 2·4849$$

EXPONENTIAL AND HYPERBOLIC FUNCTIONS

x	e^x	e^{-x}	sinh x	cosh x	x	e^x	e^{-x}	sinh x	cosh x
·02	1·0202	·9802	·0200	1·0002	1·0	2·7183	·3679	1·1752	1·5431
·04	1·0408	·9608	·0400	1·0008	1·1	3·0042	·3329	1·3356	1·6685
·06	1·0618	·9418	·0600	1·0018	1·2	3·3201	·3012	1·5095	1·8107
·08	1·0833	·9231	·0801	1·0032	1·3	3·6693	·2725	1·6984	1·9709
·10	1·1052	·9048	·1002	1·0050	1·4	4·0552	·2466	1·9043	2·1509
·11	1·1163	·8958	·1102	1·0061	1·5	4·4817	·2231	2·1293	2·3524
·12	1·1275	·8869	·1203	1·0072	1·6	4·9530	·2019	2·3756	2·5775
·13	1·1388	·8781	·1304	1·0085	1·7	5·4739	·1827	2·6456	2·8283
·14	1·1503	·8694	·1405	1·0098	1·8	6·0497	·1653	2·9422	3·1075
·15	1·1618	·8607	·1506	1·0113	1·9	6·6859	·1496	3·2682	3·4177
·16	1·1735	·8521	·1607	1·0128	2·0	7·3891	·1353	3·6269	3·7622
·17	1·1853	·8437	·1708	1·0145	2·1	8·1662	·1225	4·0219	4·1443
·18	1·1972	·8353	·1810	1·0162	2·2	9·0250	·1108	4·4571	4·5079
·19	1·2092	·8270	·1911	1·0181	2·3	9·9742	·1003	4·9370	5·0372
·20	1·2214	·8187	·2013	1·0201	2·4	11·023	·0907	5·4662	5·5569
·21	1·2337	·8106	·2115	1·0221	2·5	12·182	·0821	6·0502	6·1323
·22	1·2461	·8025	·2218	1·0243	2·6	13·464	·0743	6·6947	6·7690
·23	1·2586	·7945	·2320	1·0266	2·7	14·880	·0672	7·4063	7·4735
·24	1·2712	·7866	·2423	1·0289	2·8	16·445	·0608	8·1919	8·2527
·25	1·2840	·7788	·2526	1·0314	2·9	18·174	·0550	9·0596	9·1146
·26	1·2969	·7711	·2629	1·0340	3·0	20·085	·0498	10·018	10·068
·27	1·3100	·7634	·2733	1·0367	3·1	22·198	·0450	11·076	11·121
·28	1·3231	·7558	·2837	1·0395	3·2	24·532	·0408	12·246	12·287
·29	1·3364	·7483	·2941	1·0423	3·3	27·113	·0369	13·538	13·575
·30	1·3499	·7408	·3045	1·0453	3·4	29·964	·0334	14·965	14·999
·31	1·3634	·7335	·3150	1·0484	3·5	33·115	·0302	16·543	16·573
·32	1·3771	·7261	·3255	1·0516	3·6	36·598	·0273	18·285	18·313
·33	1·3910	·7189	·3360	1·0550	3·7	40·447	·0247	20·211	20·236
·34	1·4050	·7118	·3466	1·0584	3·8	44·701	·0224	22·339	22·362
·35	1·4191	·7047	·3572	1·0619	3·9	49·402	·0202	24·691	24·711
·36	1·4333	·6977	·3678	1·0655	4·0	54·598	·0183	27·290	27·308
·37	1·4477	·6907	·3785	1·0692	4·1	60·340	·0166	30·162	30·178
·38	1·4623	·6839	·3892	1·0731	4·2	66·686	·0150	33·336	33·351
·39	1·4770	·6771	·4000	1·0770	4·3	73·700	·0136	36·843	36·857
·40	1·4918	·6703	·4107	1·0811	4·4	81·451	·0123	40·719	40·732
·41	1·5068	·6636	·4216	1·0852	4·5	90·017	·0111	45·003	45·014
·42	1·5220	·6570	·4325	1·0895	4·6	99·484	·0100	49·737	49·747
·43	1·5373	·6505	·4434	1·0939	4·7	109·95	·00910	54·969	54·978
·44	1·5527	·6440	·4543	1·0984	4·8	121·51	·00823	60·751	60·759
·45	1·5683	·6376	·4653	1·1030	4·9	134·29	·00745	67·141	67·149
·46	1·5841	·6313	·4764	1·1077	5·0	148·41	·00674	74·203	74·210
·47	1·6000	·6250	·4875	1·1125	5·1	164·02	·00610	82·008	82·014
·48	1·6161	·6188	·4986	1·1174	5·2	181·27	·00552	90·633	90·639
·49	1·6323	·6126	·5098	1·1225	5·3	200·34	·00499	100·17	100·17
·50	1·6487	·6065	·5211	1·1276	5·4	221·41	·00452	110·70	110·71
·60	1·8221	·5488	·6367	1·1855	5·5	244·69	·00409	122·34	122·35
·70	2·0138	·4966	·7586	1·2552	5·6	270·43	·00370	135·21	135·21
·80	2·2255	·4493	·8881	1·3374	5·7	298·87	·00335	149·43	149·43
·90	2·4596	·4066	1·0265	1·4331	5·8	330·30	·00303	165·15	165·15
					5·9	365·04	·00274	182·52	182·52
					6·0	403·43	·00248	201·71	201·72

$$\cosh x = \tfrac{1}{2}(e^x + e^{-x}), \quad \sinh x = \tfrac{1}{2}(e^x - e^{-x}).$$

SINES, COSINES AND TANGENTS OF ANGLES IN DEGREES AND RADIANS

0° to 90° by steps of 1°
100° to 360° by steps of 20°

Degrees	Radians	Sine	Cosine	Tangent	Degrees	Radians	Sine	Cosine	Tangent
0	.000	.0000	1.0000	.0000	53	.925	.7986	.6018	1.3270
1	.017	.0175	.9998	.0175	54	.942	.8090	.5878	1.3764
2	.035	.0349	.9994	.0349	55	.960	.8192	.5736	1.4281
3	.052	.0523	.9986	.0524	56	.977	.8290	.5592	1.4826
4	.070	.0698	.9976	.0699	57	.995	.8387	.5446	1.5399
5	.087	.0872	.9962	.0875	58	1.012	.8480	.5299	1.6003
6	.105	.1045	.9945	.1051	59	1.030	.8572	.5150	1.6643
7	.122	.1219	.9925	.1228	60	1.047	.8660	.5000	1.7321
8	.140	.1392	.9903	.1405	61	1.065	.8746	.4848	1.8040
9	.157	.1564	.9877	.1584	62	1.082	.8829	.4695	1.8807
10	.175	.1736	.9848	.1763	63	1.100	.8910	.4540	1.9626
11	.192	.1908	.9816	.1944	64	1.117	.8988	.4384	2.0503
12	.209	.2079	.9781	.2126	65	1.134	.9063	.4226	2.1445
13	.227	.2250	.9744	.2309	66	1.152	.9135	.4067	2.2460
14	.244	.2419	.9703	.2493	67	1.169	.9205	.3907	2.3559
15	.262	.2588	.9659	.2679	68	1.187	.9272	.3746	2.4751
16	.279	.2756	.9613	.2867	69	1.204	.9336	.3584	2.6051
17	.297	.2924	.9563	.3057	70	1.222	.9397	.3420	2.7475
18	.314	.3090	.9511	.3249	71	1.239	.9455	.3256	2.9042
19	.332	.3256	.9455	.3443	72	1.257	.9511	.3090	3.0777
20	.349	.3420	.9397	.3640	73	1.274	.9563	.2924	3.2709
21	.367	.3584	.9336	.3839	74	1.292	.9613	.2756	3.4874
22	.384	.3746	.9272	.4040	75	1.309	.9659	.2588	3.7320
23	.401	.3907	.9205	.4245	76	1.326	.9703	.2419	4.0108
24	.419	.4067	.9135	.4452	77	1.344	.9744	.2250	4.3315
25	.436	.4226	.9063	.4663	78	1.361	.9781	.2079	4.7046
26	.454	.4384	.8988	.4877	79	1.379	.9816	.1908	5.1445
27	.471	.4540	.8910	.5095	80	1.396	.9848	.1736	5.6713
28	.489	.4695	.8829	.5317	81	1.414	.9877	.1564	6.3137
29	.506	.4848	.8746	.5543	82	1.431	.9903	.1392	7.1154
30	.524	.5000	.8660	.5774	83	1.449	.9925	.1219	8.1443
31	.541	.5150	.8572	.6009	84	1.466	.9945	.1045	9.5143
32	.559	.5299	.8480	.6249	85	1.484	.9962	.0872	11.4300
33	.576	.5446	.8387	.6494	86	1.501	.9976	.0698	14.3006
34	.593	.5592	.8290	.6745	87	1.518	.9986	.0523	19.0811
35	.611	.5736	.8192	.7002	88	1.536	.9994	.0349	28.6361
36	.628	.5878	.8090	.7265	89	1.553	.9998	.0175	57.2892
37	.646	.6018	.7986	.7536	90	1.571	1.0000	.0000	
38	.663	.6157	.7880	.7813	100	1.745	.9848	−.1736	−5.6713
39	.681	.6293	.7771	.8098	120	2.094	.8660	−.5000	−1.7321
40	.698	.6428	.7660	.8391	140	2.443	.6428	−.7660	−.8391
41	.716	.6561	.7547	.8693	160	2.793	.3420	−.9397	−.3640
42	.733	.6691	.7431	.9004	180	3.142	.0000	−1.0000	.0000
43	.750	.6820	.7314	.9325	200	3.491	−.3420	−.9397	.3640
44	.768	.6947	.7193	.9657	220	3.840	−.6428	−.7660	.8391
45	.785	.7071	.7071	1.0000	240	4.189	−.8660	−.5000	1.7320
46	.803	.7193	.6947	1.0355	260	4.538	−.9848	−.1736	5.6713
47	.820	.7314	.6820	1.0724	280	4.887	−.9848	.1736	−5.6713
48	.838	.7431	.6691	1.1106	300	5.236	−.8660	.5000	−1.7321
49	.855	.7547	.6561	1.1504	320	5.585	−.6428	.7660	−.8391
50	.873	.7660	.6428	1.1918	340	5.934	−.3420	.9397	−.3640
51	.890	.7771	.6293	1.2349	360	6.283	.0000	1.0000	.0000
52	.908	.7880	.6157	1.2799					

Symbols Index

(See also p. 16)

(See pages as listed above for correct form of symbols)

Index